SELECTIVE SENTINEL LYMPHADENECTOMY FOR HUMAN SOLID CANCER

Cancer Treatment and Research
Steven T. Rosen, M.D., *Series Editor*

Sugarbaker, P. (ed): *Peritoneal Carcinomatosis: Principles of Management.* 1995. ISBN 0-7923-3727-1.
Dickson, R.B., Lippman, M.E. (eds.): *Mammary Tumor Cell Cycle, Differentiation and Metastasis.* 1995. ISBN 0-7923-3905-3.
Freireich, E.J, Kantarjian, H.(eds):*Molecular Genetics and Therapy of Leukemia.* 1995. ISBN 0-7923-3912-6.
Cabanillas, F., Rodriguez, M.A.(eds): *Advances in Lymphoma Research.* 1996. ISBN 0-7923-3929-0.
Miller, A.B. (ed.): *Advances in Cancer Screening.* 1996. ISBN 0-7923-4019-1.
Hait , W.N. (ed.): *Drug Resistance.* 1996. ISBN 0-7923-4022-1.
Pienta, K.J. (ed.): *Diagnosis and Treatment of Genitourinary Malignancies.* 1996. ISBN 0-7923-4164-3.
Arnold, A.J. (ed.): *Endocrine Neoplasms.* 1997. ISBN 0-7923-4354-9.
Pollock, R.E. (ed.): *Surgical Oncology.* 1997. ISBN 0-7923-9900-5.
Verweij, J., Pinedo, H.M., Suit, H.D. (eds): *Soft Tissue Sarcomas: Present Achievements and Future Prospects.* 1997. ISBN 0-7923-9913-7.
Walterhouse, D.O., Cohn, S. L. (eds.): *Diagnostic and Therapeutic Advances in Pediatric Oncology.* 1997. ISBN 0-7923-9978-1.
Mittal, B.B., Purdy, J.A., Ang, K.K. (eds): *Radiation Therapy.* 1998. ISBN 0-7923-9981-1.
Foon, K.A., Muss, H.B. (eds): *Biological and Hormonal Therapies of Cancer.* 1998. ISBN 0-7923-9997-8.
Ozols, R.F. (ed.): *Gynecologic Oncology.* 1998. ISBN 0-7923-8070-3.
Noskin, G. A. (ed.): *Management of Infectious Complications in Cancer Patients.* 1998. ISBN 0-7923-8150-5.
Bennett, C. L. (ed.): *Cancer Policy.* 1998. ISBN 0-7923-8203-X.
Benson, A. B. (ed.): *Gastrointestinal Oncology.* 1998. ISBN 0-7923-8205-6.
Tallman, M.S., Gordon, L.I. (eds): *Diagnostic and Therapeutic Advances in Hematologic Malignancies.* 1998. ISBN 0-7923-8206-4.
von Gunten, C.F. (ed): *Palliative Care and Rehabilitation of Cancer Patients.* 1999. ISBN 0-7923-8525-X
Burt, R.K., Brush, M.M. (eds): *Advances in Allogeneic Hematopoietic Stem Cell Transplantation.* 1999. ISBN 0-7923-7714-1.
Angelos, P. (ed.): *Ethical Issues in Cancer Patient Care* 2000. ISBN 0-7923-7726-5.
Gradishar, W.J., Wood, W.C. (eds): *Advances in Breast Cancer Management.* 2000. ISBN 0-7923-7890-3.
Sparano, Joseph A. (ed.): *HIV & HTLV-I Associated Malignancies.* 2001. ISBN 0-7923-7220-4.
Ettinger, David S. (ed.): *Thoracic Oncology.* 2001. ISBN 0-7923-7248-4.
Bergan, Raymond C. (ed.): *Cancer Chemoprevention.* 2001. ISBN 0-7923-7259-X.
Raza, A., Mundle, S.D. (eds): *Myelodysplastic Syndromes & Secondary Acute Myelogenous Leukemia* 2001. ISBN: 0-7923-7396.
Talamonti, Mark S. (ed.): *Liver Directed Therapy for Primary and Metastatic Liver Tumors.* 2001. ISBN 0-7923-7523-8.
Stack, M.S., Fishman, D.A. (eds): *Ovarian Cancer.* 2001. ISBN 0-7923-7530-0.
Bashey, A., Ball, E.D. (eds): *Non-Myeloablative Allogeneic Transplantation.* 2002. ISBN 0-7923-7646-3.
Leong, Stanley P.L. (ed.): *Atlas of Selective Sentinel Lymphadenectomy for Melanoma, Breast Cancer and Colon Cancer.* 2002. ISBN 1-4020-7013-6.
Andersson , B., Murray D. (eds): *Clinically Relevant Resistance in Cancer Chemotherapy.* 2002. ISBN 1-4020-7200-7.
Beam, C. (ed.): *Biostatistical Applications in Cancer Research.* 2002. ISBN 1-4020-7226-0.
Brockstein, B., Masters, G. (eds): *Head and Neck Cancer.* 2003. ISBN 1-4020-7336-4.
Frank, D.A. (ed.): *Signal Transduction in Cancer.* 2003. ISBN 1-4020-7340-2.
Figlin, Robert A. (ed.): *Kidney Cancer.* 2003. ISBN 1-4020-7457-3.
Kirsch, Matthias; Black, Peter McL. (ed.): *Angiogenesis in Brain Tumors.* 2003. ISBN 1-4020-7704-1.
Keller, E.T., Chung, L.W.K. (eds): *The Biology of Skeletal Metastases.* 2004. ISBN 1-4020-7749-1.
Kumar, Rakesh (ed.): *Molecular Targeting and Signal Transduction.* 2004. ISBN 1-4020-7822-6.
Verweij, J., Pinedo, H.M. (eds): *Targeting Treatment of Soft Tissue Sarcomas.* 2004. ISBN 1-4020-7808-0.
Finn, W.G., Peterson, L.C. (eds.): *Hematopathology in Oncology.* 2004. ISBN 1-4020-7919-2.
Farid, N., (ed): *Molecular Basis of Thyroid Cancer.* 2004. ISBN 1-4020-8106-5.
Khleif, S., (ed): *Tumor Immunology and Cancer* Vaccines. 2004. ISBN 1-4020-8119-7.
Balducci, L., Extermann, M. (eds.): *Biological Basis of Geriatric Oncology.* 2004. ISBN 0-387-23961-8.
Abrey, L., Chamberlain, M., Engelhard, H. (eds.): *Leptomeningeal Metastases.* 2005. ISBN 0-387-24198-1.
Platanias, L.C., (ed.): *Cytokines and Cancer.* 2005. ISBN 0-387-24360-7.
Leong, Stanley P.L., Kitagawa, Y., Kitajima, M. (eds.): *Selective Sentinel Lymphadenectomy for Human Solid Cancer* 2005. ISBN 0-387-23603-1.

SELECTIVE SENTINEL LYMPHADENECTOMY FOR HUMAN SOLID CANCER

edited by

STANLEY P. L. LEONG, MD, FACS
Professor and Director of Sentinel Lymph Node Program
University of California San Francisco Medical Center
at Mount Zion
San Francisco, CA, USA

YUKO KITAGAWA, MD, PhD, FACS
Assistant Professor of Surgery
Keio University School of Medicine
Tokyo, Japan

MASAKI KITAJIMA, MD, FACS
Professor and Chairman of Surgery
Keio University School of Medicine
Tokyo, Japan

Springer

Stanley P. L. Leong
Department of Surgery
University of California
Medical Center at Mount Zion
1600 Divisadero Street
San Francisco, CA 94143
leongs@surgery.ucsf.edu

Yuko Kitagawa / Masaki Kitajima
Department of Surgery
Keio University
School of Medicine
35 Shinanomachi, Shinjuku-ku
Tokyo 160-8582, Japan
kitagawa@sc.itc.keio.ac.jp
kitajima@sc.itc.keio.ac.jp

Selective Sentinel Lymphadenectomy for Human Solid Cancer

A C.I.P. Catalogue record for this book is available
from the Library of Congress.

ISBN 1-4899-8869-6 ISBN 0-387-23604-X (eBook)

Softcover re-print of the Hardcover 1st edition 2005

9 8 7 6 5 4 3 2 1 SPIN 11052487

springeronline.com

CONTENTS

PREFACE

Lymph node (LN) status is the most important prognostic indicator for the clinical outcome of patients in human solid cancer. Recent developments in sentinel lymph node (SLN) concept and technology have resulted in the application of this revolutionary approach to determine if cancer has metastasized to the regional nodal basin. The underlying thesis in solid cancer biology is that metastasis generally starts in an orderly progression, often spreading through the lymphatic channels to the SLNs, the first lymph node or nodes to receive the metastatic cancer cells. Thus, the logical approach is to harvest that specific SLN for thorough analysis. Because a tumor-free SLN is usually associated with a negative residual LN basin, a negative SLN is an excellent indication that micrometastasis has not occurred in the regional LNs. When the SLN is involved, it is unknown whether or not metastasis is limited only to the SLN or if the disease has spread to the remainder of the nodal basin. For this reason, if an SLN is positive, a complete LN dissection is recommended. Therefore, selective sentinel lymphadenectomy (SSL) should be considered as a staging procedure so that patients with negative SLNs (about 80%) may be spared an extensive LN dissection.

Malignant melanoma has been proven to be the most ideal tumor model to study the role of SLN. Subsequently, SSL has been applied to breast cancer, colon cancer, and other types of solid cancer. The multidisciplinary approach encompassing the surgeon, nuclear medicine physician, and pathologist is the key to such a successful procedure. Such a team can be readily formed with appropriate training. Beyond the technical aspects of harvesting the SLN, the implication of micrometastasis remains to be defined. Follow-up of melanoma and breast cancer patients after SSL is crucial. Therefore, for both melanoma and breast cancer, ongoing clinical trials are in progress to determine the biological and clinical significance of SLNs. Although the concept of SLN is viable in other types of cancer, such as gastrointestinal, lung, urologic, gynecologic and head & neck cancers, the technical aspects of the procedure need to be perfected and verified.

The most exciting possibility of SSL is that it will lead to early diagnosis of micrometastasis in regional LNs. Early diagnosis makes it useful as a clinical staging procedure, and opens up new opportunities to study micrometastasis and its evolution within the SLNs. New molecular and genetic tools may be used to dissect the mechanisms of lymphatic and hematogenous routes of metastasis. Multifaceted aspects of micrometastasis including differentiation of different clones with respect to the primary tumor, the acquisition of adhesion molecules, host interaction with the microscopic tumor, and so forth will shed new light on the biology and mechanism of early metastasis. If such mechanisms can be understood, new therapeutic advances may be developed to prevent the process of micrometastasis. In addition, clinical trials can be developed for high risk patients following definitive surgical resection, rather than using it in treating large tumor burdens, such as in Stage IV disease. SSL is a standard staging procedure for patients with melanoma and is rapidly evolving into a standard staging procedure for breast cancer as well. The techniques of harvesting SLNs are being developed in other solid cancers as mentioned above.

We are extremely delighted to be the editors of this exciting book on Selective Sentinel Lymphadenectomy for Human Solid Cancer. The historical background and rationale of SSL will be summarized by Dr. Wong. The role of lymphoscintigraphy for SSL will be addressed by Dr. Uren and his associates. SSL for cutaneous cancer, including malignant melanoma, Merkel cell carcinoma, and squamous cell carcinoma of the skin will be discussed by Dr. Leong. The role of SSL for breast cancer will be updated by Dr. Cox and his team. Dr. Saha and his group will show how the techniques of SSL apply to colorectal cancer. Dr. Kitagawa and his associates will present their extensive experience on SSL for upper gastrointestinal cancer. Exciting application of SSL in lung cancer will be summarized by Dr. Liptay, genitourinary cancer by Dr. Cabanas, and gynecological cancer by Dr. Levenback. SSL has been utilized to head and neck squamous carcinoma and this will be addressed by Dr. Werner. Pathological evaluation of SLNs will be discussed by Dr. Cochran and his co-workers. The application of molecular detection of micrometastasis of SLNs will be presented by Dr. Hoon and his group. Multidisciplinary approach in the performance of SSL will be discussed by Dr. Kitajima and his colleagues. The past, present, and future of SSL will be addressed by Dr. Thompson and his associates.

SSL allows us to identify lymph nodes with micrometastasis in a more selective fashion. With the advances in molecular, genetic, and immunological techniques, micrometastasis as detected by SSL can finally be studied in its detail. When mechanisms of early metastasis are fully understood, potential treatment modalities can be developed to either prevent or eliminate micrometastasis in the early stage of lymph node involvement.

Stanley P. L. Leong, MD, FACS
Department of Surgery
UCSF Comprehensive Cancer Center
San Francisco, California 94143-1674

Yuko Kitagawa, MD, FACS
Department of Surgery
Keio University School of Medicine
Shinjuku-ky Tokyo, Japan

Masaki Kitajima, MD, FACS
Department of Surgery
Keio University School of Medicine
Shinjuku-ky Tokyo, Japan

FOREWORD

During the mid-1970s my colleagues and I conceptualized cutaneous lymphoscintigraphy as a method to identify the lymph basin at risk of receiving cancer cells metastasizing from a primary melanoma in the trunk or other sites with ambiguous lymphatic drainage, such as the scalp or the shoulder. During the 1980s we formulated the necessary surgical and pathologic concepts and developed sensitive techniques to determine which nodes *within* that nodal basin drained a particular primary cutaneous site. In 1990 I presented the concept of intraoperative lymphatic mapping and sentinel lymphadenectomy for patients with primary cutaneous melanoma at the annual meeting of the Society of Surgical Oncology. Although publication of the seminal study was delayed by skeptical reviewers at several prominent journals, its eventual appearance in the April 1992 issue of the *Archives of Surgery* heralded a seismic change in the number and profile of published studies on cancer staging. A recent search of the National Library of Medicine's PubMed database for *sentinel lymph node* yielded 13 citations from 1980 to 1990 (all relating to penile cancer), 1554 citations from 1991 to 2001, and a remarkable 1689 citations from 2002 to the present!

The sentinel node is the first nodal target of lymph from the primary tumor site and therefore the node most likely to receive metastatic cells from the primary tumor. Because this node is defined by its function rather than a fixed anatomic location, the sentinel node concept is applicable to primary neoplasms of the skin, breast, colon, lung, or gastrointestinal tract – any tumor that that spreads via the lymphatics. Sometimes an anatomically high-risk node will prove to be the sentinel node. For example, the node of Cloquet can assume the role of the sentinel node in patients whose superficial inguinal lymph nodes drain through Cloquet's node to the iliac/obturator nodes. Similarly, the lymph node adjacent to the inferior epigastric vein may become the primary drainage node for lymphatic flow from the penis. But, as many investigators have observed for cancer of the penis, reliance on anatomically based nodal sampling leads to clinically unacceptable rates of nodal recurrence. The *true* sentinel node can only be identified by lymphatic mapping because its location will vary with the site of the primary tumor and with the patient's lymphatic anatomy.

Although the concept of a functionally identified sentinel node is relatively simple, the definitive identification and accurate immunohistochemical/molecular evaluation of a sentinel lymph node require careful teamwork and close communication among oncologic specialists. *Selective Sentinel Lymphadenectomy for Human Solid Cancer*, edited by three internationally known surgical oncologists, admirably delineates each component of the interdisciplinary process – from preoperative lymphoscintigraphy, to intraoperative probe-guided and dye-directed mapping, to assessment of the sentinel nodes for micrometastatic disease. It shows that the surgeon's responsibilities are matched and in some cases determined by efforts of the nuclear medicine physician and the pathologist.

The book's 14 chapters are information-dense; they offer a comprehensive overview of sentinel node mapping for solid cancers, with meticulous attention to the relative importance of each multidisciplinary component in each cancer. For example, preoperative lymphoscintigraphy is invaluable in patients with melanoma but, as discussed in the excellent chapter on gynecologic cancer, is of limited use for cervical cancer. A useful overview chapter on lymphoscintigraphy emphasizes the variability of drainage patterns from patient to patient. A chapter on histologic assessment not only provides a step-by-step outline of immunohistochemical assessment but also offers an intriguing immunologic assessment to confirm the identity of the sentinel node. The state-of-the-art chapter on molecular assessment emphasizes the importance of multimarker RT-PCR and introduces real-time PCR of paraffin-embedded sentinel node tissue. Elsewhere in the book is a provocative discussion of magnetic resonance spectroscopy for in vivo assessment of sentinel node status.

Given the rapidly changing technology for cancer assessment and staging, particularly the increasing use of molecular markers as prognostic indices, I am impressed by this text's ability to balance definitive statements with cautionary notes. Authors are careful to emphasize the absence of standardized techniques and training. Indeed, one of the primary goals of the recently formed International Sentinel Node Society is the standardization of sentinel node technology through periodic international meetings, interdisciplinary interchange of knowledge and information, education on best practices, and cooperative trials across the full range of suitable neoplasms.

Yet, while many applications of sentinel node mapping require further investigation, the sentinel node hypothesis has withstood all challengers. This excellent text clearly describes the rationale, indications, technical variations, and outcomes of sentinel node mapping for solid malignancies. It concisely reviews the field and summarizes areas for future research. Its wealth of practical information reflects each author's extensive experience in surgical oncology, nuclear medicine, pathology, and/or molecular oncology. *Selective Sentinel Lymphadenectomy for Human Solid Cancer* is a welcome addition to the sentinel node literature and will be a useful reference guide for oncologic specialists.

Donald L. Morton, MD, FACS
John Wayne Cancer Institute
Santa Monica, California

ACKNOWLEDGEMENTS

This work was supported in part by a grant from the Eva B. Buck Charitable Trust and Tyco Health Care in Japan.

CONTRIBUTORS

• *Foreword*

Donald L. Morton, MD, FACS
Medical Director
Surgeon-in-Chief
John Wayne Cancer Institute
Santa Monica, CA 90404 USA

• *The Development of Lymphatic Mapping and Selective Lymphadenectomy: A Historical Perspective*

Jan H. Wong, MD, FACS
Professor of Surgery
Cancer Research Center of Hawaii
John A. Burns School of Medicine
University of Hawaii at Manoa
Honolulu, Hawaii, USA

• *Role of Lymphoscintigraphy for Selective Sentinel Lymphadenectomy*

Roger F Uren, MD, FRACP, DDU
Clinical Associate Professor
Discipline of Medicine
University of Sydney
Sydney, NSW, Australia

Director
Nuclear Medicine and Diagnostic Ultrasound
Suite 206, RPAH Medical Centre
100 Carillon Ave
Newtown, NSW, 2042 Australia

Robert Howman-Giles, MD, FRACP, DDU
Clinical Associate Professor
Discipline of Medicine
University of Sydney
Sydney, NSW, Australia

David Chung, FRACP, DDU
Consultant Physician
Nuclear Medicine and Diagnostic Ultrasound
Suite 206, RPAH Medical Centre
100 Carillon Ave
Newtown, NSW, 2042, Australia

• *Selective Sentinel Lymphadenectomy for Malignant Melanoma, Merkel Cell Carcinoma, and Squamous Cell Carcinoma*

Stanley P. L. Leong, MD, FACS
Professor and Director, Sentinel Lymph Node Program, Department of Surgery, University of California, San Francisco Medical Center at Mount Zion; and Member, UCSF Comprehensive Cancer Center, San Francisco, California, USA

• *Selective Sentinel Lymphadenectomy for Breast Cancer*

Charles E. Cox, MD, FACS
Professor of Surgery, University of South Florida College of Medicine
Director Comprehensive Breast Cancer Program
H. Lee Moffitt Cancer Center and Research Institute
Tampa, Florida USA

Elizabeth S. Weinberg, MD
Breast Surgical Oncology Fellow: Comprehensive Breast Cancer Program
H. Lee Moffitt Cancer Center and Research Institute
Tampa, Florida USA

Ben T. Furman, MD
Assistant Professor of Surgery,
University of South Florida College of Medicine
Surgical Oncologist: Comprehensive Breast Cancer Program
H. Lee Moffitt Cancer Center and Research Institute
Tampa, Florida USA

Laura B. White, BS
Senior Research Intern: Comprehensive Breast Cancer Program
H. Lee Moffitt Cancer Center and Research Institute
Tampa, Florida USA

Daniel C. Dickson, BS
Research Intern: Comprehensive Breast Cancer Program
H. Lee Moffitt Cancer Center and Research Institute
Tampa, Florida USA

Jeff King, BA/BS
Departmental Systems Specialist: Comprehensive Breast Cancer Program
H. Lee Moffitt Cancer Center and Research Institute
Tampa, Florida USA

Jayesh Patel
Research Intern: Comprehensive Breast Cancer Program
H. Lee Moffitt Cancer Center and Research Institute
Tampa, Florida USA

• *Sentinel Lymph Node Mapping in Colon and Rectal Cancer: Its Impact on Staging, Limitations, and Pitfalls*

Sukamal Saha, MD, FRCS (C)
Assistant Professor of Surgery and Anatomy, Michigan State University College of Human Medicine; and the Department of Surgery, McLaren Regional Medical Center, Flint, Michigan USA

Adrian G. Dan, MD
Michigan State University
East Lansing, Michigan USA

Carsten T. Viehl, MD
Professor of Surgery,
Dept of Surgery at Kantonsspital Olten
Olten, Switzerland

Markus Zuber, MD
Professor of Surgery,
Dept of Surgery at Kantonsspital Olten
Olten, Switzerland

David Wiese, MD
Dept of Pathology at McLaren Regional Medical Center
Flint, Michigan USA

• *Sentinel Lymph Node Mapping in Esophageal and Gastric Cancer*
Yuko Kitagawa, MD, FACS
Assistant Professor
Department of Surgery
Keio University School of Medicine
Tokyo, Japan

• *Sentinel Lymph Node Mapping in Lung Cancer*
Michael J. Liptay, MD, FACS
Chief, Division of Thoracic Oncology
Evanston Northwestern Healthcare
Assistant Professor of Surgery
Feinberg School of Medicine
Northwestern University
Chicago, Illinois USA

• *Lymphatic Mapping and Sentinel Lymphadenectomy in Urology*
Ramon M. Cabanas, MD
Attending Surgeon
Victory Memorial Hospital
Brooklyn, New York 11228 USA

• *Selective Sentinel Lymphadenectomy for Gynecological Cancer*
Charles F. Levenback, MD
Professor and Deputy Chairman
Department of Gynecologic Oncology
The University of Texas M. D. Anderson Cancer Center
Houston, TX 77030 USA

• *Selective Sentinel Lymphadenectomy for Head and Neck Squamous Cell Carcinoma*
Jochen A. Werner, MD
Professor and Chairman of the Dept. of Otolaryngology
Head and Neck Surgery
Philipps University of Marburg
Deutschhausstr. 3
35037 Marburg, Germany

- *Accurate Evaluation of Nodal Tissues for the Presence of Tumor is Central to the Sentinel Node Approach*

Alistair J. Cochran, MD, FRCP (Glasg.), FRCPath.
Professor of Pathology and Surgery
Department of Pathology and Laboratory Medicine
David Geffen School of Medicine,
University of California Los Angeles
Los Angeles, CA USA

Alice A. Roberts, MD, PhD
UCLA Department of Pathology and Laboratory Medicine
David Geffen School of Medicine
University of California Los Angeles
Los Angeles, California, USA

Duan-Ren Wen, MD
UCLA Department of Pathology and Laboratory Medicine
David Geffen School of Medicine
University of California Los Angeles
Los Angeles, California, USA

Rong-Rong Huang, MD
UCLA Department of Pathology and Laboratory Medicine
David Geffen School of Medicine
University of California Los Angles
Los Angeles, California, USA

Eijun Itakura, MD
UCLA Department of Pathology and Laboratory Medicine
David Geffen School of Medicine
University of California Los Angeles
Los Angeles, California, USA

Frank Luo, MD
UCLA Department of Pathology and Laboratory Medicine
David Geffen School of Medicine
University of California Los Angeles
Los Angeles, California, USA

Scott W. Binder, MD
Professor and Chief of Dermatopathology
UCLA Department of Pathology and Laboratory Medicine
David Geffen School of Medicine
University of California Los Angeles
Los Angeles, California, USA

• *Molecular Diagnosis of Micrometastasis in the Sentinel Lymph Node*

Dave S.B. Hoon, MSc, PhD, Member
Director Dept. Molecular Oncology
John Wayne Cancer Institute
Santa Monica, CA 90404 USA

Hiroya Takeuchi, MD, PhD
Dept. Molecular Oncology
John Wayne Cancer Institute
Santa Monica, CA 90404 USA

Robert A. Wascher, MD
Dept. Molecular Oncology
John Wayne Cancer Institute
Santa Monica, CA 90404 USA

Christine Kuo, BS, PSyD
Dept. Molecular Oncology
John Wayne Cancer Institute
Santa Monica, CA 90404 USA

Roderick R. Turner, MD
Division of Surgical Pathology
Saint Johns Health Center
John Wayne Cancer Institute
Santa Monica, CA 90404 USA

• *Credentialing of Nuclear Medicine Physicians, Surgeons and Pathologists as a Multidisciplinary Team for Selective Sentinel Lymphadenectomy*

Masaki Kitajima, MD, FACS
Dean, School of Medicine
Professor and Chairman, Department of Surgery
Keio University School of Medicine
Tokyo, Japan

Hirofumi Fujii, MD
Assistant Professor
Department of Radiology
Keio University School of Medicine
Tokyo, Japan

Makio Mukai, MD
Associate Professor
Division of Diagnostic Pathology
Keio University School of Medicine
Tokyo, Japan

Atsushi Kubo, MD
Professor, Department of Radiology
Keio University School of Medicine
Tokyo, Japan

• *Selective Sentinel Lymphadenectomy: Progress to Date and Prospects for the Future*

John F. Thompson, MD, FRACS, FACS
Director, The Sydney Melanoma Unit Sydney Cancer Centre
Royal Prince Alfred Hospital
Professor of Melanoma and Surgical Oncology
The University of Sydney
Sydney, Australia

Jonathan Stretch, MBBS, D.PHIL (OXON), FRACS
Deputy Director, Sydney Melanoma Unit, Sydney Cancer Centre
Royal Prince Alfred Hospital
Senior Lecturer (Melanoma and Surgical Oncology)
The University of Sydney
Sydney, Australia

Richard Scolyer, MBBS, FRCPA
Staff Specialist in Anatomical Pathology &
Director of MASCRI Pathology Research
Royal Prince Alfred Hospital
Sydney, Australia

Chapter 1

THE DEVELOPMENT OF LYMPHATIC MAPPING AND SELECTIVE LYMPHADENECTOMY:

A Historical Perspective

Jan H. Wong

John A. Burns School of Medicine & Clinical Sciences Program, Cancer Research Center of Hawaii, University of Hawaii at Manoa

INTRODUCTION

Intraoperative lymphatic mapping and sentinel lymphadenectomy (ILM/SL) is a novel surgical technique that has substantially impacted on the way cutaneous melanoma and breast cancer are now being staged and managed. Originally described as a method to identify individuals with cutaneous melanoma who could potentially benefit from therapeutic regional lymphadenectomies,[1] ILM/SL is now routinely utilized in the staging of patients with cutaneous melanoma and invasive breast cancer and is being explored as an adjunct to routine pathologic analysis of the regional lymphatics in a number of other solid neoplasms. The development of ILM/SL represents one specialized aspect in the evolution of surgical care of the cancer patient as a diagnostic, adjunctive, and curative therapy.

THE LYMPHATICS AND CANCER

The relevance of the lymphatic system in human cancer has long been recognized. Since the original descriptions of the lymphatics by a number of independent investigators in the 17th century,[2-4] a continued examination of the importance of the lymphatics in human disease has been vigorously pursued. In a comprehensive atlas published in 1786, Cruikshank[5] laid the foundation of the modern knowledge of the lymphatics describing among many observations, reddened lymphatics associated with cutaneous infections and enlargement of lymph nodes associated with acute and chronic infections. Utilizing injection techniques and meticulous dissection, Marie Philibert Constant Sappey published an atlas of the lymphatic anatomy that was notable for its detailed illustrations of the dermal lymphatics and which served as the foundation for the anatomic understanding of the lymphatics. [6]

With relatively few exceptions, all cancer eventually metastasizes if left untreated. The observation that the lymphatics represent one of the primary routes for the development of metastatic disease, however, is relatively new in the conceptual history of cancer. Although Henry-Francois Le Dran described the spread of cancer via the lymphatics to regional lymph nodes in the 18th century, it was founded on the lymph theory of cancer which implicated "fermenting and degenerating lymph" as the etiology of cancer.[7] It was not until the late 19th century that the concept of cellular metastases from a local disease to a systemic disease through an initial group of regional nodes was developed.[8] Regional lymph nodes were viewed as biologic barriers to the dissemination of disease and resection of the regional lymphatics has been a routine part of the surgical management of most solid malignancies.

Although the concept that early in its natural history, cancer is a systemic disease has dominated the current conceptual paradigm of cancer care,[9-11] management of the regional lymphatics remains an integral part of the surgical treatment of cancer. Few would argue with the prognostic importance of accurate staging and the regional control of disease obtained following lymphadenectomy. The impact on overall survival, however, following regional lymphadenectomy continues to generate considerable debate, most notably in cutaneous melanoma and breast cancer in which the associated morbidity of a regional lymphadenectomy may not be insignificant and the number of "nontherapeutic" procedures are considerable. It was within this conceptual framework that alternative approaches to surgical management of the regional lymphatics have evolved.

THE CLINICAL PROBLEM

One of the most controversial topics in the surgical management of cutaneous melanoma has been the therapeutic value of immediate lymphadenectomy in the clinically node negative individual. This controversy is not new. In 1892, Herbert Snow[12] noted that "the danger lies in the diffusion of malignant cells....These always implicate the nearest lymph glands.... Palpable enlargement of these glands is, unfortunately, but a late symptom of deposits therein....We see the paramount importance of securing the perfect eradication of these lymph glands which will necessarily be first infected."

Although numerous single institutional trials have all suggested improved survival in patients who undergo immediate lymphadenectomy when compared with those who undergo lymphadenectomy for clinically evident disease,[13-17] three prospective randomized clinical trials have failed to confirm these retrospective analyses.[18-20] These prospective randomized trials have raised the possibility that the presence of regional nodal metastases is an indicator of systemic disease rather than a manifestation of the orderly progression of disease from the primary tumor to the regional lymph nodes.

Given the apparent absence of an overall survival advantage in individuals undergoing immediate lymphadenectomy and the morbidity associated with regional lymphadenectomy,[21] many have questioned the continued routine use of this surgical modality in both melanoma[18] and breast cancer.[22] It had been generally well recognized that a significant number of individuals would undergo an operative procedure for what ultimately would prove to be node negative disease. These individuals would suffer the morbidity associated with a radical regional lymphadenectomy without any potential for survival benefit in order to identify a minority of individuals who were found to have microscopically involved nodes and who might have improved survival due to a timely intervention.

Although a number of alternative explanations for the lack of benefit observed in these trials were proposed, perhaps the most compelling reason for failing to demonstrate any potential improvement in survival was the inability to accurately stage individuals. It is apparent that the only patients who could potentially enjoy improved survival with an immediate lymphadenectomy were individuals who were node positive but who had not developed concomitant distant metastatic disease. Natural history studies indicate that these patients represent a relatively small percentage of the populations that were studied and raised the possibility that these trials might have had insufficient statistical power to identify a survival advantage.

IMPROVING THE RISK/BENEFIT RATIO

The recognition that not all individuals with cutaneous melanoma would benefit from an immediate regional lymphadenectomy led to a number of strategies to maximize the ability to accurately predict the presence or absence of nodal disease. In 1969, Clark and co-workers[23] and in 1970, Breslow[24] reported on the prognostic significance of microstaging of the primary tumor, demonstrating that the more deeply invasive the primary tumor, the higher the risk for developing metastatic disease. Utilizing the microstaging techniques of Clark[23] and Breslow,[24] individuals could be characterized as being at increased high risk for harboring regional metastatic disease and could rationally be offered an immediate lymphadenectomy.[25, 26]

Additionally, the recognition that the dermal lymphatics, particularly in melanomas located on the trunk, could have substantial variability from that originally described by Sappey, led to the development of cutaneous lymphoscintigraphy to define the regional lymphatic basins that were at risk for harboring metastatic disease.[25] This anatomic information along with microstaging of the primary tumor could identify which regional node basin in patients at increased risk for harboring regional node metastatic disease might require surgical intervention. Although these approaches could predict with reasonable accuracy the individuals at increased risk for harboring metastatic nodal disease and significantly reduced the number of node negative regional lymphadenectomies, the routine practice of regional lymphadenectomy even for high-risk cutaneous melanoma continued to result in substantial numbers of individuals undergoing nontherapeutic, staging procedures. However, until recently, the only method to identify regional node metastases was a complete lymph node dissection.

THE SENTINEL NODE CONCEPT

The origin of the concept that the lymphatics of a given organ site drain preferentially to a given group of nodes is unclear. In 1963, Busch and Sayegh[27] described a preliminary experience with direct cannulation of the lymphatics of the testis to perform lymphangiography and reported on a consistent drainage pattern to regional lymph nodes between the levels of the lumbar spine L4 and L2. These observations raised the possibility that this anatomic information might be utilized to determine the extent of the lymphadenectomy in testicular cancer. It was noted that the radiopaque substances in use during that era, Thorotrast and Diodrast, were not useful in "indirect" lymphangiography in man because of the inadequate absorption of the injected dye.[28]

Although it has been well accepted that solid tumors regularly metastasized to the regional lymphatics, the concept that a primary tumor would drain via the lymphatics preferentially to a specific lymph node and the status of the lymph node would reflect the histology of the entire regional lymphatics was extremely novel. Faced with a similar clinical

dilemma to that in cutaneous melanoma of identifying individuals requiring regional lymphadenectomy, Cabanas[29] hypothesized that when carcinoma of the penis metastasized, it most commonly would metastasize to a node that was located medially and superiorly to the saphenofemoral junction in each groin. This hypothesis was the result of extensive anatomic studies utilizing lymphangiograms obtained by cannulation of the dorsal lymphatics of the penis. These studies demonstrated a consistent drainage to a particular superficial node in the groin, prior to drainage to the deep inguinal nodes. Cabanas coined the term "sentinel node" to describe this node and suggested that only if the sentinel node was found to have metastatic disease would the patient require a formal lymphadenectomy. Conversely, and just as importantly, if the sentinel node did not have metastatic disease, the likelihood of metastatic disease being present in the lymphatic basin was low and no further resection was necessary.

Based upon his lymphangiographic studies, Cabanas intimated that the sentinel node was constant in location and described an operative technique in which anatomic landmarks were utilized to identify the site of the sentinel lymph node. Through a 5-cm incision and "by inserting the finger under the upper flap toward the pubic tubercle, the SLN is encountered."[29] Initial clinical data supported the sentinel node concept .[30] However, others were unable to reproduce these results and the validity of this concept was considered controversial[31-33] and fell into some disrepute.

Independent of Cabanas, the Division of Surgical Oncology at UCLA [1, 34] hypothesized that the lymphatic drainage from a cutaneous melanoma would drain to a specific lymph node that was termed the sentinel lymph node. However, in distinct contrast to Cabanas, the UCLA group proposed that the lymphatic drainage might vary from individual to individual and from anatomic site to anatomic site, and therefore, was not necessarily fixed in anatomic location. For this reason, to reproducibly identify the sentinel lymph node, intraoperative techniques would be required to define the lymphatic drainage of each individual patient rather than an operative approach that was dependent upon anatomic landmarks.

We performed initial studies in a feline model[34] testing the feasibility of a number of compounds to map the dermal lymphatics in an effort to develop an operative approach to identifying the sentinel lymph node. While most animals have a single large node in the axilla or groin and were not suitable to examine the sentinel node hypothesis, we found that the cat had three lymph nodes in the groin. We believed this to be analogous to the anatomy of humans in which regional node basins had multiple lymph nodes and selected this as our animal model to explore intraoperative lymphatic mapping techniques.

The vital blue dye, isosulfan blue, proved to be the most useful lymphatic dye. Following injection of the vital blue dye, an incision was made in the groin and after careful elevation of the skin flaps, an inguinal node dissection was performed. The specimen was oriented and examined for the presence or absence of blue dye-stained lymph nodes. Rapid uptake of isosulfan blue was observed and allowed for ready visualization of the lymphatic channels and lymph nodes, which were stained blue. These studies, in a feline model, demonstrated that the intradermal injection of a lymphatic dye, isosulfan blue, would result in the uptake of the dye in the dermal lymphatics. With meticulous dissection, the dermal lymphatics could then be visualized and utilized to map the lymphatic drainage of the skin to a sentinel lymph node.

We utilized the skin of the hind limb, abdomen, and perineum as sites for the intradermal injection of isosulfan blue. The location of lymph nodes that were stained blue was determined. From these observations, a predictable pattern of lymphatic drainage emerged from the various anatomic sites in which intradermal injections were performed. Specific areas of skin would drain only to the medial, middle or lateral lymph nodes. These results, most importantly, demonstrated that certain areas of skin would reproducibly drain to a specific lymph node and suggested that a primary tumor arising in a particular area of skin would indeed drain to a "sentinel" node and supported the feasibility of an operation that was termed selective lymphadenectomy[1].

CLINICAL INVESTIGATIONS IN CUTANEOUS MELANOMA

Based upon the hypothesis that operative techniques, developed to identify the lymphatic drainage, could be utilized to identify lymph nodes within the lymphatic basin that would be the primary drainage of a primary tumor, studies in 223 consecutive patients with cutaneous melanoma were performed at UCLA .[1] These studies involved the intradermal injection of isosulfan blue either around the tumor if the tumor remained in situ or most commonly around the biopsy scar. An incision over the regional lymphatic basin at risk for harboring metastatic disease that was defined either by cutaneous lymphoscintigraphy[35] or by anatomic guidelines was made and a blue-stained lymph node or nodes were removed.

The technique of ILM/SL evolved from a blunt dissection of the regional lymph basin to identify blue-stained lymph nodes to a very refined technique. After the skin flap closest to the primary tumor was carefully elevated, gentle dissection through the subcutaneous fat in an area where the blue-stained afferent lymphatic channels were predicted to most likely enter the regional lymphatic basin was performed. Once identified, the blue-stained lymphatic channels were then meticulously traced through the regional nodal basin to a blue-stained node. Identifying and dissecting the fine afferent lymphatic channel could be extremely difficult at times. For this reason, ILM/SL proved to be technically challenging particularly in the axilla because of the three-dimensional aspects of that lymphatic basin and the head and neck where the lymphatic channels were particularly fine in caliber. Because isosulfan blue travels rapidly through the lymphatic channels, disruption of the afferent lymphatic channels would result in the inability to identify a blue-stained lymph node. The overall success rate of identifying a blue-stained sentinel lymph node during the development of ILM/SL was 82% and was clearly experience dependent.

This initial report clearly demonstrated that when cutaneous melanoma metastasizes to the regional lymphatics, it most commonly will do so to the sentinel lymph node. Of 48 lymphadenectomy specimens with metastatic tumor identified, all but 2 had tumor present in the sentinel node, a demonstrated false-negative rate of approximately 5%. These initial findings subsequently have been duplicated by a number of other institutions both with immediate completion node dissection and with completion node dissection only when the sentinel node was positive (Table 1).

Table 1

Author	No. of Pts	Complete LND	SN Pos (%)	False Neg (%)*
Morton[1]	223	Y	22	5
Reintgen[42]	42	Y	19	0
Thompson[60]	118	Y	21	2
Albertini[41]	106	N	15	
Leong[40]	163	N	18	
Lingam[61]	35	N	26	
Morton[62]	72	N	15	

*Documented False Negative by completion node dissection.

PATHOLOGIC ANALYSIS OF THE SENTINEL LYMPH NODE

It is well recognized that conventional hematoxylin–eosin examination of the regional lymph nodes underestimates the extent of nodal metastases.[36] Although this is not surprising, since only a fraction of the nodal tissue submitted is routinely examined, it has been an accepted practice in the pathologic analysis of apparently normal lymph nodes. It was not feasible due to cost and labor constraints to perform a more thorough analysis of multiple lymph nodes from the regional node basin.

The development of an S-100 protein as a marker for melanocytic tumors as well as the availability of a number of antibodies to melanoma associated epitopes has provided the necessary tools to examine regional lymph nodes in a more thorough and sensitive fashion. Immunohistochemical techniques can identify a single tumor cell in a background of approximately 10^5 lymphocytes, a far more sensitive technique than routine hematoxylin–eosin staining. Utilizing these tools, occult tumor cells have been identified in approximately 30% of apparently node negative melanoma patients.[36]

Despite the apparent utility of immunohistochemical staining in upstaging cutaneous melanoma, no cost-effective alternative had been defined until the implementation of lymphatic mapping and selective lymphadenectomy. The sentinel lymph node is now reproducibly defined by lymphoscintigraphy and lymphatic mapping with isosulfan blue and a radioactive marker. The convergence of surgical technique and sensitive immunohistochemical markers for melanoma and melanocytic tumors provided the unique opportunity to reexamine the role of immediate therapeutic lymphadenectomy in cutaneous melanoma through the Multicenter Selective Lymphadenectomy Trial.[37]

One of the key elements that have evolved from the sentinel node concept was the opportunity to evaluate a small volume of lymph node tissue more thoroughly. The technique represents a substantial improvement in the ability to more accurately stage the regional lymphatics. For this reason, the surgical pathologist has become a critical partner in the implementation of a successful sentinel lymph node program.

RADIOGUIDED APPROACHES TO SENTINEL NODE HARVESTING

Because of the technical difficulties associated with ILM/SL the feasibility of this approach in less than high-volume settings has been questioned.[38] The development of a number of radiopharmaceuticals with appropriate particle size provided the opportunity for the development of cutaneous lymphoscintigraphy. In contrast to previous radiopaque agents that could not be absorbed by the dermal lymphatics,[28] these newer radiolabeled agents are readily absorbed into the dermal lymphatics and are actively taken up by antigen-presenting cells.[39] This allowed for the identification of the regional node basins at risk for harboring metastatic disease in sites of ambiguous lymphatic drainage, a surprisingly frequent occurrence.[35] For this reason, cutaneous lymphoscintigraphy had become a routine component of the management of most melanoma patients.[35]

With increasing attention to the details of cutaneous lymphoscintigraphy, it became apparent that the actual sentinel node(s) could be visualized with appropriate camera positioning. With careful positioning of the patient beneath a gamma camera at the time of lymphoscintigraphy, it became possible to identify an area of increased radioactivity that has been demonstrated to correlate with the blue-stained sentinel lymph node.[40,41] Utilizing a hot marker, the nodes that had uptake of the radiocolloid were marked on the skin to aid the surgeon in selecting the surgical approach to the lymphatic basin.[42,43] The suggestion that cutaneous lymphoscintigraphy identified nodes that were sentinel nodes opened up a new avenue to identify and harvest the sentinel node.

The use of radioguided techniques in the care of the cancer patient originated with the development of gamma detection devices that could be transported into the operating room[44] and identify tissue that had been marked by a radionuclide. Initially utilized for radioimmunoguided surgery,[44-46] it was only a matter of time before the technology was applied to the identification and harvesting of sentinel lymph nodes identified by cutaneous lymphoscintigraphy.

With the aid of a hand-held gamma probe, Alex and co-workers[47] described first in a feline model and subsequently in melanoma patients that technetium-99m-labeled colloid would localize in a regional lymph node after an intradermal injection and that these lymph nodes could be readily identified and subsequently resected. Increasing evidence has supported that the hot lymph node correlates with a sentinel lymph node.[40,41,48] Albertini and co-workers[41] demonstrated that the combined use of isosulfan blue along with intraoperative use of a hand held-gamma probe could improve the ability to harvest a sentinel lymph node. There results have been reproduced in the Multicenter Selective Lymphadenectomy Trial.[37]

THE SENTINEL NODE CONCEPT IN BREAST CANCER

As in melanoma, the value of regional lymphadenectomy in breast cancer remains controversial. Axillary node dissection is widely viewed as a staging procedure without inherent therapeutic value.[9,10] For this reason, a minimally invasive procedure to accurately stage the axilla is particularly appealing. The possibility that the sentinel node concept was applicable to breast cancer was initially investigated by Giuliano and co-workers.[49] Utilizing the techniques that had been refined in cutaneous melanoma patients from the same institution, Giuliano demonstrated the feasibility of ILM/SL in breast cancer. However, important differences emerged between melanoma and breast cancer. Increasing volumes of isosulfan blue were required to map the breast lymphatics, which were less profuse than the dermal lymphatics. Additionally, care was required to inject isosulfan blue around the tumor and/or biopsy cavity to successfully map the lymphatics of the breast. In general, this technique was found to be more difficult to perform in the breast cancer patient. As in cutaneous melanoma, this approach requires substantial experience[49,50] but substantial and increasing evidence now strongly supports the diagnostic accuracy of ILM/SL in breast cancer.

The most compelling evidence supporting the sentinel node hypothesis was published by Turner and co-workers.[51] In order to address the possibility that the likelihood of identifying metastatic disease was an artifact related to a more thorough analysis of the sentinel lymph node, Turner and co-workers examined all lymph nodes, both sentinel and nonsentinel, in an identical fashion with standard hematoxylin–eosin staining and immunohistochemical staining if negative by routine hematoxylin–eosin staining. When the sentinel lymph node was negative by both hematoxylin–eosin and immunohistochemical staining, then the probability of a non-sentinel node being involved with metastatic disease was <0.1% despite the more intensive examination of these nonsentinel lymph nodes providing compelling evidence that the sentinel lymph node is indeed the most likely node to harbor metastatic tumor.

LYMPHATIC MAPPING IN SOLID NEOPLASMS OTHER THAN MELANOMA AND BREAST CANCER

It was inevitable that investigations of the applicability of ILM/SL in other solid neoplasms would be undertaken in an effort to obtain the benefits of improved staging information observed in cutaneous melanoma and breast cancer. Like cutaneous melanoma and breast cancer, regional nodal metastases present the single most important prognostic factor in most solid neoplasms and often represent the primary indication for adjuvant systemic therapy. Additionally, it is well recognized that although individuals who are node negative in many solid neoplasms have an excellent prognosis, a substantial number of these individuals do ultimately recur and die of disease. The possibility that this might represent understaging of the disease has been raised. ILM/SL in these settings is being explored in an effort to examine these issues. Lymphatic mapping and sentinel node staging has now been explored in a number of cutaneous tumors including Merkel cell carcinoma[52] and squamous cell cancer,[53] and in gastrointestinal tumors including the colon[54, 55] and rectum,[55] pancreas,[56] and stomach.[56, 57]

ILM/SL for many common neoplasms, particularly of the gastrointestinal tract, may prove to be useful as an adjunct to standard hematoxylin–eosin staging. In contrast to cutaneous melanoma and breast cancer in which avoiding a complete lymphadenectomy has substantial impact on morbidity, a complete mesenteric lymph node dissection in patients with most gastrointestinal cancers does not significant increase the morbidity of these procedures. However, the improvements in staging may lead to refinement of adjuvant treatments that could translate into improved outcomes.

CONCLUSIONS

Intraoperative lymphatic mapping and selective lymphadenectomy is a revolutionary concept that, in its very short history, has shown the potential to dramatically alter the management of many patients with solid neoplasms. The rapid embrace of this approach by the surgical oncology community to staging of solid neoplasms has resulted in an explosion of data on this subject. Initially described as a surgical technique in which each surgeon has to climb an individual learning curve, ILM/SL is now recognized as being a multidisciplinary surgical, nuclear medicine, pathologic approach to the management of the patient with cutaneous melanoma and breast cancer. The potential utility of ILM and SLND is now being vigorously examined in numerous other solid neoplasms as is discussed in other chapters.

Despite lack of standardization of this technique, debate regarding the operative definition of a sentinel node,[58] and even the appropriateness of this approach outside of research settings,[59] all reports from a variety of clinical settings support the original sentinel node hypothesis. Important unresolved issues remain including standardization issues and the biologic relevance of immunohistochemical findings. However, it is apparent that ILM/SL provides greater diagnostic accuracy and lower morbidity as substantial numbers of truly node negative patients with cutaneous melanoma and breast cancer can be spared the morbidity of a regional node dissection that has no potential therapeutic value. Even if ILM/SL does not ultimately prove to improve survival, this approach may provide biologically relevant information that can be utilized to improve outcomes in patients with solid neoplasms.

REFERENCES

1. Morton DL, Duan-Ren W, Wong JH, et al. Technical details of intraoperative lymphatic mapping for early stage melanoma. Archives of Surgery 1992; 127(4):392-399.
2. Bartholin T. De lacteis thoracicis in homine brutisque. Hafniae: M. Martzan, 1653.
3. Glisson F. Anatomia hepatis...subjiciuntur nonnulla de lymphae-ductibus nuper repertis. Londini: Typ. Du-Gardianis, 1654.

4. Rudbeck O. Nova exercitatio anatomica, exhibens ductus hepaticos aquosos, et vasa glandularum serosa. Arosiae: ecus. E. Lauringerus, 1653.
5. Cruikshank W. The anatomy of the absorbing vessels of the human body. London: G. Nicol, 1786.
6. Sappey M. Anatomie, physiologie, pathologie, des vaisseaux lymphatiques consideres ches l'homme et les vertebres. Paris, 1874.
7. Haagensen C. An exhibit of important books, papers, and memorabilia illustrating the evolution of the knowledge of cancer. American Journal of Cancer 1933; 18:42-126.
8. Kardinal C, Yarbro J. A conceptual history of cancer. Seminars in Oncology 1979; 6:396-408.
9. Fisher B, Jong-Hyeon J, Anderson S, et al. Twenty-five year follow-up of a randomized trial comparing radical mastectomy, total mastectomy and total mastectomy followed by irradiation. New England Journal of Medicine 2002; 347(8):567-575.
10. Fisher B, Anderson S, Bryant J, et al. Twenty-year follow-up of a randomized trail comparing total mastectomy, lumpectomy, and lumpectomy plus irradiation for the treatment of invasive breast cancer. New England Journal of Medicine 2002; 347(16):1233-1241.
11. Veronesi U, Cascinelli N, Mariani L, et al. Twenty-year follow-up of a randomized study comparing breast-conserving surgery with radical mastectomy for early breast cancer. New England Journal of Medicine 2002; 347(16):1227-1232.
12. Snow H. Melanotic cancerous disease. Lancet 1892; 2:872.
13. Roses DF, Provet JA, Harris MN, et al. Prognosis of patients with pathologic stage II cutaneous malignant melanoma. Annals of Surgery 1985; 201:103-107.
14. McNeer G, Das Gupta TK. Prognosis in malignant melanoma. Surgery 1964; 56:512-518.
15. Balch CM, Soong S-J, Murad TM, et al. A multifactorial analysis of melanoma III. Prognostic factors in melanoma patients with lymph node metastases (Stage II). Annals of Surgery 1981; 193:377-388.
16. Morton DL, Wanek L, Anne Nizze JA, et al. Improved long-term survival after lymphadenectomy of melanoma metastatic to regional nodes: Analysis of prognostic factors in 1134 patients from the John Wayne Cancer Clinic. Annals of Surgery 1991; 214(4):491-501.
17. Cohen MH, Ketcham AS, Felix EL, et al. Prognostic factors in patients undergoing lymphadenectomy for malignant melanoma. Annals of Surgery 1976; 186(5):635-642.
18. Veronesi U, Adamus J, Bandiera DC, et al. Delayed regional lymph node dissection in stage I melanoma of the skin of the lower extremities. Cancer 1982; 49(11):2420-2430.
19. Sim FH, Taylor WF, Pritchard DJ, Soule EH. Lymphadenectomy in the management of stage I malignant melanoma: A prospective randomized study. Mayo Clinic Proceedings 1986; 61(3):697-705.
20. Balch CM, Soong S-J, Bartolucci AA, et al. Efficacy of an elective regional lymph node dissection of 1 to 4 mm thick melanomas for patients 60 years of age and younger. Annals of Surgery 1996; 224(3):255-266.
21. Hack T, Cohen L, Katz J, et al. Physical and psychological morbidity after axillary lymph node dissection for breast cancer. Journal of Clinical Oncology 1999; 17:143-149.
22. Cady B. Is axillary lymph node dissection necessary in routine management of breast cancer? No. Principles & Practice of Oncology, Update 1998; 12(7):1-12.
23. Clark WH, From L, Bernardino EA, Mihm MC. The histogenesis and biologic behavior of primary human malignant melanoma of the skin. Cancer Research 1969; 29(3):705-727.
24. Breslow A. Thickness, cross-sectional areas and depth of invasion in the prognosis of cutaneous melanoma. Annals of Surgery 1970; 172:902-907.

25. Holmes E, Moseley H, Morton DL, et al. A rational approach to the surgical management of melanoma. Annals of Surgery 1977; 186:481-490.
26. Wanebo H, Fortner J, Woodruff J, et al. Selection of the optimum surgical treatment of Stage I melanoma by depth of microinvasion: Use of the combined microstage technique (Clark-Breslow). Annals of Surgery 1975; 182:302-315.
27. Busch F, Sayegh E. Roentgenographic visualization of human testicular lymphatics: A preliminary report. Journal of Urology 1963; 89(1):106-110.
28. Gergely R. The roentgen examination of the lymphatics in man. Radiology 1958; 71:59-68.
29. Cabanas RM. An approach for the treatment of penile carcinoma. Cancer 1977; 39:456-466.
30. Fowler JE Jr., Sentinel lymph node biopsy for staging penile cancer. Urology 1984; 23(4):352-354.
31. Bouchot O, Bouvier S, Bochereau G. Cancer of the penis: the value of systematic biopsy. Progres en Urologie 1993; 2:228-233.
32. Perinetti E, Crane DB, Catalona WJ. Unreliability of sentinel lymph node biopsy for staging penile carcinoma. Urology 1984; 23:352-355.
33. Persky L, deKernion J. Carcinoma of the penis. Cancer 1986; 36:258-273.
34. Wong JH, Cagle LA, Morton DL. Lymphatic drainage of skin to a sentinel lymph node in a feline model. Annals of Surgery 1991; 214(5):637-641.
35. Norman J, Cruse CW, Espinosa C, et al. Redefinition of cutaneous lymphatic drainage with the use of lymphoscintigraphy for malignant melanoma. American Journal of Surgery 1991; 162:432-437.
36. Cochran AJ, Wen DR, Morton DL. Occult tumor cells in the lymph nodes of patients with pathological stage I malignant melanoma. An immunohistological study. American Journal of Pathology 1988; 12:612-618.
37. Morton DL, Thompson JF, Essner R, et al. Validation of the accuracy of intraoperative lymphatic mapping and sentinel lymphadenectomy for early-stage melanoma. A multicenter trial. Annals of Surgery 1999; 230(4):453-465.
38. Morton DL. Commentary: Intraoperative lymphatic mapping and sentinel lymphadenectomy: community standard of care or clinical investigation? The Cancer Journal 1997:328-330.
39. Faries MB, Bedrosian I, Reynolds C, et al. Active macromolecule uptake by lymph node antigen-presenting cells: A novel mechanism in determining sentinel lymph node status. Annals of Surgical Oncology 2000; 7(2):98-105.
40. Leong SPL, Steinmetz I, Habib FA, et al. Optimal selective sentinel lymph node dissection in primary malignant melanoma. Archives of Surgery 1997; 132(6):666-673.
41. Albertini JJ, Cruse CW, Rapaport D, et al. Intraoperative radiolymphoscintigraphy improves sentinel lymph node identification for patients with melanoma. Annals of Surgery 1996; 223(2):217-224.
42. Reintgen D, Cruse CW, Wells K, et al. The orderly progression of melanoma nodal metastases. Annals of Surgery 1994; 220(6):759-767.
43. Wong JH, Terada K, Ko P, Coel MN. Lack of effect of particle size on the identification of the sentinel node in cutaneous malignancies. Annals of Surgical Oncology 1998; 5(1):77-80.
44. Arnold M, Young D, Hitchcock C, et al. Radioimmunoguided surgery in primary colorectal carcinoma: An intraoperative prognostic tool and adjuvant to traditional staging. American Journal of Surgery 1995; 170:315-318.

45. Cote R, Houchens D, Hitchcock C, et al. Intraoperative detection of occult colon cancer micrometastases using 125-I-radiolabeled monoclonal antibody CC49. Cancer 1996; 77:613-620.
46. Greenson JK, Isenhart CE, Rice R, et al. Identification of occult micrometastases in pericolic lymph nodes of Dukes' B colorectal cancer patients using monoclonal antibodies again cytokeratin and CC49. Cancer 1994; 73(3):563-569.
47. Alex JC, Weaver DL, Fairbank JT, Krag DN. Gamma-probe-guided lymph node localization in malignant melanoma. Surgical Oncology 1993; 2:303-308.
48. Krag DN, Meijer SJ, Weaver DL, et al. Minimal-access surgery for staging of malignant melanoma. Archives of Surgery 1995; 130(6):654-658.
49. Giuliano AE, Kirgan DM, Guenther JM, Morton DL. Lymphatic mapping and sentinel lymphadenectomy for breast cancer. Annals of Surgery 1994; 220(3):391-401.
50. Guenther JM, Krishnamoorthy M, Tan LR. Sentinel lymphadenectomy for breast cancer in a community managed care setting. The Cancer Journal 1997; 3(6):336-340.
51. Turner RR, Ollila DW, Krasne DL, Giuliano AE. Histopathologic validation of the sentinel lymph node hypothesis for breast carcinoma. Annals of Surgery 1997; 226(3):271-278.
52. Rodrigues L, Leong S, Kashani-Sabet M, Wong JH. Early experience with sentinel lymph node mapping for Merkel cell carcinoma. Journal of the American Academy of Dermatology 2001; 45:303-308.
53. Terada KY, Coel MN, Ko P, Wong JH. Combined use of intraoperative lymphatic mapping and lymphoscintigraphy in the management of squamous cell cancer of the vulva. Gynecologic Oncology 1998; 70:65-69.
54. Saha S, Wiese D, Badin J, et al. Technical detail of sentinel lymph node mapping in colorectal cancer and its impact on staging. Annals of Surgical Oncology 2000; 7(2):120-124.
55. Wong JH, Steinemann S, Calderia C, et al. Ex vivo sentinel node mapping in carcinoma of the colon and rectum. Annals of Surgery 2001; 233(4):515-521.
56. Bilchik AJ, Guiliano AE, Essner R, et al. Universal application of intraoperative lymphatic mapping and sentinel lymphadenectomy in solid neoplasms. The Cancer Journal 1998; 4(6):351-358.
57. Kitagawa Y, Fujii H, Mukai M, et al. The role of the sentinel lymph node in gastrointestinal cancer. Surgical Clinics of North America 2000; 80:1799-1809.
58. Morton DL, Bostick PJ. Editorial: Will the true sentinel node please stand? Annals of Surgical Oncology 1999; 6(1):12-14.
59. Morton DL, Chan AD. Current status of intraoperative lymphatic mapping and sentinel lymphadenectomy for melanoma: is it standard of care? Journal American College of Surgeons 1999:214-222.
60. Thompson JF, McCarthy WH, Bosch CM, et al. Sentinel lymph node status as an indicator of the presence of melanoma in the regional lymph nodes. Melanoma Research 1995; 5(4):255-260.
61. Lingam MK, Mackie RM, McKay AJ. Intraoperative identification of sentinel node dissection in patients with malignant melanoma. British Journal of Surgery 1997; 75:1505-1508.
62. Morton DL, Wen DR, Foshag LJ, et al. Intraoperative lymphatic mapping and selective cervical lymphadenectomy for early-stage melanomas of the head and neck. Journal of Clinical Oncology 1993; 11(9):1751-1756.

Chapter 2

ROLE OF LYMPHOSCINTIGRAPHY FOR SELECTIVE SENTINEL LYMPHADENECTOMY

Roger F. Uren, Robert B. Howman-Giles, David Chung, John F. Thompson*

Nuclear Medicine and Diagnostic Ultrasound, RPAH Medical Centre and Discipline of Medicine, The University of Sydney, Sydney, NSW, Australia and The Sydney Melanoma Unit, Royal Prince Alfred Hospital, Camperdown, NSW and Discipline of Surgery, The University of Sydney, Sydney, NSW, Australia*

Abstract: An essential prerequisite for a successful sentinel node biopsy (SNB) procedure is an accurate map of the pattern of lymphatic drainage from the primary tumor site. The role of lymphoscintigraphy(LS) in SNB is to provide such a map in each patient. This map should indicate not only the location of all sentinel nodes but also the number of SNs at each location. Such mapping can be achieved using ^{99m}Tc-labeled small particle radiocolloids, high-resolution collimators with minimal septal penetration, and imaging protocols that detect all SNs in every patient regardless of their location. This is especially important in melanoma patients, since high-quality LS can identify the actual lymphatic collecting vessels as they drain into each SN. The SN is not always found in the nearest node field and is best defined as "any lymph node receiving direct lymphatic drainage from a primary tumor site."

Reliable clinical prediction of lymphatic drainage from the skin or breast is not possible. Patterns of lymphatic drainage from the skin are highly variable from patient to patient, even from the same area of the skin.

Unexpected lymphatic drainage has been found from the skin of the back to SNs in the triangular intermuscular space and in some patients through the posterior body wall to SNs in the para-aortic, paravertebral, and retroperitoneal areas. Lymphatic drainage from the head and neck frequently involves SNs in multiple node fields, and can occur from the base of the neck up to nodes in the occipital or upper cervical areas or from the scalp down to nodes at the neck base, bypassing many other node groups. Lymphatic drainage from the upper limb can be directly to SNs above the axilla. Drainage to the epitrochlear region from the hand and arm is more common than was previously thought as is drainage to the popliteal region from the foot and leg.

Interval nodes, which lie along the course of a lymphatic vessel between a melanoma site and a recognised node field, are not uncommon especially on the trunk. Drainage across the midline of the body is quite frequent on the trunk and in the head and neck region.

In breast cancer, although dynamic imaging is usually not possible, an early postmassage image will also often visualize the lymphatic vessels leading to the SN allowing them to be differentiated from any second tier nodes. Small radiocolloid particles are also needed to achieve migration from peritumoral injections sites and LS allows accurately detection of SNs outside the axilla, which occur in about 50% of patients. These nodes may lie in the internal mammary chain, the supraclavicular region, or the interpectoral region. Intramammary interval nodes can also be SNs in some patients. The location of the cancer in the breast is not a reliable guide to lymphatic drainage, since lymph flow often crosses the center line of the breast.

Micrometastatic disease can be present in any SN regardless of its location, and for the SNB technique to be accurate all true SNs must be identified and removed in every patient. LS is an important first step in ensuring that this goal is achieved.

LYMPHOSCINTIGRAPHY, CANCER, SENTINEL LYMPH NODE BIOPSY

There is now general consensus that accurate SNB requires close cooperation between nuclear medicine physician, surgeon and histopathologist. Nuclear medicine's role in this technology is to provide an accurate map of the pattern of lymphatic drainage from the primary tumor site so that the location of every SN can be marked on the overlying skin in each patient, regardless of the location of the node. The pursuit of this goal has led to the discovery of several new lymphatic drainage pathways from the skin[1-5] and a better understanding of the patterns of lymph drainage from the breast. Several factors are critical if such an accurate map of lymphatic drainage is to be obtained. These include an understanding of the physiology of lymphatic flow, the use of an appropriate small particle radiocolloid, the use of high-resolution collimators or other methods to reduce septal penetration from the activity at the injection site and the application of imaging protocols that will enable the detection of all true SNs in every patient even though SNs may lie in unexpected places.

PHYSIOLOGY OF LYMPHATIC FLOW

We know that there are several factors in the clinical setting that increase lymphatic flow and several that decrease it. Lymph flow is increased by heat, massage, inflammation, movement of the part, and an increase in hydrostatic pressure within the lumen of the lymphatic collecting vessel.[6] Lymph flow is decreased by cold, lack of movement, and external pressure.[1] When performing SNB some of these factors may affect the accuracy of the lymphatic drainage map obtained on LS and after blue dye injection at surgery. The patient must be kept warm in the operating theatre to encourage movement of the blue dye and massage can be a very useful intervention to enhance flow. In the breast, which is not as richly served with lymphatics as the skin, massage is a vital post-injection intervention to ensure entry of the radiocolloid into the initial lymphatic capillary and subsequent visualization of the SN. Even light external pressure dramatically reduces lymph flow so that any swab placed over the injection site should be only lightly applied and patients should be encouraged to exercise the relevant part of their body between the early and delayed images to further enhance flow. The increased intraluminal hydrostatic pressure in lymphatics of the lower limb which accompanies standing also increases lymph flow from this area.[6]

It should also be remembered that the velocity of lymphatic flow is not uniform throughout the body and in fact varies systematically from different areas of the skin.[7]

Table 1. Lymph Flow Rates From Cutaneous Sites

Region	Average Flow(cm/min)
Head and neck	1.5
Anterior trunk	2.8
Posterior trunk	3.9
Arm and shoulder	2.0
Forearm and hand	5.5
Thigh	4.2
Leg and foot	10.2

This information can be useful in timing blue dye injection prior to surgery and is also relevant in terms of the incidence of tracer movement to second tier nodes beyond the SN.[8] The faster the lymph flow, the more second tier nodes are seen. Second tier nodes are thus more common in the groin than elsewhere in the body since the fastest lymph flows are seen from the leg and foot.

Lymph nodes are not passive mechanical filters and radiocolloids are trapped and retained in SNs by an active physiological process which involves opsonization of the colloid and causes it to be recognized as foreign. This process may occur in the collecting vessel itself or in the subcapsular sinus of the SN. The opsonized radiocolloid is then phagocytosed by the macrophages and tissue histiocytes which line the subcapsular sinus and other sinuses of the lymph node.[9] These processes take time and can be overwhelmed if too many radiocolloid particles reach the SN per unit time. When this occurs it will be apparent on dynamic imaging that there is movement of tracer on to second tier nodes. This process occurs in the first 10 to 15 minutes after radiocolloid injection, when the initial bolus of particles reaches the SN. In most patients there is very little further migration of the radiocolloid particles from this point on and the pattern of uptake seen at 15 minutes is essentially the same as it is at 2 hours and 24 hours. This is not a function of particle size. The frequent assertion that large particles stay in the SN while small ones do not is incorrect. Even with the small particles we have used in our patients, ^{99m}Tc antimony sulfide colloid, the SN remains the only "hot" node in many patients and this is so up to 24 hours postinjection.

As a guide, there is usually a correlation between the number of lymphatic collecting vessels seen on dynamic or early imaging and the number of SNs present in that patient.[1] This is not always the case, however, and a single lymphatic collecting vessel sometimes divides to reach two or more SNs. This occurs especially in the groin for leg lesions. The reverse may also occur and two or more collecting vessels may converge to meet a single SN. This occurs most often in the axilla.

Figure 1.
(A) Summed 10 minute-dynamic sequence in the anterior projection over the right groin following intradermal injection of ^{99m}Tc antimony sulfide colloid at a melanoma excision biopsy site on the right leg. A single lymphatic collecting vessel passes to the right groin where it bifurcates to meet two SNs. A faint second lymph vessel joins this dominant vessel just below the groin. Some second tier nodes are also seen above the two SNs. (B) The summed dynamic sequence in the anterior projection following the intradermal injection of tracer at a melanoma excision biopsy site over the left costal margin. Three lymphatic collecting vessels pass to the left axilla where they converge to meet a single SN.

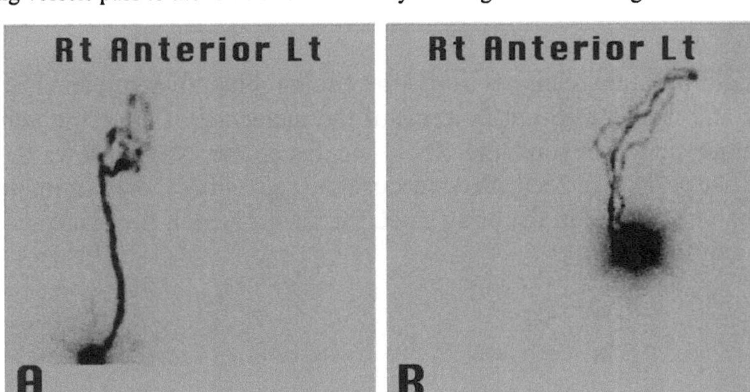

The path taken by a collecting vessel on its way to a draining node field varies from patient to patient and from skin site to skin site. These pathways can sometimes be extremely complex and tortuous.[1] The collecting vessels usually travel in the subcutaneous fat layer and generally do not penetrate the deep fascia until a node field such as the groin or axilla is reached.

THE SENTINEL NODE

Definition: "A sentinel lymph node is any lymph node which receives lymph drainage directly from a tumor site." [1]

An SN is not just the first node seen on dynamic imaging, since there may be multiple separate lymph channels that have different rates of lymph flow. If they drain to different nodes these are all SNs, regardless of the time taken for the lymph containing the radiocolloid to reach them. An SN is also not necessarily the closest node to the primary site. Lymphatic vessels can bypass many nodes and even whole node fields before reaching an SN.

The best way to identify an SN on LS is therefore to see the lymphatic collecting vessel on dynamic imaging as it drains directly to the SN (Fig. One). This is the same lymphatic collecting vessel that the surgeon sees, stained blue, in the operative field during SN surgery. In order to visualize the lymphatic collecting vessels there must be adequate numbers of radiocolloid particles in the lymph fluid during the early dynamic phase, and this requires the use of small particle radiocolloids as previously emphasized.

APPROPRIATE RADIOCOLLOID

A radiocolloid must gain access to the lumen of the initial lymphatics under physiological conditions to allow accurate mapping of lymphatic drainage. The ideal radiocolloid for LS and SNB is one which readily enters the initial lymphatic capillary following interstitial injection, and moves freely through the lymphatic vessels to the draining SN where it is retained. If this occurs, the SN can be detected at the time of surgery if this is within 24 hours. Beyond that time the radioactivity in the SN will become undetectable using a gamma detecting probe due to radioactive decay.

When the microanatomy of the lymphatic vessels is considered, it is apparent that small particle radiocolloids best enter the lymphatic capillaries. The lymphatic endothelial cells which line the walls of the initial lymphatic capillaries overlap each other over a significant distance and there is a 10 to

25 nm gap[10] between the cells through which material can freely pass to enter the lumen of the lymphatic. Small particle radiocolloids such as ^{99m}Tc antimony sulfide colloid (particle size 5–15 nm),[1] nanocolloid of albumin labeled with ^{99m}Tc(particle size 3–80 nm),[11] filtered ^{99m}Tc sulfur colloid(100 nm filter, particle size 5–100 nm)[12] and ^{99m}Tc rhenium sulfide colloid(particle size around 50 nm)[13] will all pass through this gap to some degree under physiological conditions. The gap between the endothelial cells can be increased by massage and this will allow some larger particles to enter the lumen of the lymphatic but usually in insufficient numbers to allow visualization of the lymphatic vessel itself. This is an important part of dynamic LS as the SN can be clearly identified if the lymphatic collecting vessel can be seen passing directly to it. Visualizing only a series of "hot spots" without seeing the vessels makes identification of the true SN problematic and largely speculative. This then leads to definitions of the SN based on the activity in the node compared to background or to other "hot" nodes in the node field. This is imprecise and usually leads to some second tier nodes being removed as SNs, an undesirable result when one of the rationales for the SNB technique is the reduced morbidity associated with minimal surgery.

The poor migration from the injection site that occurs with large particle radiocolloids means that a larger percentage of patients will not have an SN identified on LS. This is particularly the case in the breast with peritumoral injections. Faced with this dilemma and with no small particle colloid available as an alternative, many began injecting away from the tumor in order to radiolabel a node in the axilla. This is intuitively an undesirable approach. Intradermal or subdermal injections over the tumor site or peri-areolar injections do make the radiolabeling of an axillary node more likely when using large particle colloids compared with peritumoral injections. There is also evidence that the same node in the axilla will usually be radiolabeled regardless of the site of injection,[14] though this may not always be the case. However, these injection sites away from the tumor certainly do not provide a full map of the pattern of lymphatic drainage from the breast cancer because the skin rarely drains to the nonaxillary sentinel nodes such as those in the internal mammary and supraclavicular regions, or to intramammary interval nodes and interpectoral nodes. Our data suggest that SNs are seen in these areas in almost 50% of patients with breast cancer.[1] Thus, to obtain an accurate map of lymphatic drainage and therefore allow the identification of all true SNs in every patient we recommend small particle radiocolloids and peritumoral injections (or injection around the excision biopsy site) for both melanoma and breast cancer.

At the SN2002 conference in Yokohama, data were presented that raised questions about the best particle size to use when performing LS and SNB on visceral organs such as those in the gastrointestinal tract. Using ^{99m}Tc phytate(with a particle size of 500 nm) and Kitajima[15] showed that the detected SNs accurately staged the regional node fields with an average of about five SNs being seen for colon and stomach cancer. When using smaller particles they found extra nodes were radiolabeled. The disadvantage of the large particles was that a 2-hour delay was required between tracer injection and LS or surgery with a gamma detecting probe. This meant that tracer injection had to be performed endoscopically at a different time from blue dye, which was injected during surgery. It is possible that lymph nodes draining visceral structures have a functional anatomy that is different from that found in peripheral lymph nodes. Such nodes may be less efficient at retaining radiocolloid particles, perhaps because their phagocytic capacity is less well developed. This may mean that larger particles are required for SNB in these areas. We have noticed that interval nodes tend to be more "porous" to small particle radiocolloid than other lymph nodes and in our breast cancer patients it is routine to see a string of second tier internal mammary nodes superior to the sentinel node which is seen directly receiving the lymphatic collecting vessel. Ege[16] and Kaplan et al.[17] years ago showed that almost the full chain of internal mammary nodes could be displayed using an injection of ^{99m}Tc antimony sulfide colloid in the upper posterior rectus sheath (an observation that was probably the source of the erroneous assumption that small particle radiocolloids always pass rapidly through the first node they meet–the SN). There is thus considerable evidence that lymph nodes throughout the body vary in their ability to trap radiocolloid particles and it is therefore possible that larger particles will prove preferable for SNB in patients with cancer of the visceral organs.

HIGH RESOLUTION COLLIMATORS

Regardless of the radiocolloid used, the majority of the injected dose for lymphatic mapping will remain at the site of injection. Even the best small particle colloids such as ^{99m}Tc antimony sulfide colloid show only 5–8% migration to the sentinel node so that 92–95% remains at the injection site while with ^{99m}Tc sulfur colloid 99% remains at the injection site.[18] Quite often in melanoma patients and almost always in breast cancer and other tumors this means that the injected activity remains in the field of view. Since the SN contains a small amount of activity compared with the injection site in order to visualize the sentinel nodes the image will need to be digitally enhanced so that even the faintest uptake is seen. With many high resolution collimators, especially folded metal collimators, this digital enhancement of the image will cause star artifact to become apparent which may obscure possible SNs. This collimator star artifact is caused by septal penetration of the collimator. When using digital enhancement, which is necessary when trying to highlight small areas of low activity, this "star" can bloom on the image and completely obscure true sentinel nodes in the field.

To avoid this we use a superhigh-resolution collimator. This is microcast and not made using the folded metal approach. Such collimators minimize star artifact since septal penetration is less than 1% at an energy of 140 keV, the energy of the gamma ray emitted by ^{99m}Tc. If a superhigh-resolution collimator is unavailable we would recommend using a medium-energy collimator. Though this will result in loss of resolution it will prevent star artifact and should allow better detection of sentinel nodes in areas outside the axilla especially in breast cancer patients.

An alternate approach in melanoma and breast cancer patients who have an accessible site of injection is to attempt to shield this activity using lead sheets. This will be effective if carefully performed but is cumbersome and time consuming and thus not a practical solution for most busy nuclear medicine departments. It is also not an option in most cancers of visceral origin with the exception of cervical cancer.

A low level of septal penetration is especially important in LS for patients with visceral organ cancer. Such patients require tomographic imaging and any star artifact will completely obscure SNs near the injection site. This is a common situation in stomach, colon, prostate, and cervical cancer. If no superhigh-resolution microcast collimator is available, it would be preferable to use the medium-energy collimator.

IMAGING PROTOCOLS

Imaging protocols for LS should be designed to detect all SNs in every patient. In breast cancer patients this is relatively straightforward, since anterior and lateral views will suffice in all except those with a lower outer quadrant lesion in whom posterior views should also be obtained to detect the rare occurrence of drainage to posterior intercostal nodes. In melanoma patients, however, the situation is more complex and requires a full understanding of the unusual patterns of lymphatic drainage that can occur from the skin.[1] In the trunk, posterior and lateral views are required for back lesion sites and a check should be made for intra-abdominal drainage. The head and neck region, particularly the nape of the neck area can also be challenging and superior oblique or vertex views are usually required to ensure that SNs are not obscured by the injected activity, a situation which is common on straight AP views in this part of the body.

In patients with cancer of the GI tract or other visceral organs, three-dimensional SPECT imaging will be required and even just displaying a movie of the raw projection data will allow determination of the best angle to view the SN separate from the injection site when the two are close to each other. Star artifact during SPECT imaging will be further reduced using a continuous rotation acquisition rather than step and shoot and by using OSEM during reconstruction rather than the back projection method.

LYMPHOSCINTIGRAPHY METHOD

MELANOMA

At the Sydney Melanoma Unit, LS to locate SNs in patients with melanoma involves the intradermal injection of a radiocolloid around the melanoma site or excision biopsy site[1,19] Injections of 5–10 MBq in 0.05–0.1 ml/injection are used and typically four injections are required, though this will depend on the primary melanoma size. Following tracer injection, dynamic imaging is performed to follow the lymphatic collecting vessels until they reach the draining SNs. An image should be acquired as the vessels reach the node field so that SNs directly receiving the channels can be identified and distinguished from any second tier nodes that may be seen. This phase of the study usually takes 10–20 minutes.

Delayed scans are performed 2–2.5 hours later, at which time all regions that could possibly drain the primary melanoma site are examined with 5 to10-minute static images. Appropriate lateral, posterior, oblique or vertex views are also acquired as necessary to define the exact location of all sentinel nodes. We routinely use a transmission source on all delayed images to highlight the body outline and these images are especially useful when performing a retrospective review of the scans. We often repeat delayed scans without the transmission source however, as in some patients a faint sentinel node in a new node field will be obscured by the scattered activity from the source. (Most of the scans used as illustrations in this article have been acquired without the transmission source for this reason, and the body outlines have been added later.)

The surface location of all SNs is marked on the overlying skin with an "X" of indelible ink. A permanent point tattoo of carbon black can also be applied and is a useful locator to guide clinical or ultrasound follow up over subsequent years. The depth of the sentinel node from the skin mark is measured in an orthogonal view with a radioactive marker placed on the skin mark. The depth can then be measured off the film directly or by using electronic calipers. Some centers use a gamma probe in the nuclear medicine suite to further aid localization of the sentinel node. In whatever fashion the patient and the scan data are presented to the operating surgeon, it is essential that the method of presentation is completely understood. The surgeon must be familiar with the appearance of your scans so that reference to them can be made while searching for the SN during surgery. This very close communication and understanding between nuclear medicine and surgical colleagues is invaluable if the SNB method is to be accurate, and we regularly have communication directly from the operating suite between surgeon and nuclear medicine physician if there is an unusual lymphatic drainage pattern to be clarified.

The pattern of drainage seen in an individual patient is surprisingly reproducible and in the small number of patients who have had the study repeated we have invariably seen exactly the same SNs though there has been some variation in the relative intensity of tracer uptake by the nodes.

Figure 2.
(A) Anterior and posterior 2-hour postinjection delayed LS images performed on two occasions 3 days apart on a patient with an upper back melanoma. The same drainage pattern is seen with SNs in the axilla bilaterally though there are slight differences in the intensity of the nodal uptake. (B) Two-hour postinjection delayed LS images anteriorly over the groin and posteriorly over the popliteal fossa in the same patient on two occasions 7 days apart. The lesion site was on the lower right thigh laterally. A single SN is seen in the right groin on both scans though it is much fainter on the second study and faint second tier nodes are seen on the first scan in the groin above the SN.

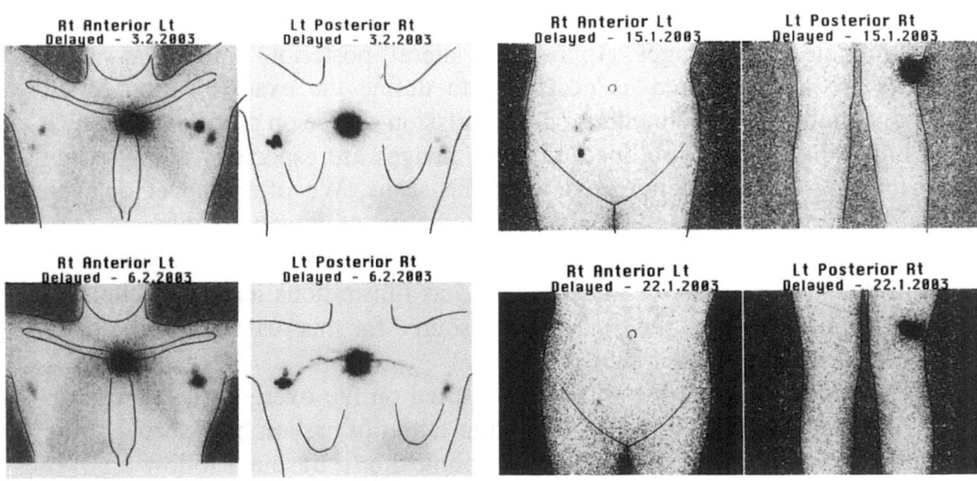

This is the protocol we have successfully used in over 3000 patients with cutaneous melanoma. More detailed descriptions of our technique and imaging protocols are recorded elsewhere.[1,19]

Whenever possible the lymphatic mapping should be done prior to wide local excision of the primary melanoma, as this disrupts lymph drainage pathways and may cause nonmigration of the tracer or the identification of lymph nodes that are not true SNs.

BREAST CANCER

In breast cancer we use ultrasound to locate the tumor and inject at four points at 3, 6, 9, and 12 o'clock around it at the depth of the center of the mass. Each injection contains 5–20 MBq of ^{99m}Tc antimony sulfide colloid in a volume of 0.2ml, with the higher activity being used if surgery is to be performed the following day. The patient then performs massage in a rotary fashion for 5 minutes, thus we do not acquire a dynamic sequence in breast cancer patients. Immediately postmassage, 5 to10-minute anterior and lateral static images are acquired, and will often show the lymphatic collecting vessel as it drains directly to the SN or SNs. A posterior view is also performed for lower outer quadrant lesions to check for SNs in the posterior intercostal region. If no movement of tracer is seen on these early images, a further 5 minutes of massage is performed by the patient. Delayed static images for 5–10 minutes are performed 2 hours later in the anterior and lateral projections. The surface location of all SNs is then marked on the skin as described previously for melanoma patients.

With our protocol in about 3% of patients, no movement of tracer from the peritumoral injection site is seen on the delayed 2-hour images and we then place a single intradermal injection of 5 MBq ^{99m}Tc antimony sulfide colloid in the skin overlying the tumor. Imaging is then performed over the following 20–30 minutes until a radiolabeled axillary node is observed. The surface location of this node is then marked on the skin as the likely SN in the axilla.

LYMPHATIC DRAINAGE OF THE SKIN

In 1984 the Sydney Melanoma Unit began performing lymphatic mapping using ^{99m}Tc antimony sulfide colloid to find the draining node fields in patients with intermediate thickness melanomas located in the so-called "ambiguous zones" prior to elective dissection of the relevant node field. Over a 6-year period we performed about 200 studies.[19]

As soon as Morton and colleagues described successful SNB in melanoma patients using injection of blue dye[20] we began to apply the method described above to locate the SNs using LS the day before surgery. This meant that all patients with intermediate thickness melanomas were studied, regardless of the site of the lesions on the skin. Since our examinations required us to track down every SN and not just to image in standard positions we began to observe drainage to lymph nodes in completely unexpected places.[1] Some were in new node fields not previously known to drain the skin. We quickly began to appreciate that there was unambiguous drainage from very few sites on the skin, and that without preoperative LS, accurate SNB was simply not possible in many patients. This variability in lymph drainage and drainage to SNs in unexpected places has also been observed by others.[21-23]

We have performed lymphatic mapping in 3280 patients with cutaneous melanoma up to October 2002, and have accumulated a large body of data relating to common and uncommon cutaneous lymphatic drainage pathways. All of these studies were undertaken by a small group of nuclear medicine physicians and were not performed by trainees. The surgical correlation and SNBs were all performed by a group of specialist melanoma surgeons. The following is a detailed description of the patterns of lymphatic drainage that we have observed.

PATTERNS OF LYMPH DRAINAGE FROM THE SKIN

Posterior Trunk

Melanoma sites on the posterior trunk included axillary drainage in 91% of 1086 patients. Flow to the groin occurred in 11% of patients with back lesions. Drainage across the midline of the patient to contralateral SNs occurred in 35% of patients with back melanomas, and 20% showed drainage over the shoulders to SNs in the neck.

Further unexpected drainage that was seen included lymphatic pathways draining to the triangular intermuscular space(TIS) lateral to the scapula, behind the axilla,[24] and pathways that passed through the posterior body wall directly to SNs in the retroperitoneal, paravertebral and intercostal areas.[25]

The most common of these unexpected pathways is drainage from the skin of the back to an SN in the TIS.[24] We have observed this drainage pathway in 11% of our patients with back melanomas. The lymphatic pathway then passes anteriorly, following the course of the circumflex scapular vessels, into the posterior part of the axilla. This will mean that in some patients tracer will pass on from an SN in the TIS to a second tier node in the axilla. We have seen this occur in several patients. Without accurate lymphatic mapping with LS this could lead to a radiolabeled second tier node being mistakenly identified as the SN and removed from the axilla while the true SN in the TIS remained in the patient. Histological examination of this radiolabeled axillary node will give a false picture of the lymph node status in this patient. This would occur if a gamma probe-only approach was used to find and remove radiolabeled nodes from the axilla, or if the LS imaging protocol was inadequate. Older protocols called only for anterior views of the axilla, but posterior and lateral views are required to identify the SNs in this unexpected location since attenuation of the photons as they pass through the patient's body will mean that nodes in the TIS may not be seen at all in an anterior view. Drainage to an SN in the TIS often occurs along with drainage to an SN in another node field, but we have seen eight patients with exclusive drainage to a SN in this unexpected location.

The second unexpected lymphatic drainage pathway that we have observed draining the skin of the back is one which passes directly through the posterior body wall to SNs in the paravertebral, para-aortic, retroperitoneal, or intercostal areas.[25] This drainage pattern is usually to intra-abdominal sites, but we have also seen paravertebral nodes and intercostal nodes in the thorax as SNs draining the skin of the back. The skin sites which may drain via this unexpected pathway are concentrated mainly in the posterior loin area. We have observed this pathway in 3% of patients with back melanomas, making it much less common than the pathway draining to the TIS. If we consider only the posterior loin area, however, we find drainage via this pathway in 24% of patients. Again drainage to SNs in these unexpected areas is usually accompanied by drainage to SNs in expected node fields (the axilla and/or groin) but we have encountered four patients who had exclusive drainage to SNs in these areas with no drainage whatsoever to axillary or groin nodes.[26] The importance of identifying drainage to SNs in the paravertebral, para-aortic, retroperitoneal, and intercostal areas is that metastatic disease in one of these nodes represents locoregional metastasis, not systemic disease.

Most patients with melanoma sites on the posterior trunk however, do drain to SNs in the expected node fields (the axilla and/or groin), but drainage to combinations of node fields is also very common and will be missed without detailed preoperative lymphatic mapping with LS(Figure 3). Careful imaging is required, including vertex or lateral oblique views, to ensure all SNs are identified around the base of the neck, since such nodes are often obscured by injection site activity in straight anterior or posterior views.

Figure 3. Summed dynamic sequence (top left) and 2-hour delayed scans in the anterior, posterior, and left lateral projection following the injection of ^{99m}Tc antimony sulfide colloid around the melanoma excision biopsy site on the back just to the left of midline. SNs are present in the left axilla but a separate SN is also seen in the left infraclavicular area.

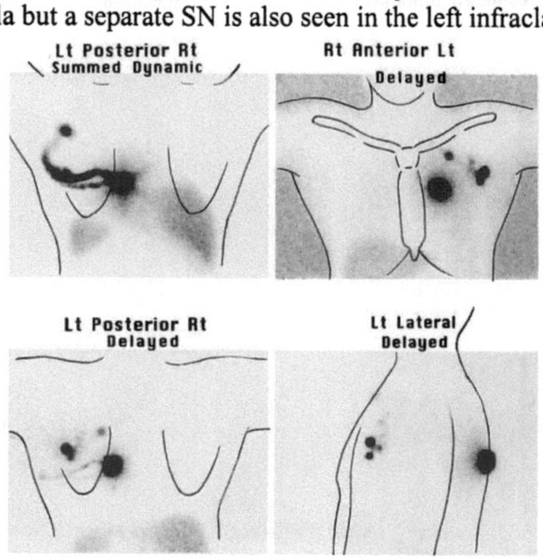

Interval nodes, which are nodes that lie along the course of a lymphatic collecting vessel between a primary site and a draining node field, were seen as SNs more commonly on the back than elsewhere in our patients with melanoma.

Anterior Trunk

Lymphatic drainage from the skin of the anterior trunk is generally to expected node fields and there tends to be less frequent passage of lymph vessels across the midline than on the posterior trunk. In 244 anterior trunk melanoma patients, 83% included drainage to the axilla and 19% included drainage to the groin. Contralateral drainage occurred in 20% of patients. Lymph drainage also occurs to neck nodes from the anterior trunk, just as it occurs from the posterior trunk (Figure 4). Drainage to interval nodes is less common than on the back.

We did detect one new unexpected drainage pathway which passes from the periumbilical skin to an SN which lies in the subcutaneous fat over the costal margin.[27] The lymphatic pathway then passes medially and through the chest wall to internal mammary nodes on the same side as the costal margin node. Thus the SN in these patients is the costal margin node with an internal mammary node receiving drainage as a second tier node. In fact, we have seen an internal mammary node as an SN for the skin of the anterior trunk in only two patients. One had undergone lymph node dissection of his ipsilateral axilla 20 years earlier as treatment for lymphoma. This presumably caused an alternative lymphatic drainage pathway to open up. The other patient had undergone an extensive excision biopsy of a melanoma in the epigastrium and showed drainage to an SN in the right internal mammary chain as well as a left axillary SN.

Figure 4. Summed dynamic and 2 hour delayed images in two patients who had melanomas over the manubrium and upper sternum. The patient in panel A shows a right axillary and right lower cervical SN, while the patient in panel B shows a left axillary and left midcervical SN from the same skin site.

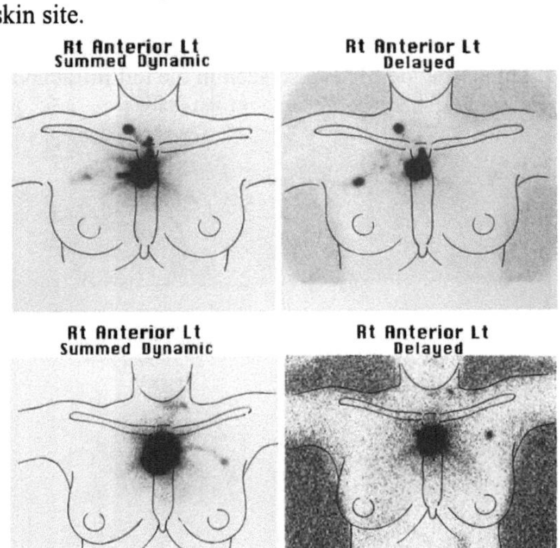

Head and Neck

The head and neck is a challenging area for accurate lymphatic mapping, both for nuclear medicine physicians and for surgeons. Drainage to multiple SNs is common[1,28] and the nodes are often small. The draining SNs often lie very near or sometimes immediately beneath the melanoma site. Detection of such nodes is thus extremely difficult on LS and sometimes impossible. However, if care is taken and such limitations are understood, accurate lymphatic mapping and reliable SNB can be achieved in the head and neck region just as elsewhere in the body.

Lymphatic drainage from the skin of our 578 head and neck melanoma patients is shown in Table 2. As we have found elsewhere, clinical prediction of lymphatic drainage in the head and neck is unreliable and 33% of patients drain to node sites discordant with clinical prediction.[28]

Table 2. Head and neck melanoma– sentinel node sites (*n*=578)

Location of SN		%
Cervical	Level I	20
	Level II	55
	Level III	13
	Level IV	9
	Level V	33
	(Supraclavicular)	10
Occipital		8
Parotid		33
Postauricular		17
Interval node		5
Contralateral		10

This is often to postauricular nodes from the skin of the face and anterior scalp. Such nodes are not usually excised in elective neck dissections for melanoma. Drainage also occurs across the midline and we have seen this in 10% of patients with head and neck melanomas. Such a contralateral node can in the occasional patient be the only site of micrometastatic disease. Lymph drainage also may occur from the base of the neck upwards to SNs in the upper cervical or occipital area. Again we have seen patients with this pattern in whom the only positive SN was an occipital node even though other SNs were present in the axilla, upper cervical area and lateral neck base. Drainage is also seen regularly from the upper scalp directly down to SNs at the base of the neck or in the supraclavicular region. Lymphatic vessels reaching these SNs are thus completely bypassing all the nodes in the upper and midcervical areas as well as the preauricular (parotid) nodes, occipital and postauricular nodes. This reinforces the important concept that the SN is not simply the closest node to the primary melanoma site.

Upper Limb

Lymph drainage from the skin of the upper limb is to the axilla, as expected, in almost all patients. However, that is often not the complete picture. Drainage to SNs in the epitrochlear region is more common than previously thought and we observed drainage to this site in 20% of patients with melanomas located on the forearm and hand. We also have detected direct drainage to nonaxillary SNs (in the supraclavicular region, interpectoral region, lateral neck base, and TIS) in 6% of our 608 patients with upper limb melanomas.[1] These patients also usually had an SN in the axilla and the lymph drainage to these unexpected sites occurred via a separate, discrete lymph vessel. Relying exclusively on gamma probe guided removal of axillary SNs in these patients would very likely have missed these other SNs. Accurate lymphatic mapping with LS is thus imperative.

An "interval" SN is regularly seen lying medially in the arm about half way between the shoulder and elbow. We have seen one patient who had drainage exclusively to this interval node in the mid inner arm, so that it was the only SN.

Lower Limb

In our 764 patients with lower limb melanomas, drainage was always to the ipsilateral groin unless there had been prior surgery to the groin nodes. In this circumstance drainage to the contralateral groin may occur and we have found micrometastases in such contralateral groin SNs.[29]

Lymph drainage from the foot and leg may also occur to popliteal SNs and we have observed this in 38 of 518(7%) patients with melanomas in these areas (Figure 5). The melanoma sites draining to popliteal SNs are quite variable and it is not just the skin of the lateral heel which drains here, as was previously thought.[30] Skin sites on the posterior calf as well as the dorsum and sole of the foot can drain here. The anterior leg less commonly drains to the popliteal fossa.

Figure 5. (A) Summed dynamic and 2-hour delayed images in a patient with a melanoma on the right upper shin. Drainage occurs to a single SN in the right popliteal fossa and to several SNs in the right groin. (B) Summed dynamic image anteriorly over the knees with an early image anteriorly over the groin and a 2-hour delayed posterior image over the popliteal area and anterior image over the groin in a patient with a melanoma excision biopsy site on the left upper shin. An interval node is seen in the left leg as well as nodes in the left popliteal fossa and a single SN in the left groin (see upper right early image). Both of these patients show second tier nodes in the groin above the SNs and the patient in panel B has an unusually large amount of tracer in these second tier nodes. This is related to rapid lymph flow.

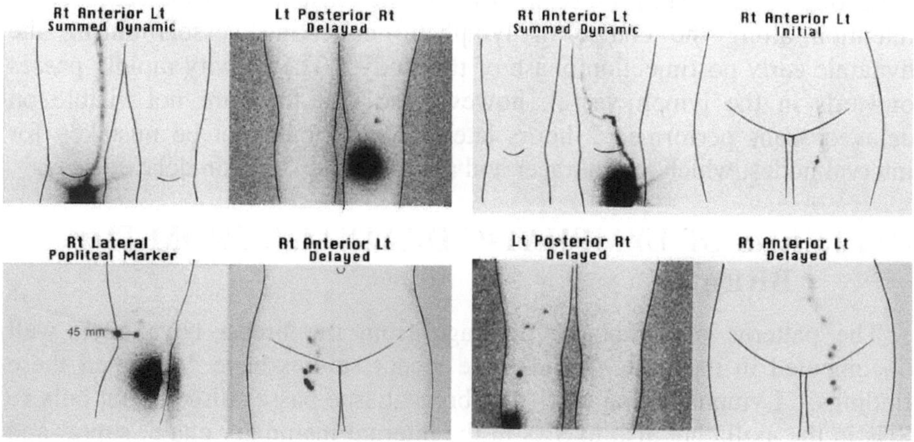

Interval Nodes

Interval nodes can be SNs and we have seen 10 patients in whom they were the only SNs. When present they must be detected and removed if an SNB procedure is to be accurate. We have shown these interval nodes, when SNs, contain micrometastases with the same incidence as SNs found in standard node fields.[31] We found interval nodes in 7% of patients overall and they are more common on the trunk(12% posterior trunk and 8% anterior trunk) than in the head and neck(5%) or upper limb(4%), while they are rare in the lower limb(0.5%). In a large multicenter study McMasters and colleagues[32] also found that in melanoma patients interval nodes were positive for metastases with the same frequency as SNs in standard node fields. In their 13 patients with a positive interval node it was the only positive SN in 11 patients (85%).

Although interval nodes may be found at any point along the course of a lymphatic collecting vessel they are more common in certain locations, such as the midaxillary line, the upper back, and the medial aspect of the mid upper arm.

Interval nodes remain "hot" on delayed scans as they retain the radiocolloid, though it is noticeable that much of the radiocolloid reaching an interval node passes on almost immediately to second tier nodes. They thus seem to be more "porous" to radiocolloids than SNs in standard node fields or in other unexpected node sites.

Lymphatic Lakes

Unlike interval nodes, lymphatic lakes do not need to be examined during the SNB procedure, because they are simply focal dilatations of lymphatic collecting vessels. They are seen during LS as focal areas of increased tracer retention along the course of lymphatic collecting vessels during the dynamic early postinjection phase of the study.[1] The activity rapidly passes onwards in the lymph vessel, however, so that they are not visible on delayed scans performed 2 hours later. These should not be mistaken for interval nodes, which retain tracer and are therefore "hot" on delayed scans.

PATTERNS OF LYMPHATIC DRAINAGE FROM THE BREAST

The patterns of lymphatic drainage from the breast have been well documented in the past[33,34] and more recent studies have confirmed these findings.[35] Lymphatic drainage from breast tissue passes directly not only to SNs in the axilla but also to SNs in the internal mammary chain, supra- and infraclavicular regions, interpectoral region or to intramammary interval nodes. Flow to posterior intercostal nodes has also been described[33] although we have not observed this phenomenon.

In our 640 patients with breast cancer the primary tumors were located as shown in Figure 6. The location of the SNs is shown in Table 3. Most patients (94%) displayed an SN in the axilla and these patients had an average

Table 3. Breast cancer—sentinel node sites

Location	Number (%)
Axilla	578 (94%)
Internal mammary	249 (40%)
Supraclavicular	048 (7.8%)
Infraclavicular	007 (1.1%)
Interpectoral	008 (1.2%)
Interval node	053 (8.6%)
SN outside axilla	286 (46 %)
Exclusive nonaxillary SN	030 (5 %)
No drainage	022 (3.4%)

of 1.45 SNs in the axilla. It is noteworthy that 46% of patients showed drainage to an SN outside the axilla (Figure 7). The demonstration of such lymph flow to SNs outside the axilla is one of the important contributions LS makes to patients with breast cancer. The commonest nonaxillary site for SNs is the internal mammary chain where we have found SNs in 40% of patients overall. This figure is higher than that generally reported for internal mammary node drainage but is almost identical to the 38% of internal mammary drainage found by Shimazu and colleagues (36) when they used subtumoral injections of radiocolloid.

Figure 6. The location of primary breast cancers.

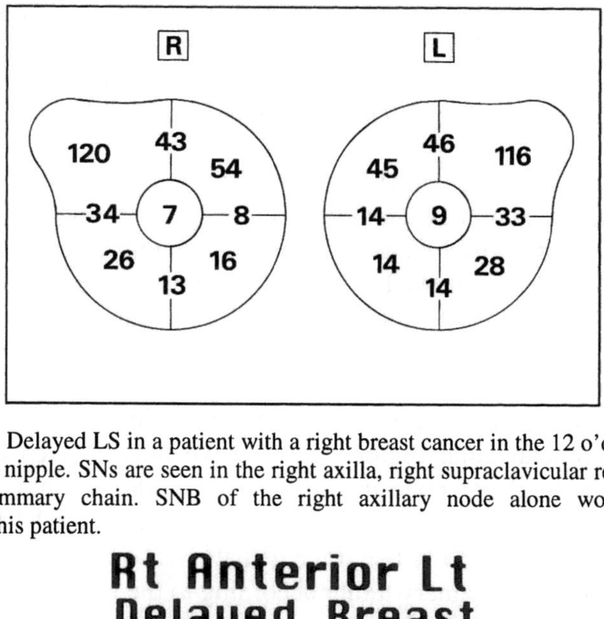

Figure 7. Delayed LS in a patient with a right breast cancer in the 12 o'clock position 8 cm from the nipple. SNs are seen in the right axilla, right supraclavicular region, and right internal mammary chain. SNB of the right axillary node alone would potentially understage this patient.

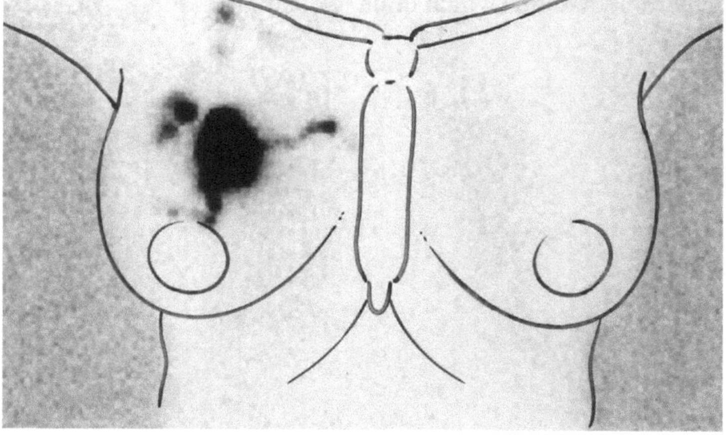

We also believe the depth of injection is critically important in obtaining a true map of lymph drainage from the tumor site. Our injections are given under ultrasound control with the needle tip at the depth of the center of the lump so that the tracer is deposited at this depth or slightly deeper. Injections given more superficially will not demonstrate drainage to internal mammary SNs because the initial lymphatic capillaries that drain to internal mammary nodes lie in the posterior part of the mammary gland. Clearly, if the SNB method is to be accurate, all true SNs in every patient must be examined. An SNB procedure that targets only axillary SNs, based on our data, potentially understages 46% of breast cancer patients. The status of the internal mammary nodes in breast cancer is the second most important prognostic indicator and a positive internal mammary SN has an adverse effect on prognosis regardless of axillary node status.[37] Excision biopsy of SNs found in the internal mammary chain is associated with low morbidity and has been shown to improve staging and change treatment strategies.[38,39]

Like others, we have found that the pattern of lymphatic drainage in a particular patient cannot be predicted clinically on the basis of the location of the tumor in the breast tissue. Tumors that were located entirely in outer quadrants of the breast showed drainage to internal mammary SNs in 29% of cases, while tumors located entirely in inner quadrants drained to SNs in the axilla in 86%. Thus, lymph flowed across the centerline of the breast in 46% of patients. We have observed flow across the midline of the patient to contralateral nodes that were second tier nodes in the internal mammary chain and supraclavicular region but we have not yet seen drainage to a contralateral second tier node in the opposite axilla. We have also not yet seen drainage to a sentinel node on the side contralateral to the primary breast cancer. Table 4 shows the drainage patterns seen in 419 patients based on the location of the primary tumor according to the four breast quadrants.

As mentioned earlier, when internal mammary drainage was observed there was usually a string of second tier nodes seen above the SN, reinforcing our view that "visceral" lymph nodes inside body cavities have a different physiology and do not retain radiocolloid as effectively as do nodes in the standard node fields which drain the skin.

Table 4. Lymph flow patterns by breast quadrant (419 patients)

	Site of breast cancer			
SN location	UOQ (*n*=236)	UIQ (*n*=99)	LOQ (*n*=54)	LIQ (*n*=30)
Axilla	227 (98%)	79 (86%)	54 (100%)	25 (89%)
Internal mammary	054 (23%)	60 (65%)	28 (52%)	14 (50%)
Supraclavicular	022 (9%)	07 (8%)	01 (2%)	02 (7%)
Infraclavicular	003 (1%)	01 (1%)	00 (0%)	00 (0%)
Interpectoral	002 (1%)	02 (2%)	00 (0%)	01 (3%)
Interval node	013 (6%)	06 (6%)	05 (9%)	01 (3%)
SN outside axilla	072 (31%)	60 (65%)	30 (56%)	16 (57%)
No drainage	005 (2%)	07 (7%)	00 (0%)	02 (7%)

SN,sentinel node; U,upper; L,lower; O,outer; I,inner.

CONCLUSIONS

Lymphatic drainage of the skin is highly variable from patient to patient, even when the same region of the body is being examined. The path taken by lymphatic collecting vessels is unpredictable, as is the ultimate location of the draining SN or SNs as several recent studies have confirmed.[40-42] Lymphatic drainage of the breast is also not clinically predictable and passes to SNs outside the axilla in a significant number of patients.

Preoperative LS with small particle radiocolloids allows lymphatic vessels to be visualized as they drain directly to SNs. Careful imaging technique will thus allow all true SNs to be identified in each patient, even if these SNs lie outside standard node fields or are interval SNs lying between the primary site and a node field. By providing more accurate nodal staging this is an important contribution to the management of patients with cancer.

We now know that clinical prediction of the pattern of lymph drainage in an individual patient is unreliable and inaccurate. We also know that we now have an accurate method of mapping lymph drainage in every patient, which can make the difficulties associated with clinical prediction irrelevant. This technique which provides an accurate map of lymph drainage in each patient can thus have a direct and important impact on the clinical management of patients with solid tumors that drain to lymph nodes. The technique has proven accurate in melanoma and breast cancer and is now being applied to an increasing number of other solid tumors.

ACKNOWLEDGMENTS

The authors would like to thank all the nuclear medicine technologists whose skill and dedication were so important to the success of our lymphatic mapping studies. These include Kim Ioannou, Nicholas Trpezanovski, Angelique Ngyuen, Tracey Smith, Sally Raymond, and Ian Dyer. We thank the other nuclear medicine physicians who have added their enthusiasm to our work, including Drs. Robert Mansberg, John Roberts, Reginald Hutcherson, and Elizabeth Bernard. We also thank the surgeons of the Sydney Melanoma Unit for referring their patients and providing the surgical correlation and validation of the lymphatic drainage patterns we have documented, including Professor William McCarthy, Dr. Michael Quinn, Dr. Kerwin Shannon, Associate Professor Christopher O'Brien, Dr. Andrew Spillane, Dr. Robyn Saw and Dr. Jonathan Stretch and also the breast surgeons who have collaborated with us including Professor David Gillett, Associate Professor Stuart Renwick, Dr. Andrew Spillane, Dr. Owen Ung, Dr. Hugh Carmalt, Dr. Fred Niesche, Associate Professor Richard West and Dr. Robert Claxton.

REFERENCES

1. Uren RF, Thompson JF, Howman-Giles RB: Lymphatic drainage of the skin and breast: Locating the sentinel nodes. Amsterdam, Harwood Academic Publishers, 1999.
2. Thompson JF, Uren RF, Shaw HM, et al: The location of sentinel lymph nodes in patients with cutaneous melanoma. New insights into lymphatic anatomy. J Am Coll Surg 1999; 189: 195-206.
3. McMasters KM, Chao C, Wong SL, et al: Interval sentinel lymph nodes in melanoma. Arch Surg 2002; 137:543-549.
4. O'Toole GA, Hettiaratchy S, Allan R, et al: Aberrant sentinel nodes in malignant melanoma. Br J Plast Surg 2000; 53: 415-417.
5. Statius Muller MG, Hennipman FA, van Leeuwen PAM, et al: Unpredictability of lymphatic drainage patterns in melanoma patients. Eur J Nucl Med 2002; 29: 255-261.
6. Sjoberg T, Steen S: Contractile properties of lymphatics from the human lower leg. Lymphology 1991; 24: 16-21.
7. Uren RF, Howman-Giles RB, Thompson JF: Variation in cutaneous lymphatic flow rates. Ann Surg Oncol 1997; 4: 279-280.

8. Uren RF, Howman-Giles RB, Thompson JF: Demonstration of second tier lymph nodes during preoperative lymphoscintigraphy for melanoma: Incidence varies with primary tumour site. Ann Surg Oncol 1998; 5: 517-521.
9. Nopajaroonsri C, Simon GT: Phagocytosis of colloidal carbon in a lymph node. Am J Pathol 1971; 65: 25-42.
10. Leak LV: Lymphatic vessels, in Cardiovascular system, lymphoreticular and hematopoietic system. Johannessen, JV (ed). New York, McGraw-Hill, pp159-183,1980.
11. Kapteijn BAE, Nieweg OE, Muller SH, et al: Validation of gamma probe detection of the sentinel node in melanoma. J Nucl Med 1997; 38: 362-366.
12. Alazraki NP, Eshima D, Eshima LA, et al: Lymphoscintigraphy, the sentinel node concept, and the intraoperative gamma probe in melanoma, breast cancer, and other potential cancers. Semin Nucl Med 1997; 27: 55-67.
13. Bergqvist L, Strand S-E, Persson BRR: Particle sizing and biokinetics of interstitial lymphoscintigraphic agents. Semin Nucl Med 1983; 8: 9-19.
14. Maza S, Valencia R, Geworski L, Zander A, Guski H, Winzer KJ, Munz DL. Peritumoural versus subareolar administration of technetium-99m nanocolloid for sentinel lymph node detection in breast cancer: preliminary results of a prospective intra-individual comparative study. Eur J Nucl Med Mol Imaging 2003; 30:651-656.
15. Kitagawa Y, Kitajima M. Gastrointestinal cancer and sentinel node navigation surgery. J Surg Oncol 2002; 79: 188-193.
16. Ege GN. Internal mammary lymphoscintigraphy in breast carcinoma: A study of 1072 patients. Int J Radiat Oncol Biol Phys1977; 2:755-761.
17. Kaplan WD, Andersen JW, Siddon RL, et al. The three dimensional localization of internal mammary lymph nodes by radionuclide lymphoscintigraphy. J Nucl Med 1988; 29:473-478.
18. Strand SE, Persson BRR: Quantitative lymphoscintigraphy I: basic concepts for optimal uptake of radiocolloids in the parasternal lymph nodes of rabbits. J Nucl Med 1979; 20: 1038-1046.
19. Uren RF, Howman-Giles RB, Shaw HM, et al: Lymphoscintigraphy in high risk melanoma of the trunk: predicting draining node groups, defining lymphatic channels and locating the sentinel node. J Nucl Med 1993; 34: 1435-1440.
20. Morton DL, Wen D-R, Wong JH, et al: Technical details of intraoperative lymphatic mapping for early stage melanoma. Arch Surg 1992; 127: 392-399.
21. Norman J, Cruse W, Espinosa C, et al: Redefinition of cutaneous lymphatic drainage with the use of lymphoscintigraphy for malignant melanoma. Am J Surg 1991; 162: 432-437.
22. Eberbach MA, Wahl RL: Lymphatic anatomy: functional nodal basins. Ann Plast Surg 1989; 22: 25-31.
23. Leong SP, Achtem TA, Habib FA, et al: Discordancy between clinical predictions versus lymphoscintigraphic and intraoperative mapping of sentinel lymph node drainage of primary melanoma. Arch Dermatol 1999; 135: 1472-1476.
24. Uren RF, Howman-Giles RB, Thompson JF, et al: Lymphatic drainage to triangular intermuscular space lymph nodes in melanoma on the back. J Nucl Med 1996; 37: 964-966.
25. Uren RF, Howman-Giles RB, Thompson JF: Lymphatic drainage from the skin of the back to intra-abdominal lymph nodes in melanoma patients. Ann Surg Oncol 1998; 5: 384-387.

26. Uren RF, Howman-Giles RB, Thompson JF, et al: Exclusive lymphatic drainage from a melanoma on the back to intraabdominal lymph nodes. Clin Nucl Med 1998; 23: 71-73.
27. Uren RF, Howman-Giles RB, Thompson JF, et al: Lymphatic drainage from periumbilical skin to internal mammary nodes. Clin Nucl Med 1995; 20: 254-255.
28. O'Brien CJ, Uren RF, Thompson JF, et al: Prediction of potential metastatic sites in cutaneous head and neck melanoma using lymphoscintigraphy. Am J Surg 1995; 170: 461-466.
29. Thompson JF, Saw RP, Colman MH, et al: Contralateral groin node metastasis from lower limb melanoma. Eur J Cancer 1997; 33: 976-977.
30. Clouse ME, Wallace S, eds. Lymphatic Imaging: Lymphography, computed tomography and scintigraphy. 2nd ed. Williams & Wilkins: Baltimore. 15-21, 1985.
31. Uren RF, Howman-Giles R, Thompson JF, et al: Interval nodes. The forgotten sentinel nodes in patients with melanoma. Arch Surg 2000; 135:1168-1172.
32. McMasters KM, Chao C, Wong SL, et al: Interval sentinel lymph nodes in melanoma. Arch Surg 2002; 137:543-549.
33. Turner-Warwick RT: The lymphatics of the breast. Br J Surg 1959; 46:574-582 .
34. Vendrell-Torne E, Setain-Quinquer J, Domenech-Torne FM: Study of normal mammary lymphatic drainage using radioactive isotopes. J Nucl Med 1972; 13:801-805.
35. Uren RF, Howman-Giles RB, Thompson JF et al: Mammary lymphoscintigraphy in breast cancer. J Nucl Med 1995; 36: 1775-1780.
36. Shimazu K, Tamaki Y, Taguchi T, et al. Lymphoscintigraphic visualization of internal mammary nodes with subtumoral injection of radiocolloid in patients with breast cancer. Ann Surg 2003; 237: 390-398.
37. Veronesi U, Marubini E, Mariani L, Valagussa P, Zucali R: The dissection of internal mammary nodes does not improve the survival of breast cancer patients. 30-year results of a randomized trial. Eur J Cancer 1999; 35:1320-1325.
38. Tanis PJ, Nieweg OE, Valdes Olmos RA, Peterse JL, Rutgers EJ, Hoefnagel CA, Kroon BB. Impact of non-axillary sentinel node biopsy on staging and treatment of breast cancer patients. Br J Cancer 2002; 87: 705-710.
39. Noguchi M. Relevance and practicability of internal mammary sentinel node biopsy for breast cancer. Breast Cancer 2002; 9: 329-336.
40. Thompson JF, Uren RF, Shaw HM, et al. The location of sentinel lymph nodes in patients with cutaneous melanoma. New insights into lymphatic anatomy. J Am Coll Surg 1999; 189: 195-206.
41. O'Toole GA, Hettiaratchy S, Allan R, Powell BWEM. Aberrant sentinel nodes in malignant melanoma. Br J Plast Surg 2000; 53: 415-417.
42. Statius Muller MG, Hennipman FA, van Leeuwen PAM, Pijpers R,Vuylsteke RJCLM, Meijer S.Unpredictability of lymphatic drainage patterns in melanoma patients, Eur J Nucl Med . 2002; 29: 255-261.

Chapter 3

SELECTIVE SENTINEL LYMPHADENECTOMY FOR MALIGNANT MELANOMA, MERKEL CELL CARCINOMA, AND SQUAMOUS CELL CARCINOMA*

Stanley P. L. Leong
University of California San Francisco

Abstract: To date, selective sentinel lymphadenectomy (SSL) should be considered a standard approach for staging patients with primary invasive melanoma greater than or equal to 1 mm. It is imperative that the multidisciplinary team master the techniques of preoperative lymphoscintigraphy, intraoperative lymphatic mapping, and postoperative pathologic evaluation of the sentinel lymph nodes (SLNs). An SLN is defined as a blue, "hot" and any subsequent lymph node greater than 10% of the ex vivo count of the hottest lymph node. Any enlarged or indurated lymph node in the nodal basin should be excised. Frozen sections are not recommended. For extremity melanoma, delayed SSL may be performed. Preoperative lymphoscintigraphy for extremity melanoma may be done the night before so that the surgery can be scheduled as the first case of the following day. Every surgeon who uses blue dye should be aware of the potential adverse reaction to isosulfan blue and treatment for such a potential fatal reaction. A complete lymph node dissection is done if the SLN is found to be positive. Elective lymph node dissection (ELND) should not be done if an SSL can be performed as a staging procedure. SSL has further been applied to stage the nodal basin for Merkel cell carcinoma and high-risk squamous cell carcinoma. It is important for investigators involved with the SSL to follow the clinical outcome of these patients, so that the role of SSL can be further defined.

Keywords: selective sentinel lymphadenectomy, melanoma, Merkel cell carcinoma, squamous cell carcinoma

INTRODUCTION

Over the past 5 years or so, SSL for primary invasive melanoma has replaced ELND for several reasons: (1) several prospectively randomized studies showed that there was no notable benefit.[1-4] Since most patients with primary melanoma do not harbor nodal metastases, it is difficult to demonstrate survival benefit in prospective and randomized studies because of the dilutional effect[5,6]; (2) ELND may result in more postoperative morbidity such as limb edema with marginal benefit[6]; (3) SSL is an ideal procedure because it is minimally invasive, yet powerful enough to select the relevant lymph node of the nodal basin, without a complete radical lymph node dissection; 4) SSL yields fewer lymph nodes and the harvested nodes can be processed meticulously to look for occult micrometastasis. Thus, SSL provides a suitable alternative to ELND in assessing patients with primary melanoma for the occurrence of micrometastasis.

HISTORICAL PERSPECTIVES OF SLNs

The phenomenon of metastasis of cancer cells to regional nodes was well documented by Seaman and Powers.[7] Within the nodal basin, the first node that received the cancer cells was coined by Gould et al. in 1960[8] and further studied by Cabanas.[9,10] Both the feline model[11] and the melanoma work by Morton et al,[5] based on the blue-stained lymphatics and lymph node, were independently conceptualized and proven as a physiological mechanism of metastasis of cancer cells from a primary site through that individual's specific lymphatic channel to a specific "SLN",[11] rather than the more anatomical definition of the SLN in the relatively fixed anatomical location being medially and superiorly to the saphenofemoral junction in each groin as proposed by Cabanas.[9] Thus, both studies by Wong and Morton imply that a functional study is required to identify the SLN for each primary site. A false negative rate of approximately 5% by this study has subsequently been substantiated by a number of other studies.[12-15] If the blue-stained SLN is negative for metastatic melanoma, the incidence of micrometastasis in the remaining lymph node basin is less than 1–2%.[5] Using the blue dye technique in melanoma, relatively larger skin flaps are needed and a considerable amount of time is needed to dissect along these lymphatic channels to reach the blue lymph node. In about 20% of the cases, a blue lymph node may not be found.[5] In the identification of regional lymph node involvement by melanoma, a separate study again by Morton's group, approximately 25 years ago, first demonstrated the utility of cutaneous lymphoscintigraphy to define the lymphatic drainage of ambiguous skin sites.[16] In addition to the blue dye technique, Alex and Krag[17] devised another approach to identify the SLN using the principles of lymphoscintigraphy. Following intradermal injection of the melanoma primary site with radiocolloid, an intraoperative lymphatic mapping technique using a hand-held gamma probe was successfully applied to the identification of SLNs. The application of radiocolloid material as a marker for the SLN and a hand-held gamma counter as an intraoperative mapping device has revolutionized the identification of SLNs, in which the radiocolloid material within the lymph node may be identified and a small incision can be made at the site of radioactivity and the "hot" SLNs can be harvested.[17,18] Thus, the controversy between the blue SLN versus the "hot" SLN becomes an issue. A compromise was reached that both techniques would be used since identification of SLNs was enhanced by using both methods.[19]

Morton and Bostick maintain that the blue dye lymph node is the true SLN.[20] To date, although the controversy whether a blue-stained lymph node or a radioactive lymph node should be considered the SLN has not been fully settled, most investigators are comfortable calling an SLN either by the blue dye technique or the radiocolloid technique or by both techniques. Despite these various techniques being available, the relatively simple concept that cancer cells from a primary site will drain to its respective SLN first rather than randomly to any node in the regional nodal basin prior to dissemination to other sites has been well established in melanoma.[21] This concept has been further validated in breast cancer[22] and colon cancer[23-25] and is currently under investigation in other types of human solid cancers[21,26] such as upper gastrointestinal cancer[27] penile cancer,[28] gynecological,[29-31] lung cancer,[32] Merkel cell carcinoma,[33,34] head and neck cancer,[35-38] and prostate cancer.[39] The historical perspective of cancer metastasis from the primary site to the regional nodes and especially to SLNs, has been elegantly reviewed by Borgstein and Meijer.[40]

The validation of the SLN concept in human solid cancer is definitely a turning point in the management of human solid cancer and in particular for melanoma. The rapid adoption of this technique by surgical oncologists at large has quickly made the debate whether an ELND should be done versus watchful observation at the time when the primary invasive melanoma is at least 1 mm or greater irrelevant. Although the therapeutic role of SSL in melanoma has not been determined and the conclusions will await the completion of the multicenter SSL trial by Morton et al., [15] the practical significance is that it is being applied widely as a staging procedure so that a negative SLN can spare a patient a radical regional lymph node dissection and thus the associated morbidity of such a procedure.

TECHNIQUES OF SSL FOR MELANOMA

A detailed account of the techniques has been published elsewhere.[41] A CD-ROM accompanying this book will illustrate the techniques in the actual operating room setting. Several major steps may be summarized in Table 1.

Table 1. Steps for selective sentinel lymphadenectomy

1.	Preoperative lymphoscintigraphy Injection of radioisotope Identification of lymphatic basins
2.	Anesthesia: local vs. general
3.	Intraoperative mapping technique Injection of lymphazurin Intraoperative mapping with hand-held gamma probe
4.	Identification of SLNs
5.	Pathological examination of SLNs by H&E and IHC

Briefly, preoperative lymphoscintigraphy is a prerequisite for identifying nodal basins for melanoma. Our recent study has found that discordancy between lymphoscintigraphic and clinically defined nodal basins is 5% for lower extremity, 14% for upper extremity, 25% for truncal melanoma, and 48% for head and neck. The overall discordancy rate is 19.5%.[42] Because of discordance between clinical predictions and lymphatic drainage as determined by preoperative lymphoscintigraphy, it is a prerequisite to perform the preoperative imaging study to determine the lymphatic drainage pattern in patients with primary melanoma especially for sites such as the head and neck as well as the trunk before SSL.[42] Our studies are in agreement with other studies.[13,43-45] Because of potential lymphatic drainage disruption by wide local reexcision, it is preferred to have reexcision performed in the same setting as the SSL. For the sake of argument even if no disruptions were made by initial wide local reexcisions, consideration should be given to the patient so that reexcision can be done at the same time of SSL.[46,47] For patients who have had a wide local reexcision, a delayed SSL may be performed if the primary melanoma is in the extremities.[48] Therefore, it is important to have a narrow biopsy of any suspected pigmented lesion without a wide local excision. If the histological diagnosis is confirmed to be melanoma and fits the criteria for the SSL—such as Breslow thickness of at least 1 mm, transection of the melanoma without definitive thickness, regression and ulceration—wide local reexcision should be delayed until the time of SSL. At UCSF Melanoma Center at Mount Zion, we have developed a close working relationship between the nuclear medicine physician and the surgical staff. The imaging information is communicated to the surgeon prior to SSL. This practice gives the surgeon a greater reliability in localizing the lymph node. In-transit nodes and other basins for consideration are noted. The sulfur colloid is made by a hydrogen sulfide technique,[49] which makes the particles much smaller than the standard thiosulfate method.[49] The radiocolloid is filtered through a 22-micron filter to remove any large particles. The average injected dose of Tc-99m in our series of patients was 20.7 MBq (range, 3.7–74 MBq). The time from radioisotope injection to surgical incision ranged from 60 to 413 minutes (mean time, 139 minutes). Lymphatic basins at risk are identified by the nuclear medicine physician, and the location of the highest radioisotope uptake is marked to indicate the presence of the SLN in each of the basins. In most of the cases the lymphatic channels are visualized leading to the SLN. We have learned that it may be necessary to cover the injection site with lead to visualize the lymphatic channels, especially if the injection site is in the field of view with the SLN such as in head and neck sites.[50] Intraoperative mapping technique consists of Lymphazurin injection and detection of "hot" SLNs by a hand-held gamma probe (Neoprobe 2000, Neoprobe Corporation, Dublin, OH). Lymphazurin is injected intradermally prior to the procedure around the primary melanoma site ranging from 1 to 5 ml. In general, 1.5 to 2 ml is adequate. The surgical wound is then prepared. One should be aware of any adverse reactions such as urticaria, respiratory and hemodynamic changes which usually occur in the first 10 to 20 minutes.[51] The patient should be instructed that his or her urine may become blue for several days, as the blue dye also enters the circulatory system. General anesthesia has been used preferentially (77.5%), as compared to monitored anesthesia care (17.2%), regional (4.6%), and local (0.7%). Smidt et al. recently proposed that SLN biopsy could be performed under local anesthesia.[52] Based on our extensive experience, especially with multiple nodal sites and deep axillary SSL, general anesthesia is preferred. In general, the colloid or the blue dye will travel through the lymphatics to the appropriate SLNs within 5–15 minutes. A 2 to 3-cm incision is made over the marked area of greatest activity as detected by the hand-held gamma probe. The incision is carried down through the subcutaneous fat in a tunnel-like fashion, and the fascia is incised. The lymph nodes usually reside beneath the fascia. Using the gamma probe, the SLNs can be located by detecting increased radioactivity in counts per second. This often results in the identification of blue dye-stained lymphatics that otherwise would require a more extensive dissection to detect. The combination of the blue dye and radioisotope mapping allows harvesting of the SLNs with minimal extent of dissection which should be as close to the SLN as possible to avoid injury to nerves and vessels. In general, the SLN may be identified using a gamma probe, blue dye, or both. After the removal of the SLN, the resection bed count is taken to ensure that no residual elevated radioactivity is present. Further exploration is carried out if the resection bed count remains high.[53] In general, the presence of residual SLNs in the basin should be considered if the resection bed-to-background ratio remains above 3:1 or if the node shows an in situ count >10% hottest node.[54] The author always does a "roaming count" at 8 positions of the clock to make sure that the entire operative field is of low background count. The resection bed count is the count where the lymph node has been harvested and therefore it should be to normal background or at least significantly drops down unless there is an adjacent "hot" lymph node. On the other hand, roaming counts may be elevated despite the fact that the resection bed count is low because an elevated roaming count indicates a separate SLN away from the resection bed. Prior to closure, a digital exploration is warranted to make sure that no suspicious nodes are left behind. When an SLN is totally replaced by tumor cells, it may not pick up the blue dye or radiocolloid, presumably due to blockage of the tracer from entering into the lymph node. The intraoperative hand-held gamma probe directs the surgeon to the area of greatest radioactivity with pinpoint accuracy. In general, the primary melanoma site would be widely excised. Therefore, retention of the blue dye in the original melanoma or biopsy site is not a problem. Furthermore, the dye usually dissipates in weeks if, indeed, there is some residual dye still left in the skin following wide excision. After SSL, the superficial fascia is closed with interrupted 3-0 Dexon (Davis & Geek Manati, PR) sutures, and the skin with running subcuticular sutures of 4-0 Dexon. Particularly in the axilla, placement of too deep a suture may entrap the nerves. Drains are not usually placed. After changing gloves and instruments, the primary site is excised according to the thickness of the primary melanoma. Most of the time, the primary melanoma resection site is closed primarily, and only occasionally are split-thickness skin grafts used. If the blue dye is not used, the wide local reexcision may precede SSL, especially if the primary injection site is close to the SLN nodal basin to avoid the shine-through effect. Most patients are discharged from the hospital either on the day of surgery or the day after. It is important to dissect the SLN from the non-SLN or lymphatic tissue within the resected specimen on a separate table using the gamma probe and inspection for blue coloration so that each lymph node is correctly labeled with respect to blue coloration and radioactive counts for pathologic evaluation. It is important to remember that an SLN is initially imaged by a nuclear medicine physician. It is the surgeon's responsibility to harvest and identify it for the pathologist for detailed examinations.

For pathological evaluation, we have followed a protocol by which the SLN is bivalved, on each half of the SLN, multiple sections were cut with each of the two sections of each half of the lymph node being used for H&E

staining. If these are negative, then additional sections being obtained will be used for immunohistochemical staining using monoclonal antibodies against S100 and HMB45 markers.[55] Monoclonal antibodies against chromogranin A and chromogranin B as well as anti-cytokeratin 20 monoclonal antibody are used for the identification of Merkel cell carcinoma. For squamous cell carcinoma, monoclonal antibodies AE 1/3 and CAM 5.2 (antikeratin antibodies) are used to stain for keratin proteins.

A recent study by Tanis et al. on the effect of frozen section investigation of the SLN in malignant melanoma and breast cancer[56] examined a total of 177 SLNs from 99 melanoma patients and 444 SLNs from 262 breast cancer patients. Each lymph node was bisected and a complete crossection was obtained for frozen section. Step sections at three levels were made of the remaining lymphatic tissue and were stained with H&E and S100/HMB45 for melanoma. Frozen section investigation revealed metastasis in 8 of 17 node-positive melanoma patients with a sensitivity of 41% and the specificity was 100%. The authors conclude that frozen section analysis is not recommended in patients with melanoma.

For detailed preoperative lymphoscintigraphy, operative procedures, and pathologic evaluation of SLNs, readers are referred to the author's recent publication.[41] It is important for surgeons, nuclear medicine physicians, and pathologists to be competent and work together as a multidisciplinary team. False-negative results from SSL are summarized in Table 2.

Table 2. False-negative results from SSL for melanoma

Failed preoperative lymphoscintigraphy including injection techniques and interpretation of the lymphoscintigraphy
Failed intraoperative lymphatic mapping
Failed pathological evaluation
Skip metastasis
Too few cells only detectable by PCR

BLUE DYE AND RADIOISOTOPE TECHNIQUE

As mentioned above, intraoperative localization of the SLN is accomplished by injection of two tracer agents at the primary site: technetium-99m sulfur colloid and Lymphazurin or blue dye.

In a group of 163 melanoma patients, we have found that the success rate of harvesting the SLN by blue dye alone is 82%, by radiotracer mapping is 94%, and by combination method is 98. Using combined technique, we reported that about 27% showed no blue dye visualization.[53] SLN exploration would have been unsuccessful if the gamma probe was not used.[57] When SLNs by blue dye staining and/or radioactivity determination are negative for micrometastasis, the remainder of the lymph node basin is usually negative.[5,12,13,18,19,58] Different types of radiocolloid have been used such as Tc-99m sulfur colloid with human serum albumin, Tc-99m antimony sulfur colloid, and Tc-99m sulfur colloid for identification of SLNs.[59] The ideal radiotracer is one that, after injection, moves rapidly to the regional lymph node and concentrates in that node without leakage. This allows the patient to be transported to the operating room within a reasonable period of time for successful intraoperative mapping using a hand-held gamma probe without contaminating the rest of the nodal basin. Based on the studies by Albertini et al.,[19] the Tc-99m sulfur colloid has been shown to concentrate in the regional lymph node within at least 3–6 hours. Comparisons have been made between the radioactivity of the SLN being harvested immediately following injection of the radiocolloid material and after 3–4 hours of injection. The radioactivity of the delayed SLN (n=16) was much higher than that of the immediate group (n=90) (p<0.01). This result indicated that Tc-99m on injection would migrate quickly to the SLN and concentrate within it for at least 4 hours without significant leakage. In our study, this phenomenon of sustained concentration of radioisotope in the SLN has been substantiated.[53] The average time of imaging between radiocolloid injection and lymph node identification by lymphoscintigraphy was 55 minutes (range 1–165 minutes) and an additional delay of 139 minutes (range 60–413 minutes) to the time of surgery. Furthermore, we have demonstrated that Tc-99m can be detected in SLNs up to nearly 7 hours without significant leakage of the radioisotope to the adjacent lymph nodes or the adjacent lymphatic tissue. A recent study has demonstrated no significant discordancy between immediate and overnight patterns of lymphoscintigraphy.[60] We have performed delayed SSL in over 30 cases for patients with extremity melanoma. Lymphoscintigraphy on the day before and the next day prior to surgery showed a concordancy rate of almost 100% (data not shown). This is in contrast with the study by Glass et al.,[61] which showed that delayed imaging of 2–4 hours later resulted in increased "hot" lymph nodes using ^{99m}Tc-albumin colloid, ^{99m}Tc-human serum albumin, and ^{99m}Tc-sulfur colloid. Their definition of an SLN was being the first "hot" node appearing on the scan. Therefore, any additional "hot" nodes that appear in 2–4 hours are not considered SLNs.[61] However, "hot" non-SLNs were not studied, whether they contained micrometastasis or not. Glass et al.[61] demonstrated that there was leakage following injection of the radioisotope using albumin-tagged sulfur. Using technetium sulfurcolloid, we have found that there was no significant amount of leakage following the radioisotope injection. The explanation for this discrepancy is probably due to different molecules being used in that albumin-tagged sulfur colloid tends to migrate from one lymph node to the other, while the technetium sulfur colloid, once it gets into the lymph node, stays in the lymph node without further migration as it binds to the reticular endothelial system of the cells of the lymph node.[50]

Using both the blue dye and radiocolloid technique, Martin et al.[62] studied the positive incidence of SLNs for cancer with respect to the amount of radioactivity of the lymph nodes. They concluded that "neither the presence of blue dye nor isotope count ratios of any particular threshold level consistently identified the positive SLN in all patients." They recommended "the removal of all nodes containing isotope regardless of the relative level of counts". McMasters et al.[63] maintained that these conclusions were not particularly useful for surgeons with respect to the removal of multiple "hot" lymph nodes, whether to remove the third or fourth mildly radioactive lymph nodes. On the other hand, they believed strongly that where a third or fourth lymph node was present, removing these lymph nodes would reduce the false-negative rate.[64] The authors analyzed 2285 consecutive cases of breast cancer patients who underwent SSL for breast cancer. Only 5% of patients (24/463) being positive, lymph nodes with less than a positive node were less than 10% of the radioactive count of the "hottest" node. Of these 24 patients, all but 3 had blue-stained SLNs. It was recognized that the blue dye and radiocolloid techniques provide complementary approaches to SLN identification.[65] The reason was that sometimes blue lymph nodes were not very "hot", nodes that were not blue, or a minimal amount of radioactivity might be the only site harboring metastatic disease. In the melanoma study, a total of 288 of 1184 patients (24.3%) were found to have sentinel node metastasis detected by histology or immunohistochemistry. In 40 of 306 positive nodal basins (13.1%), the most radioactive SLN was negative for tumor when another, less radioactive, SLN was positive for tumor. Based on these studies, the authors cited the "10% rule" that was validated in the University of Louisville multicenter breast cancer study[66] and in the melanoma SSL study.[67] The authors have recommended the 10% “rule” as a practical guide for surgeons to terminate a procedure without dissecting the entire nodal basin to find every possible radioactive lymph node. Furthermore, the rule states "any lymph node that is blue, any lymph node that is the hottest lymph node, and any lymph node that is 10% or greater the ex vivo radioactive count of the hottest SLN should be removed."[66,67]

We have analyzed our first 309 consecutive patients who underwent melanoma SLN mapping procedure using both tracers between 1993 and 1999. Following Lymphazurin injection, blue dye-stained lymphatics and lymph nodes could easily be visualized in 74.1% of the SLNs. The explanation as to why over 20% of lymph nodes were not stained blue grossly is twofold: (1) The blue dye has to stain a certain amount in the tissue in order to give a visual image of being blue. On the other hand, radiocolloid accumulation could be picked up more sensitively by the gamma counter. (2) Lymphazurin being a smaller molecule may leak out of the lymph node more easily. Experienced surgeons have noted that initially the lymph node may be quite blue, but the blue disappears rapidly during dissection indicating that it probably requires continuous flow of blue dye from the primary site. The leakage of blue dye from the lymph node may result in the visual impression that the blue coloration is fading away. On the other hand, radiocolloid is a larger molecule and tends to stick more avidly to the lymph node tissue resulting in a continuous detection by its radioactivity using the hand held gamma probe. When radiocolloid was used to locate SLNs, an SLN was defined as any lymph node with radioactivity greater than three times the background in vivo or 10 times the background ex vivo.[19] Using this definition, 98% of the cases of SLNs were determined using the gamma probe. In about 27% of the cases, no blue lymphatics were seen. In such cases, gamma probe detection was crucial in detecting the SLNs. Five hundred seventy seven lymph nodes were studied for blue dye intensity, radioactivity uptake (hot), and presence of blue afferent lymphatic channels. Fifty-four of the 309 patients (17.5%) were found to have SLNs positive for melanoma, and 68 of the 577 SLNs harvested (11.8%) were found to harbor micrometastasis. The distribution of blue and hot SLNs positive for micrometastasis is summarized in Table 3. Blue afferent lymphatic channels were not consistent in leading to a blue lymph node. For all the positive SLNs, the lowest ex vivo to resection bed count ratio exceeded 3:1. Using positive SLNs as relevant references, almost all SLNs (98.5%) could be detected by increased radioactivity uptake and yet only approximately 80.9% were visualized as blue. Only one SLN which was blue and not hot was shown to contain metastatic melanoma. In fact, this particular SLN was totally effaced with melanoma. This can be explained by the fact that the lymphatics to a lymph node being entirely replaced by tumor probably are blocked so that the larger molecules such as the radiocolloid rather than the smaller molecule of Lymphazurin could not enter the afferent lymphatics into the SLN. In 7 of 50 regional nodal basins (14%), a less radioactive node(s) contained micrometastasis. Thus, the data shows that in melanoma patients, the most radioactive node is not always the biologic SLN.[68] This is in concordance with a more extensive series by McMasters et al.,[67] which formed the basis for the 10% rule.

Table 3. Distributions of positive SLNs with respect to blue and "hot" nodes.[a]

Positive SLNs by tracer identification	Number	Percentage
Blue only	1	1.5
Blue and hot	54	79.4
Hot only	13	19.1
Total	68	100.0

[a]Extracted from Leong.[21]

Whether SLNs localized by radioactivity or blue dye are of any biological significance is undetermined at this time. However, 27.3% of the SLNs were detected using only the hand-held gamma probe with no blue dye staining.[53] Some radiolabeled lymph nodes were positive for micrometastasis, certainly qualifying them as SLNs. Therefore, radiocolloid detection is more sensitive than blue dye as shown in our study[53] as well as other studies.[57,69,70] Thus, we conclude that radioactive localization of SLN using gamma probe is a far superior technique than blue dye, and that in most cases, the radiotracer can replace the blue dye.[71] Several disadvantages of the blue dye include: (1) the cost is about $250.00 per injection; (2) the injection time will usually take approximately 10–15 minutes; and (3) potential anaphylactic reaction (0.7%) by Lymphazurin.[51] Based on the data presented, we conclude that preoperative lymphoscintigraphy and intraoperative mapping by radiocolloid alone is a highly reliable technique and that Lymphazurin probably would not be needed except when lymphoscintigraphy could not localize the appropriate nodal basin. Although the anaphylactic reaction is low to Lymphazurin, the severity is certainly real once anaphylaxis occurs. Therefore, for patients with a history of anaphylaxis and hypersensitivity, blue dye should be avoided if possible, particularly in view of the fact that radiocolloid material can be equally effective and highly reliable.

A recent study from Brazil using patent blue dye and gamma probe detected SLNs for primary melanoma in the neck, trunk, or extremities from a series of 64 patients with 70 lymphatic basins. Gamma probe identified the SLN in 68 basins (97%) and blue dye in 53 (76%). Both gamma probe and blue dye identified in 100% of the inguinal basins. They entitled the paper "Is intra-operative gamma probe detection really necessary for inguinal sentinel lymph node biopsy?"[72] Since the inguinal nodal basin drains both from the lower trunk and the lower extremity, it is imperative that a preoperative lymphoscintigraphy be done to determine the exact location of the inguinal SLN whether superficial or deep inguinal (external iliac). Further, in our series,[73] we have found that approximately 5% of the distal extremities will have a popliteal SLN. If, indeed, only patent blue is used to detect inguinal SLN as implied in their title, this will be inappropriate and certainly should not be accepted as a standard of practice. Since both the gamma probe and patent blue identified 100% of the time in the inguinal lymph node basin and that a preoperative lymphoscintigraphy is being done for every case anyway for the reasons mentioned above, they should have changed the title to "Is blue dye detection really necessary for inguinal SLN biopsy?" It is more appropriate to imply that the blue dye is not needed since the radiotracer will identify 100% of the time being detected by the gamma probe and that radiotracer will be used anyway for preoperative lymphoscintigraphy. Overall, there is no doubt that the gamma probe scores a much higher identification rate of 97% versus 76% for overall basins including auxiliary and cervical in addition to the inguinal. It is unfortunate that the title implies that the gamma probe may not be needed.

Let us use mathematical calculation to argue against the use of blue dye. In general, it is accepted that the overall rate of positive SLNs for invasive melanoma $\geq$ 1 mm is about 18%. If indeed the combined blue dye and radiotracer achieves 98% over 90% of radiotracer alone for SLN detection, the difference is 8%. The actual impact will be 8% x 18% = 1.4%, which is significantly lower in actually missing a positive SLN. Considering the extra cost, negligible yield to detect actual positive SLNs, and potential anaphylactic reaction, blue dye is usually not used by the author.

Blue dye may be useful when the primary injection site is very close to the SLN basin, say within 5 cm as the shine-through effect may make it difficult to localize the "hot" SLN as the radioactivity in the injection may be significantly high and mask the SLN. This is particularly important in the pre-auricular area or post-auricular sites. In another situation, blue dye may be used when preoperative lymphoscintigraphy fails to demonstrate any SLN nodal basins.

EVOLVING DEFINITION OF SLN IN MALIGNANT MELANOMA

Based on the published data on SLN and SSL for melanoma and breast cancer, the primary lymphatic drainage may involve more than one lymph node as originally proposed by Morton to be the blue lymph node.[5,20] Several studies in melanoma have shown that the number of SLNs per basin is in the range of 1.5 to 1.8. [53,57,74] Using blue dye technique, for breast cancer, Giuliano et al. reported that the mean number of SLNs identified for each breast cancer was 1.7.[22] Several other studies show the SLN to range from 1.2 to 3.6.[75] According to Albertini's study[19], an arbitrary number was used with respect to the 3-to-1 in vivo ratio and 10-to-1 ex vivo ratio to find that a lymph node was positive. McMasters et al. have further refined the definition of SLNs using the 10% rule based on an extensive database.[67] Thus, an SLN: may be (1) blue; (2) may be the "hottest"; or (3) or may be 10% or greater ex vivo radioactive count. It is also apparent that careful dissection of the specimen being removed on a separate table is essential in order to identify the SLN versus the non-SLN being contained within the SLN specimen to be submitted for pathological examination.

COMPLICATIONS

The surgical and anesthesia complications of SSL are consistent to the procedure performed. Bonenkamp et al. reported complications of 43 melanoma patients undergoing SSL. One of the axillary procedures was complicated by wound dehiscence (morbidity 4%), and 4 of the 12 (30%) inguinal procedures were complicated by lymphocele or infection with one wound. SLN dissection in the neck region had no morbidity. All these complications were treated out of the hospital.[76] A recent study detailed both major (5%) and minor (31%) complications from SSL for melanoma.[77] In a prospective fashion, Temple et al. have found that sensory morbidity following selective SLN dissection for breast cancer may be significant and persistent.[78] Based on these experiences, it is assumed that complications such as seroma, wound infection, sensory loss, and even lymphedema may occur in SSL for melanoma in the axilla and groin. We have recently conducted a prospective analysis of complications for melanoma patients undergoing SSL. The aim of our study is to collect prospective follow-up data on postoperative SSL melanoma patients to evaluate patients' complications. The subject population consisted of patients with invasive melanoma ≥ 1 mm, who underwent wide local reexcision and SSL from 2/27/2003 to 9/23/2004. Data were collected directly from patients during the pre- and initial post-operative visits (average 10–21 days). Prospective data included pain, numbness, wound separation, skin graft failure, seroma, cellulitis, limitation of limb range of motion, and lymphedema at the initial and subsequent follow-ups. A total of 92 patients were included in this study for analysis (upper extremity=37, trunk=31, lower extremity=24). All patients signed informed consent approved by the UCSF Committee on Human Research. The initial postoperative complications from the primary melanoma sites were numbness (47.8%), pain (17.4%), cellulitis (6.5%), and wound separation (3.3%). There were a total of 114 SSL procedures performed. For the SSL sites, complications consisted of numbness (38.6%), seroma (23.7%), limb motion restriction (18.5%), pain (14.9%), lymphedema (13%), and cellulitis (5.3%). No patients were admitted to the hospital for any severe complications. This prospective study of post-operative complications of SSL provides an important account of different types of complications to this recently established procedure. Understanding the potential complications of SSL may help us develop methods to prevent or treat such morbidity.

We have reported severe anaphylactic reactions from blue dye.[51] From November 1993 to August 1998, 406 patients underwent intraoperative lymphatic mapping using both isosulfan blue (1–5cm^3 injected intradermally around the primary melanoma) and radiocolloid injection at UCSF Medical Center at Mount Zion. Three cases of anaphylaxis following intradermal injection with isosulfan blue were encountered (0.7%) with various severity from urticaria, erythema, and treatable hypotension to severe cardiovascular collapse with or without bronchial spasm or urticaria. Other reports have also documented the adverse reactions to isosulfan blue.[79,81] In our series, the incidence of anaphylaxis to isosulfan blue was about 0.7%. Anaphylaxis can be fatal if not recognized and treated rapidly.

Recently Krouse and Schwarz in their letter to the editor of Annals of Surgical Oncology entitled "Blue dye for sentinel lymph node mapping: not too sensitive, but too hypersensitive?," they described a case in which a melanoma patient following blue dye injection developed blue hives.[82] They assert that the routine use of blue dye for intraoperative mapping is probably not needed when a radiolabled SLN technique is to be performed. The author agrees with their suggestion.[83] On the other hand, a total number of over 1500 patients having had preoperative lymphoscintigraphy to date at UCSF Mount Zion Medical Center have not developed a single anaphylactic reaction to the radioisotope colloid injections.

To determine the true incidence of isosulfan blue adverse reactions in patients undergoing SSL, a survey was conducted by us sending questionnaires regarding blue dye adverse reactions for both melanoma and breast cancer to the members of the Society of Surgical Oncology in the United States. This study summarized the survey results of 184 surgical oncologists from 187 institutions reporting 14,809 cases of melanoma and 16,020 cases of breast cancer from 1993 to 2002. The average volume of blue dye injection for melanoma was 1.87 ml and that for breast cancer was 4.54 ml. The overall incidence of blue dye adverse reactions based on a multi-institutional survey for melanoma and breast cancer is low but definitely present. Although multivariable modeling of the rates of blue dye adverse events require additional databases beyond this survey, it may be speculated that higher incidence of adverse reactions in breast cancer may be related to the higher volume of blue dye injection.[84] When blue dye is injected, surgeons and operating room personnel must be aware of the potential consequences and be prepared to treat anaphylaxis.

SIGNIFICANCE OF MELANOMA MICROMETASTASIS TO SLNs AND OTHER HIGH-RISK FACTORS

We have analyzed our first group of 363 melanoma patients with a median follow-up of 4.8 years. The overall incidence of patients with positive SLNs was 18%. The overall mortality rate in patients with primary cutaneous melanoma was 18.7% and 74 recurrences occurred (20.4%). The factors related to survival and disease recurrence were analyzed by Cox proportional hazard models. Mortality was significantly related to SLN status (HR = 2.06, 95% CI 1.18, 3.58), angiolymphatic invasion (HR = 2.21,

95% CI 1.08, 4.55), ulceration (HR = 1.79, 95% CI 1.02, 3.15), mitotic index (HR = 1.38, 95% CI 1.01, 1.90), and tumor thickness (HR = 2.20, 95% CI 1.21, 3.99). Factors significantly related to disease-free survival included SLN status (HR = 2.09, 95% CI 1.31, 3.34), tumor thickness (HR = 1.89, 95% CI 1.20, 2.98), and age (HR = 1.26, 95% CI 1.08, 1.47). In conclusion, SLN status is the most significant factor for melanoma recurrence and death. Other important predictors include tumor thickness, ulceration, lymphatic invasion, and mitotic index.[85]

Other studies have also identified several high risk factors of the primary melanoma to predict metastasis to SLNs.[86,87] Patients with positive SLN and tumor thickness > 2.0 mm were about twice as likely to have ulcerated lesions compared to those patients with tumor thickness $\leq$ 2.00 mm. According to several follow-up studies,[86,88] patients with positive SLNs do much worse than those with negative SLNs with respect to disease-free survival. Furthermore, since patients with SLNs free of metastasis may develop recurrence (although the recurrence rate is low), they should be carefully followed.

Outcome studies from melanoma patients undergoing SSL have shown that micrometastasis in SLNs is associated with a poorer prognosis. Cherpelis et al.[89] have found that SLN status is predictive of disease-free survival in melanoma patients with thickness over 3 mm. Based on databases of patients with thin and thick melanomas, Gershenwald et al.[86] found that the SLN status was the most important prognostic factor with respect to disease-free and disease-specific survival. Statius Muller et al.[90] have found that SLN status along with Breslow thickness, ulceration, lymphatic invasion, and age appear to have additional value in predicting a minimal 3-year disease-free period after SLN. Patients with positive SLNs have a poorer prognosis than patients with negative SLNs.[85,91,93] Starz et al. [94,95] have further defined and classified micrometastasis in melanoma SLNs. A recent report by Morton et al.[96] in 1599 melanoma patients undergoing SSL showed that the overall survival rates at 5, 10, and 15 years were 70, 65, and 65%, respectively, for 322 patients with IHC-positive SLNs. On the other hand, for 1277 patients with IHC-negative SLNs the overall survival rates were 89, 83, and 81% respectively ($p \leq 0.0001$).

CLINICAL SIGNIFICANCE OF PCR BEYOND IHC

Recently, the so-called molecular staging method using polymerase chain reaction technique to detect the tyrosinase gene messenger RNA has been shown to increase detection of submicroscopic disease.[97] Obviously, the advantage of polymerase chain reaction determination is that it examines the entire lymph node being processed via messenger RNA detection and sampling errors may be eliminated. It has enhanced our ability to detect even several cells in the SLNs. Accuracy may be increased by multiple markers. Since usually a few SLNs are involved, the cost would be much reduced as compared to application of this technique to multiple lymph nodes from ELND.

PCR molecular markers[97,98] are now available to further define the melanoma SLN-negative group by H&E and/or IHC. Both SLN- and PCR-negative patients enjoy survival approaching nearly 100%, indicating that indeed melanoma with no metastasis to the SLN(s) can be cured. Patients who are SLN negative but PCR positive have a significant recurrence rate as compared to the SLN-negative and PCR-negativegroup. In the report by Morton et al.[96] as mentioned above, when paraffin-embedded SLNs from 162 IHC-negative patients were further studied using multimarker RT-PCR, 41 (25%) showed positive signals; 5-year rates of recurrence were 40, 63, and 78% when SLNs expressed 1, 2, and ≥ 3 melanoma markers, respectively, versus only 4% for PCR-negative SLNs ($p \leq 0.001$). This difference suggests that the IHC method fails to detect 25% of SLN micrometastasis. Thus, PCR is not only more sensitive than IHC in detection of micrometastasis in SLNs, but also clinically significant for recurrence. This is consistent with the high cure rate of patients with early invasive primary melanoma. Prospective clinical follow-up of patients will further define the validity of molecular staging.[99,100]

In view of the recent finding that melanoma patients with PCR positivity in the lymph node have a worse prognosis than PCR negative patients,[96] it is possible that early dissemination of microscopic cells via the circulatory system may occur.[101] Although it has been argued that upstaging by SSL may result in a "lead time" basis, recent studies with longer follow-up suggest that the SLN status is indeed a strong and reliable prognostic indicator. Therefore, prospective and long-term follow-up of these patients is essential to further define the biology of nodal micrometastasis.

PARADIGM OF METASTASIS FOR MELANOMA BASED ON THE SLN EXPERIENCE

Although the incidence of malignant melanoma is still increasing rapidly with 1 out of 75 Americans being diagnosed with melanoma annually, the overall mortality rate has risen only slightly, indicating that most of the melanoma being diagnosed is of the thin level that can be treated effectively by surgical resection.[74] Various clinical and histological features have been utilized to predict the prognosis of primary melanoma.[102] The Clark model is about 89% accurate in predicting survival in stage I melanoma based on tumor progression.[103] Melanomas usually progress from an in situ growth to a radial growth phase in which it expands into a vertical growth phase which is associated with increased risk of metastasis. Breslow tumor thickness as measured from the stratum granulosum of the epidermis to the deepest depth of the tumor is considered the best predictor of clinical outcome and is an integral part of the pathology report.[104] The survival rate drops to single digits when metastasis is found beyond the regional lymph nodes, especially in visceral sites.[105]

In melanoma,[105,106] nodal status is the most important predictor of clinical outcome. These studies of the pre-SLN era provided strong evidence that, in general, tumor progression in a primary site resulted in metastasis to regional nodes and then to distant sites. Thus, the premise of treatment for melanoma rested on the eradication of the primary tumor and the nodal disease. Oftentimes, a regional lymph node dissection was performed in order to make sure that indeed that all the lymph nodes were harvested to stage the patient. Further, such lymph nodes would harbor microscopic disease that their removal could potentially prevent systemic metastasis.

The relationship between Breslow thickness and the sentinel node status is linearly correlated (Table 4).[71] Because of the accuracy of SSLs as a staging method, the 6th edition of the American Joint Committee on Cancer for melanoma has been revised with incorporation of the SLN status.[107] Melanoma progression can be further defined in terms of primary melanoma proliferation, metastasis to the SLNs or distant sites, progression from SLNs to non-SLNs, progression from SLNs or non-SLNs to systemic sites. The survival rate is significantly compromised as the stage of disease advances (Figure 1).

Thus, based on the literature on the pre-SLN and the SLN era, for melanoma, metastatic cells are generated as a result of proliferation (see Figure 2).

Table 4. Relationship between Breslow thickness and incidence of positive SLNs based on the first 362 melanoma patients undergoing SSL at UCSF Melanoma Center

Breslow thickness	SLN positive
0–1 mm	3%
1–2 mm	13%
2–3 mm	22%
3–4 mm	32%
> 4 mm	35%

Figure 1. Specific pattern of metastasis with corresponding survival rates for melanoma (Source: Leong.[101] Reprinted with permission.)

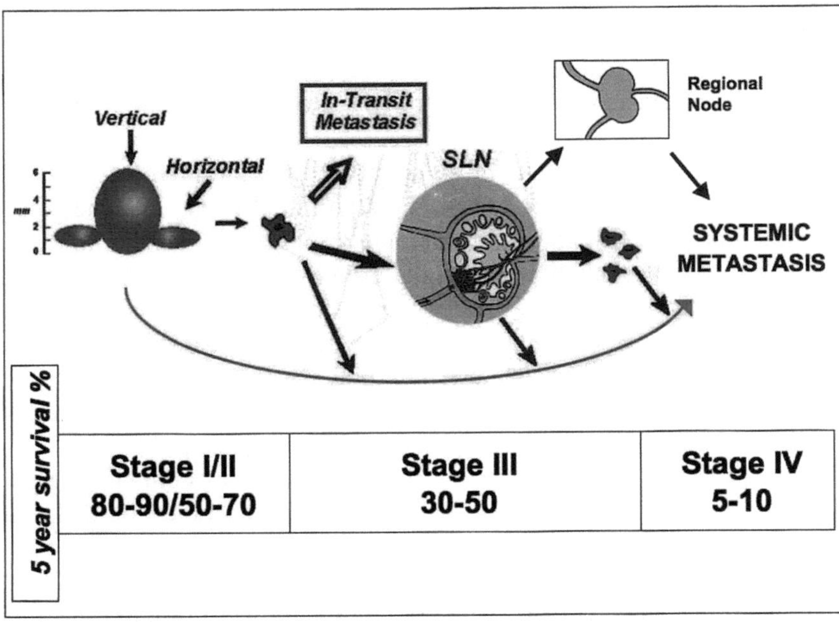

Figure 2. Paradigm of metastasis for melanoma starts as a local growth and proliferation results in more aggressive clones to metastasize to SLNs and subsequently to non-SLNs prior to systemic metastasis. Occasionally, either from the primary site, SLNs, or non-SLNs, tumor cells may spread via systemic circulation to distant sites.

Paradigm of Metastasis for Melanoma

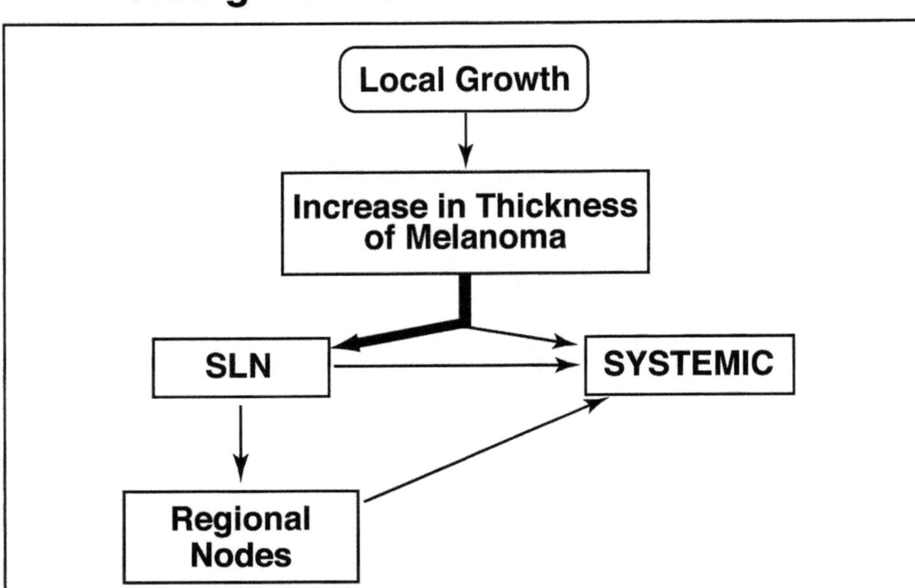

Early metastasis occurs mostly in the regional SLN and metastasis to SLN is a poor prognostic factor with respect to disease-free and overall survival. In general, the paradigm of metastasis for melanoma is characterized by initial proliferation and metastasis to SLNs and then to non-SLNs prior to systemic metastasis. In view of the recent finding that melanoma patients with PCR positivity in the lymph node have a worse prognosis than PCR-negative patients,[96] it is possible that early dissemination of microscopic cells via the circulatory system may occur. Occasionally, it is possible for the tumor cells to spread via systemic circulation to distant sites from the primary site, SLN(s), or non-SLN(s). The unresolved issue is when is the critical point of that progression such that the cancer can be arrested prior to metastasis either to the SLNs or to systemic sites? Even when only the SLNs are involved, can the removal of the positive SLNs render the patient a "cure"? In the future, molecular markers will further define the subgroups and thereby pinpoint the subgroups of patients that will require either only SSL, or completion lymph node dissection to "cure" their metastatic disease.

Thin melanomas are usually curable when treated only with wide local excision.[74] A breakthrough has been achieved in the staging of localized melanoma by SSL, although its therapeutic role remains to be defined. To date, surgical resection of early melanoma is of vital importance to control the spread of malignant melanoma and achieve a greater benefit of survival. It is critical for all melanoma surgeons to keep a computerized database so that patients undergoing SSL can be followed in a prospective fashion. Each point of follow-up is a yardstick in its correlation with molecular markers of the tumor. The extensive genetic profiles being obtained by microarray technology may be correlated with the clinical outcome in order to bring out the genes responsible for such clinical manifestations.[108] Thus, further prognostic markers and therapeutic innovations may be developed. Early diagnosis of melanoma through education and surveillance should be encouraged.[109] The challenge in the future would be to determine the mechanisms of metastasis via the lymphatic system versus the circulatory system on a molecular and genetic level. Such information will be critical to select high-risk patients for adjuvant therapy.

DIFFICULT MELANOCYTIC LESIONS

It is not uncommon to have disagreement in the diagnosis of malignant pigmented lesions.[110] The treatment of melanoma differs significantly from other skin lesions with which it may be confused histopathologically, and yet failure to correctly identify melanoma has serious clinical, medical, and legal implications. Therefore, a clinical management strategy needs to be developed so that these lesions which are not easily diagnosable with routine histological methods can be addressed adequately. Thus, SSL may be considered in patients with melanocytic neoplasms of uncertain behavior that are 1.0 mm in thickness or greater.[111] These lesions, such as Spitz nevi , some blue nevi, halo nevi, persistent (recurring) nevi, congenital nevi biopsied in infants, and nevi near genitalia and in the axilla, may be confused with the diagnosis of melanoma. Also, "dyplastic" nevi may have foci that appear very similar to evolving melanoma in situ and other processes including intraepidermal melanocytic proliferations on sun-damaged skin, and melanocytic hyperplasia within solar lentigines. Lesions that have a vacuolar degeneration of the dermoepidermal junction such as discoid lupus erythematosus and benign lichenoid keratosis may potentially be confused with melanoma in situ; further, conditions in which there is an increased pigmentation in the dermis simulating melanoma such as dermatofibrosis, postoperative scars containing iron from Monsel's, solution and processes with numerous melanophages such as regressed nevi. Occasionally melanoma may simulate several less serious benign conditions including compound, junctional, intradermal nevi, blue nevi, and even Spitz nevi. The argument is that since SSL is much less morbid than radical lymph node dissection, SSL can be used not just for the staging of melanoma, but also to determine SLN status to rule out melanoma. In this way, a relatively benign lesion can be ruled out as a potential melanoma and with minimal amount of mobility. Yet, appropriate treatment can be rendered if indeed the lymph node shows metastatic melanoma.

STAGING OF NODAL STATUS FOR PATIENTS WITH PRIMARY MELANOMA BY SSL IS NOW STANDARD OF CARE

The technique of SSL has been well described and has been reliable in several centers,[5,13,18,19,58,106] including ours.[53] Based on several studies, when SLNs by blue dye staining and/or radioisotope mapping are negative for microscopic metastasis of melanoma, the remainder of the lymph node basin does not usually contain additional lymph nodes with microscopic metastasis.[5,13,18,19,58,106] Multiple reviews have been written[12,51,73,112-118] and several books have been published[41,119-124] to attest the validity of SSL for staging melanoma. A randomized Multicenter Selective Lymphadenectomy Trial (MSLT), sponsored by the National Cancer Institute, addresses the validity of this procedure. The study is designed to determine whether intraoperative lymphatic mapping, followed by SSL and wide excision of the primary site, will effectively prolong overall and disease-free survival as compared with wide excision of the primary melanoma alone.[41] Although the therapeutic role of SLL for melanoma awaits the conclusion of the

MSLT, the staging role of SSL has been well established even without the completion of a formal clinical trial.

Clearly, the role of SSL is to provide accurate staging at the initial diagnosis of primary melanoma. In order to enhance such accuracy, it requires (1) accurate identification and localization of SLN by preoperative lymphoscintigraphy and intraoperative mapping and dissection and (2) meticulous histological evaluation. Routine histologic techniques for evaluating lymph nodes may decrease the diagnostic accuracy mainly because of sampling errors.[12] Therefore, serial sectioning with immunohistochemical staining has been incorporated to improve the detection of micrometastasis.[97,125] Serial sectioning would be too exhaustive to be performed on multiple nodes from ELND.

Several advantages of SSL for melanoma[126] include: (1) a negative SLN result will reduce the extent of surgery, cost, and morbidity for many patients with primary melanoma who might otherwise be told to have an ELND; (2) the removal of a positive SLN followed by a prophylactic lymph node dissection may provide better local control of the disease-involved lymphatic basin; (3) SSL can be considered as a staging procedure when it is positive, after which additional surgery and adjuvant treatment such as interferon α-2b [127] may be given; (4) a negative SSL may reassure the patient that the likelihood of metastatic disease to the regional lymph node is low. Therefore, it offers considerable psychological benefit. Furthermore, the follow-up studies have shown that the SLN status is a significant prognosticator for the outcome of patients with primary melanoma having no clinical adenopathy (Table 5).

To achieve a high rate of accurate and successful identification of the SLNs, it is imperative that the surgeons, nuclear medicine physicians, and pathologists work together closely as a multidisciplinary team to offer the best result to the patient. SSL in melanoma should be considered a standard approach[129-132] for staging primary malignant melanoma, provided that the surgeons, nuclear medicine physicians, and pathologists are adequately trained.[41] Because the false-negative rate is extremely low, it can be assumed that those patients with a negative SLN should have no microscopic disease in the remainder of their nodal basin. Therefore, SSL allows about 80% of patients with melanoma to be spared a formal lymph node dissection, thus avoiding the complications usually associated with that procedure. The technique of preoperative lymphoscintigraphic mapping and intraoperative SSL have evolved to become a standard staging procedure for patients with primary stage I and II malignant melanoma with Breslow thickness equal to or greater than 1 mm.[133] Numerous centers have adopted this approach as an initial approach for management of stage I and II malignant melanoma

Table 5. Summary of outcomes of melanoma patients undergoing selective sentinel lymphadenectomy[a]

Author, year	*N*	Median follow-up	Outcomes	Significant factors for Survival
Gadd 1999 [93]	89 SLN –	23 months	12% recurrence in SLN - group	None (small numbers)
Gershenwald 1999 [86]	85 SLN + 495 SLN –	40 months	3-yr disease-free survival SLN + 55.8% 3-yr disease-free survival SLN – 88.5% 3-yr survival SLN + 69.9% 3-yr survival SLN – 96.8%	Tumor thickness, Clark level > III, ulceration, and SLN status Tumor thickness, Clark level > III, and SLN status
Essner 1999 [92]	42 SLN + 225 SLN – 22 ELND + 235 ELND –	45 months SLN 169 months ELND	5-yr survival SLN + 64% 5-yr survival ELND + 45% SLN + 38% recurrence ELND + 57% recurrence SLN – 11.5 % recurrence ELND – 14.9% recurrence	N/A because matched study for age, site and tumor thickness not analyzed. The retrospective study was conducted to compare the efficiency of lymphatic mapping/ sentinel lymphadenectomy and elective lymph node dissection.
Clary 2000 [91]	31 SLN + 121 SLN – 44 ELND+ 285 ELND –	26 months SLN 79 months ELND	3-yr disease-free survival SLN 80% 3-yr disease-free survival ELND 71%	SLN: tumor thickness and age ELND: tumor thickness, ulceration, and Clark level
Cherpelis 2000 [89]	51 SLN + 150 SLN – (all > 3.0 mm)	51 months	3-yr disease-free survival SLN + 37% 3-yr disease-free survival SLN – 73% 3-yr survival SLN + 70% 3-yr survival SLN – 82%	Ulceration Age, tumor thickness, Clark level, and ulceration
Statius Muller 2001 [90]	52 SLN + 211 SLN –	48 months	3-yr disease-free survival SLN + 79% 3-yr disease-free survival SLN – 95% 5-yr survival SLN + 49% 5-yr survival SLN – 91%	SLN status, tumor thickness, ulceration lymphatic invasion and age
Wagner 2003[128]	85 SLN + 323 SLN–	31 months	31 mo disease-free survival SLN + 36.5% 31 mo disease-free survival SLN –12.1%	Tumor thickness, ulceration, SLN status and number of positive lymph nodes
Leong 2004 [85]	65 SLN + 297 SLN –	58 months	5-yr disease-free survival SLN + 38.1% 5-yr disease-free survival SLN – 68.6% 5-yr survival SLN + 59.9% 5-yr survival SLN – 68.6%	SLN status, tumor thickness, age and gender SLN status, tumor thickness, ulceration, lymphatic invasion and mitotic index

[a]Adopted from Leong SPL, et al. World J Surgery, in press

according to the recent American Joint Committee on Cancer classifications.[134] When the SLN is positive, the current recommendation is a complete lymph node dissection of the involved basin. The technique of SSL has now been learned and practiced beyond major melanoma centers and because of the many courses being given across the country, more and more community practicing surgeons are embracing this technique as an initial treatment modality for patients with primary melanoma. In fact, through library and Internet readings, most patients have concluded that they would prefer SSL rather than a prophylactic lymph node dissection unless micrometastasis is noted. It has become standard not because the removal of the positive SLNs is of clinical value, but because the majority (over 80%) of the patients may be spared a more radical procedure. Both the medical community and patients are not at this time ready to abandon lymph node dissection if indeed an SLN is involved with micrometastasis. Only future studies will be able to offer conclusive data and evidence to provide specific guidelines as to whether taking out the positive SLNs will suffice for the patient. This is the reason why this procedure has been widely accepted without waiting for the trial result of the MSLT because it has served the important purpose of selecting out those 80% of the patients to spare them a more radical lymph node dissection procedure.[133] This sentiment has been echoed eloquently by Carpenter.[135]

MERKEL CELL CARCINOMA AND SQUAMOUS CELL CARCINOMA

Merkel cells are commonly found in the dermal tissue adjacent to nerve endings; these cells were described by Merkel in 1875 and hence their name.[136] They may also be found in mucous membranes of the oral cavity. These cells are characterized by epithelial and neuroendocrine ultrastructural and immunochemical features. They are derived from the neuroendocrine system, the so-called the amine precursor uptake and decarboxylation cells system (APUD).[137,138] Thus, this cutaneous neuroendocrine carcinoma commonly called Merkel cell carcinoma (MCC) was first described by Toker in 1972 as a trabecular carcinoma.[139] Because of its relative rarity as a cutaneous carcinoma, few large series of studies have been published. Multiple case reports or smaller studies have been published, as have occasional larger reviews by pooling these studies.[140-145] From these publications, MCC is an unusual and cutaneous malignancy which has a tendency for local recurrence and occult nodal metastasis resulting in a more radical treatment approach by many investigators. Current treatment strategies consist of wide local excision with or without adjuvant radiation therapy and elective nodal dissection. In general, progression of MCC is characterized by an orderly pattern from local disease to regional nodal metastasis subsequently to distant metastasis. As the concept of SLN of malignant melanoma and breast cancer has evolved to maturity and techniques of SSL have become established, it is appropriate to apply SSL in the staging of the nodal basin for primary cutaneous MCC as shown by reports from us and others.[33,34,146] If the lymph nodes are not involved there is no need for dissection. The role of adjuvant radial therapy and chemotherapy for MCC has not been well established. In our institution, when the MCC can be widely excised locally with a negative margin and the lymph node is negative, usually no chemotherapy is given.

Cutaneous squamous cell carcinoma (SCC) has a high incidence (143,000 new cases per year in the United States) and has a definite tendency to metastasize to regional lymph node basins (ranging from 0.5-16%).[147] Size greater than 2 cm, depth of penetration to Clark level V, location of the primary tumor, recurrence of treated lesions and occurrence in previously radiated tissue are at higher risk of metastasis. Histologic features such as poor differentiation, perineural invasion, small tumor nests, acantholysis and single cell infiltration are also associated with metastasis.[147] Ulceration, inflammation and Breslow thickness do not seem to predict metastasis.[147] In patients with SCC, the management of regional lymph node basins is challenging. Complete dissection of all draining basins is probably not warranted due to morbidity and relatively low yield. In patients with clinically aggressive SCC, preoperative lymphoscintigraphy and SSL may select out those high risk patients with nodal metastasis.

CREDENTIALING OF SURGEONS FOR SSL

When a surgeon should be considered to be qualified to perform SSL has not been clearly established. It is paramount that the surgical community ensure that surgeons performing this procedure have gone through didactic training and proctoring. With respect to the credentialing issues, it has been proposed by Morton et al. that 30 cases should be done.[15] These criteria might have been appropriate at the inception of this technique, in the early 1990s. However, currently, this technique is widely available in most major melanoma centers. Surgeons wishing to learn this technique do not need to go through 30 cases with both a SSL followed by a complete lymph node dissection. Further, statistical estimation makes the learning curve an illusion rather than reality.[148] This approach is simply not practical as patients will be unwilling to undergo these additional procedures. It is prudent and ethical for a surgeon to learn this technique from scratch by taking a lymphatic mapping course, which is being given in several major melanoma centers on a yearly basis. The next step will be to scrub in with an experienced surgeon who has done these techniques on a routine basis. After several cases, the surgeon may want to pursue cases on his own with appropriate proctoring. When the surgeon feels that he is able to harvest the SLN in a reliable fashion, that he can honestly tell the patient that he has acquired enough competence to perform the case, the surgeon is then ready to do so. If he encounters difficulty, he should always have the option of having an intraoperative consultation with his more experienced colleague. Currently, there is no official credentialing process that will qualify the surgeon to do the procedure. According to the breast cases by the American Society of Breast Surgeons, 20 cases might be appropriate. Recently, Simmons has published data to indicate that 10 cases may be sufficient.[149]

CONTRAINDICATIONS OF SSL

Although SSL is an excellent staging procedure for patients with primary melanoma, it should not be considered as a simple procedure that can be performed at the drop of a hat. General anesthesia is usually used for patients undergoing this procedure. Complications have been reported, as described above. Certainly, increased operating room time is associated with the SSL procedure compared to simple wide local reexcision. If a blue dye is used, potential anaphylactic reactions may occur. SSL should not be performed in certain situations which include: (1) after a wide local reexcision of melanoma, especially with advanced flap or skin graft in the head and neck or trunk areas, as these sites are notorious for ambiguous lymphatic drainage with likelihood of disrupting the lymphatic flow and thus make the procedure inaccurate. The exception is extremity melanoma, for which it has been found to be acceptable to proceed with SSL if clinically indicated. We and others have shown that it is feasible to perform delayed SSL in patients with primary melanoma of the extremity which has been excised previously.[150-154] (2) In patients with less than 1 mm thickness through an excisional biopsy without other associated high-risk factors such as regression, microsatellitetosis, or angiogenesis. A history of transection or shave biopsy of the primary melanoma would warrant SSL since the exact nature of the melanoma cannot be determined. Therefore, it is important for dermatologists or surgeons involved with the primary biopsy of a suspicious, pigmented lesion not do a shave biopsy or transect the melanoma. (3) Melanoma below 2 mm and lacking high-risk factors with co-morbid conditions where the yield of a positive SLN may not be high, yet potential complications may occur for the patient with respect to these co-morbid conditions such as recent history of stroke, myocardial infarction, or significant cardiac or pulmonary conditions. (4) Desmoplastic melanomas may be considered as a relative contraindication. We have recently shown that desmoplastic melanoma has no involvement in SLNs in 16 cases, with a mean Breslow thickness of 3.9 mm.[155] Other studies, including Jaroszewski et al.,[156] Payne et al.,[157] and Gyorki et al.,[158] have shown very low incidence of positive SLNs in desmoplastic melanoma of 1–2%. If, this can be confirmed in a larger multi-series, SSL should probably not be indicated for desmoplastic melanoma.

TECHNICAL ISSUES FOR SSL IN GENERAL AND IN DIFFERENT ANATOMIC SITES

General

When the nuclear medicine physician recognizes an SLN, it could represent a cluster of a few lymph nodes.

A collimator may be used to minimize the "shine through effect" from the adjacent primary injection site being close to the SLN site. When a collimator is used, the field of detection is more focal and limited. For a more panoramic search, the collimator may be detached.

The lymph node is usually below the fascia (e.g., clavipectoral fascia in the axilla and Scarpa's fascia in the groin). Thus, a tunneling and not a flap type of incision should be developed to gain access to the fascia. Once the fascia is incised and the SLN is localized, an Allis clamp is usually used to grasp the adjacent tissue surrounding the SLN to lift it from deep into the operative field. Alternatively a silk stitch can be used, but the author finds that an Allis clamp is more reliable and more secured than a silk stitch, especially if the SLN is deep, for example, in the axilla. Dissection should be as close to the lymph node as possible to avoid injuries to the adjacent nerves and vessels.

The SLN may be in any portion of the wall of the cavity as the tunnel is being dissected, especially with respect to the second or third SLN. Therefore, the roaming counts are very important, particularly if the preoperative lymphoscintigraphy shows more than one SLN. Roaming counts are important to have a panoramic search for any additional SLNs. A resection bed count alone may not find additional residual SLNs.

If the reading is very focal with disappearance of counts with minimal motion of the probe, the lymph node is usually small. When the SLN is small, say 5 mm or so in a large basin such as axilla, it may be hidden away in a "blind spot" which may not be detected. It can be frustrating when the probe occasionally comes into contact with that lymph node with a transient registration of an elevated count. On the other hand, when you try to go back again, it is not there. Obviously, patience is needed to find such an SLN. If the reading disappears after retraction, use a shallower retractor. This indicates that the SLN is in a superficial plane being retracted away by a deep retractor.

Finding the first SLN has been found which is usually quite easy because at this point, tissue of dissection is limited and there is quite a bit of integrity of the tissue to help in dissecting that SLN. By the time the second or third SLN is being dissected, the cavity architecture is now loose. It makes identification by the Neoprobe of the SLN more difficult to localize it. Therefore, finding the second or third SLN takes patience and vigilance. Apply the "10%" rule of McMasters et al.[67] It should be noted that during initial encountering of the blue dye in vivo, it may appear to be 3 to 4 + blue and during dissection the blue may decrease in intensity. On the other hand, the radioisotope count on the lymph node remains stable during the in vivo and exvivo reading.

Digital exploration should always be done prior to the completion of SSL to make sure that no suspicious or enlarged lymph nodes are retained in the surgical bed as blue dye or radiocolloid may not enter a grossly metastatic lymph node. This point is best illustrated by a case of an 86 year old Caucasian woman who developed extensive local recurrence about 2 months following wide excision of her primary melanoma (11mm in thickness and 21 mm in diameter). An enlarged lymph node of about 2 cm was palpated in the right axilla. The patient's metastatic work-up including MRI of the head, CTs of the chest, abdomen and pelvis was negative except for an enlarged right axillary lymph node. She inadvertently had a preoperative lymphoscintigraphy with an opportunity to examine the traffic of radiocolloid to a metastatic lymph node showing minimal background count (109) from the radical axillary lymph node dissection. The radiocolloid had been "redirected" from the "original" SLN, which was totally replaced by melanoma to a "new" SLN at the junction of level I and II (count=2,893) and another SLN at the junction of lever II and III (count=821). Both of these SLNs were negative for metastatic melanoma. (See page 149, No. 1, Fig. 3 in color section of book and DVD)

Head and Neck

In the neck area, occasionally you have a midneck internal jugular vein SLN; it could be posterior to the sternocleidomastoid muscle. Since the incision is small, do not enter the carotid sheath anteriorly as you would do a radical neck dissection with the lifting of the sternocleidomastoid muscle, but instead split the muscle in a longitudinal fashion to open the space so that part of the muscle will be retracted anteriorly and half the muscle will be retracted posteriorly to gain access to the SLN.

For dissection of SLN in the parotid or spinal accessory nerve area, it is important to use a nerve stimulator to guide the dissection to avoid nerve injury.

Trunk

When the melanoma is in the midline back, potentially four nodal basins may be involved. In such a case it is debatable whether it is justified to do all four nodal basins. To date, my practice is limited to three nodal basins. I would proceed with a PET scan as a baseline study if more than three nodal basins are detected by lymphoscintigraphy without dissecting any one of them.

Occasionally from the lower back area, periaortic lymph nodes may be encountered, and if these are obvious from lymphoscintigrapy, then these lymph nodes are not harvested. Obviously, subsequent follow-up studies such as PET scans or CT scans may be needed if the more superficial lymph node basin is positive for metastatic melanoma.

For trunk melanoma particularly with respect to the upper back, at times, the exact imaging of the lower neck SLN by preoperative lymphoscintigraphy may be somewhat difficult whether exactly anteriorly or posteriorly. Of course, from a surgical viewpoint, it makes a difference if it is indeed anteriorly located in the supraclavicular area, for which the supine position is the best approach to harvest the SLN. On the other hand, if it is posterior to the trapezius muscle, then it will be better to approach it posteriorly in a prone position. Therefore, it is important to use an intraoperative gamma probe to determine whether it is posteriorly located or more anteriorly located in the superclavicular area prior to the incision.

Extremities

For the distal upper extremity, melanoma epitrochlear nodal basin may be detected in less than 5% by preoperative lymphoscintigraphy in addition to the axillary nodal basin. A longitudinal incision of 2 to 2.5 cm may be made overlying the "hot" spot, usually at about 3–4 cm above the elbow crease on the ulnar aspect. The lymph node is usually found underneath the superficial fascia and it may be situated in the intramuscular space. More detailed descriptions have been published elsewhere.[159,160] For the distal lower extremity melanoma, popliteal SLNs may be encountered in 5% of the cases.

It is not clear whether a deep external inguinal lymph node should be explored initially if both superficial and deep inguinal lymph nodes are identified by preoperative lymphoscintigraphy. If they are contiguous, the author's approach is to harvest the superficial inguinal nodes only. If they are positive, the patient would then undergo an iliolingual lymph node dissection. On the other hand, when a separate channel leads to a deep SLN, it will be harvested separately. No data are available on whether the deep inguinal SLN should be taken if it is contiguous with the superficial inguinal SLN. Because of the relative increase of operative time and potential morbidity, it is the author's preference at this time not to pursue the deep iliac inguinal lymph nodes if they are contiguous with the superficial ones. It is important for the nuclear medicine physician to do a scan with rotations to maximize determination of whether it is a single contiguous lymphatic channel versus separate channels. For the deep inguinal SLN dissection, when it is just proximal to the inguinal ligament, sometimes the distal external iliac SLN may be accessed just beneath the inguinal ligament into the distal external iliac vessel and the SLN can be harvested that way. Most of the time, a formal incision of about 3 cm is made through the abdominal wall muscles layer by layer to gain access into the retroperitoneal space for the harvesting of the external iliac SLNs.

For anatomical sites which are difficult to triangulate for marking preoperatively by the nuclear medicine physician including the lower neck, upper back, epitrochlear, popliteal, and any in-transit area, it is important to do a careful mapping by the hand-held gamma probe prior to making the incision.

In-Transit Nodes

The SLN is the first lymph node in the regional nodal basin to receive metastatic cells. In-transit nodes are found between the primary melanoma site and regional nodal basins. Therefore, the obvious question is whether regional "hot" SLNs should be harvested when the in-transit "hot" nodes are resected. Our retrospective database and medical records were reviewed from October 21, 1993, to November 19, 1999. Thirty (5%) out of 557 extremity and truncal melanoma patients undergoing SSL had in-transit SLNs. Three patients had positive in-transit SLNs and negative SLNs in the regional nodal basin. Two patients had positive in-transit and regional SLNs. Three patients had negative in-transit SLNs but positive regional SLNs. The remaining 22 patients were negative for in-transit and regional SLNs. In-transit SLNs may harbor micrometastasis. About 10% of the time, micrometastasis may involve the in-transit and not the regional SLN. Therefore, both in-transit and regional SLNs should be harvested.[161] The concept of the second tier lymph node not being the SLN to be harvested is subject to debate according to our study. One potential problem is that the current state of the art of lymphoscintigraphic imagery cannot absolutely distinguish one single channel draining a contiguous lymph node versus another nonvisualized channel draining a separate SLN.

For in-transit metastasis following SSL, it may be the case that in this group of patients some cells are lodged in the lymphatic system at the time of the SSL and over time, as the lymphatic channels are blocked, they may develop in-transit metastasis.

CONCLUSION

Several important tenets of metastasis can be established based on the current SLN experience: (1) The earlier the cancer is detected, the less the metastatic potential; (2) in most cases, melanoma follows an orderly progression of metastasis to the SLN; and (3) a small subgroup of patients may develop systemic dissemination without SLN involvement. Since treatments for metastatic cancer are still limited, it is imperative for oncologists to detect and resect an early cancer as soon as possible. The challenge in the future will be to dissect these different patterns of metastasis based on molecular or genetic mechanisms. Such information will be critical to select high-risk patients for adjuvant therapy.

The role of the SSL is to provide accurate staging at the initial diagnosis of primary invasive melanoma equal to or greater than 1 mm because the staging result is often accurate, the morbidity is reduced, and the cost is less. To minimize the false negative rate, it is important for the surgeons, nuclear medicine physicians, and pathologist to work together closely as a multidisciplinary team to achieve the best result for the patient. SSL for melanoma should be considered the standard of care for staging patients with primary melanoma.

ACKNOWLEDGEMENTS

* This work was supported in part by a grant from the Eva B. Buck Charitable Trust and the UCSF/Mount Zion Auxiliary Fund.

REFERENCES

1. Veronesi U, Adamus J, Bandiera DC, et al. Inefficacy of immediate node dissection in stage I melanoma of the limbs. New England Journal of Medicine 1977;297(12):627-30
2. Sim FH, Taylor WF, Ivins JC, et al. A prospective randomized study of the efficacy of routine elective lymphadenectomy in management of malignant melanoma: preliminary results. Cancer 1978;41(3):948-56
3. Balch CM, Soong SJ, Bartolucci AA, et al. Efficacy of an elective regional lymph node dissection of 1 to 4 mm thick melanomas for patients 60 years of age and younger. Annals of Surgery 1996;224(3):255-66
4. Balch CM, Soong S, Ross MI, et al. Long-term results of a multi-institutional randomized trial comparing prognostic factors and surgical results for intermediate thickness melanomas (1.0 to 4.0 mm). Annals of Surgical Oncology 2000;7(2):87-97
5. Morton DL, Wen DR, Wong JH, et al. Technical details of intraoperative lymphatic mapping for early stage melanoma. Archives of Surgery 1992;127(4):392-9
6. Karakousis CP. Surgical treatment of malignant melanoma. The Surgical Clinics of North America: Cutaneous Malignant Melanoma. Leong SP, editor. Philadelphia, WB Saunders. 1996;76(6):1299-1312
7. Seaman WB, Powers WE. Studies on the distribution of radioactive colloidal gold in regional lymph nodes containing cancer. Cancer 1955;8(5):1044-46

8. Gould EA, Winship T, Philbin PH, Kerr HH. Observations on a 'sentinel node' in cancer of the parotid. Cancer 1960;13:77-8
9. Cabanas RM. An approach for the treatment of penile carcinoma. Cancer 1977;39(2):456-66
10. Cabanas RM. Lymphatic mapping and sentinel lymphadenectomy in urology. Leong SP, Kitagawa Y, Kitajima M, editors. Selective Sentinel Lymphadenectomy for Human Solid Cancer. New York, Springer; 2005
11. Wong JH, Cagle LA, Morton DL. Lymphatic drainage of skin to a sentinel lymph node in a feline model. Annals of Surgery 1991;214(5):637-41
12. Reintgen DS, Albertini J, Berman C, et al. Accurate nodal staging of malignant melanoma. Cancer Control Journal of Moffitt Cancer Center 1995;2(5):405-14
13. Thompson JF, McCarthy WH, Bosch CM, et al. Sentinel lymph node status as an indicator of the presence of metastatic melanoma in regional lymph nodes. Melanoma Research 1995;5(4):255-60
14. Albertini JJ, Lyman GH, Cox C, et al. Lymphatic mapping and sentinel node biopsy in the patient with breast cancer. JAMA 1996;276(22):1818-22
15. Morton DL, Thompson JF, Essner R, et al. Validation of the accuracy of intraoperative lymphatic mapping and sentinel lymphadenectomy for early-stage melanoma: a multicenter trial. Multicenter Selective Lymphadenectomy Trial Group. Annals of Surgery 1999;230(4):453-63; discussion 463-5
16. Holmes EC, Moseley HS, Morton DL, et al. A rational approach to the surgical management of melanoma. Annals of Surgery 1977;186:481-90
17. Alex JC, Krag DN. Gamma-probe-guided localization of lymph nodes. Surgical Oncology 1993;2(3):137-44
18. Krag DN, Meijer SJ, Weaver DL, et al. Minimal-access surgery for staging of malignant melanoma. Archives of Surgery 1995;130(6):654-8; discussion 659-60
19. Albertini JJ, Cruse CW, Rapaport D, et al. Intraoperative radiolymphoscintigraphy improves sentinel lymph node identification for patients with melanoma. Annals of Surgery 1996;223(2):217-24
20. Morton DL, Bostick PJ. Will the true sentinel node please stand? [editorial; comment]. Annals of Surgical Oncology 1999;6(1):12-4
21. Leong SP. The role of sentinel lymph nodes in malignant melanoma. Leong SP, Wong JH, editors. Sentinel Lymph Nodes in Human Solid Cancer. The Surgical Clinics of North America 2000;80(6):1741-57
22. Giuliano AE, Kirgan DM, Guenther JM, et al. Lymphatic mapping and sentinel lymphadenectomy for breast cancer. Annals of Surgery 1994;220(3):391-8, discussion 398-401
23. Saha S. Sentinel lymph node mapping in colorectal cancer— A review. Leong SP, Wong JH, editors. Sentinel Lymph Nodes in Human Solid Cancer. Surgical Clinics of North America. Philadelphia, WB Saunders. 2000;80:1811-20
24. Paramo JC, Summerall J, Poppiti R, Mesko TW. Validation of sentinel node mapping in patients with colon cancer. Journal of Surgical Oncology 2002;9(6):550-4
25. Wood TF, Nora DT, Morton DL, et al. One hundred consecutive cases of sentinel lymph node mapping in early colorectal carcinoma: detection of missed micrometastases. Journal of Gastrointestinal Surgery 2002;6(3):322-30
26. Bilchik AJ, Giuliano A, Essner R, et al. Universal application of intraoperative lymphatic mapping and sentinel lymphadenectomy in solid neoplasms. Cancer Journal from Scientific American 1998;4(6):351-8
27. Kitigawa Y, Kubota T, Ando N, et al. The role of the sentinel lymph node in gastrointestinal cancer. Wong JH, Leong SP, editors. Sentinel Lymph Nodes in Human Solid Cancer. Surgical Clinics of North America. Philadelphia, WB Saunders. 2000;80:1799-1810

28. Tanis PJ, Lont AP, Meinhardt W, et al. Dynamic sentinel node biopsy for penile cancer: reliability of a staging technique. The Journal of Urology 2002;168(1):76-80
29. de Hullu JA, Hollema H, Piers DA, et al. Sentinel lymph node procedure is highly accurate in squamous cell carcinoma of the vulva. Journal of Clinical Oncology 2000;18(15):2811-16
30. Levenback C. Intraoperative lymphatic mapping and sentinel node identification: gynecologic applications. Recent Results in Cancer Research 2000;157:150-8
31. Lim RB, Wong JH. Sentinel lymphadenectomy in gynecologic and solid malignancies other than melanoma and breast cancer. Leong SP, Wong JH, editors. Sentinel Lymph Nodes in Human Solid Cancer. Surgical Clinics of North America. Philadelphia, WB Saunders. 2000;80:1787-98
32. Liptay MJ, Masters GA, Winchester DJ, et al. Intraoperative radioisotope sentinel lymph node mapping in non-small cell lung cancer. Annals of Thoracic Surgery 2000;70(2):384-90
33. Messina JL, Reintgen DS, Cruse CW, et al. Selective lymphadenectomy in patients with Merkel cell (cutaneous neuroendocrine) carcinoma. Annals of Surgical Oncology 1997;4(5):389-95
34. Rodrigues LK, Leong SP, Kashani-Sabet M, et al. Early experience with sentinel lymph node mapping for Merkel cell carcinoma. Journal of the American Academy of Dermatology 2001;45(2):303-8
35. Pitman KT, Johnson JT, Edington H, et al. Lymphatic mapping with isosulfan blue dye in squamous cell carcinoma of the head and neck. Archives of Otolaryngology -- Head and Neck Surgery 1998;124(7):790-3
36. Mozzillo N, Chiesa F, Bottie G, et al. Sentinel node biopsy in head and neck cancer. Annals of Surgical Oncology 2001;8(9 Suppl):103S-5S
37. Werner JA, Dünne AA, Ramaswamy A, et al. Number and location of radiolabeled, intraoperatively identified sentinel nodes in 48 head and neck cancer patients with clinically staged N0 and N1 neck. European Archives of Oto-rhino-laryngology 2002;259(2):91-6
38. Werner JA. Selective sentinel lymphadenectomy for head and neck squamous cell carcinoma. Leong SP, Kitagawa Y, Kitajima M, editors. Selective Sentinel Lymphadenectomy for Human Solid Cancer. New York, Springer; 2005
39. Wawroschek F, Vogt H, Weckermann D, et al. The sentinel lymph node concept in prostate cancer— first results of gamma probe-guided sentinel lymph node identification. European Urology 1999;36(6):595-600
40. Borgstein P, Meijer S. Historical perspective of lymphatic tumour spread and the emergence of the sentinel node concept. European Journal of Surgical Oncology 1998;24:85-9
41. Leong SP. Selective sentinel lymph node mapping and dissection for malignant melanoma. Leong SP, editor. Atlas of Selective Sentinel Lymphadenectomy for Melanoma, Breast Cancer and Colon Cancer. Boston, Kluwer Academic Publishers; 2002: 39-64
42. Leong SP, Achtem TA, Habib FA, et al. Discordancy between clinical predictions versus lymphoscintigraphic and intraoperative mapping of sentinel lymph node drainage of primary melanoma. Archives of Dermatology 1999;135(12):1472-76
43. Wanebo HJ, Harpole D, Teates CD. Radionuclide lymphoscintigraphy with technetium 99m antimony sulfide colloid to identify lymphatic drainage of cutaneous melanoma at ambiguous sites in the head and neck and trunk. Cancer 1985;55(6):1403-13
44. Uren RF, Howman-Giles RB, Shaw HM, et al. Lymphoscintigraphy in high risk melanoma of the trunk: Predicting draining node groups, defining lymphatic channels and locating the sentinel node. Journal of Nuclear Medicine 1993;34(9):1435-40
45. Berman CC, Norman J, Cruse WC, et al. Lymphoscintigraphy in malignant melanoma. Annals of Plastic Surgery 1992;28(1):29-32

46. Coldiron B. No evidence to support delay in excision of malignant melanoma. [Letter]. Archives of Dermatology 2000;136(10):1269-70
47. Leong SP. No evidence to support delay in excision of malignant melanoma. [Letter, Reply]. Archives of Dermatology 2000;136(10):1269-70
48. Leong SP, Thelmo MC, Kim RP, et al. Delayed harvesting of sentinel lymph nodes after previous wide local excision of extremity melanoma. Annals of Surgical Oncology 2002;10(2):196-200
49. Kowalsky RJ, Perry JR. Radiopharmaceuticals in Nuclear Medicine Practice. Los Altos, California, Appleton and Lange; 1987
50. Morita ET. Lymphoscintigraphy in the detection of sentinel lymph nodes. Leong SP, editor. Selective Sentinel Lymphadenectomy for Melanoma, Breast Cancer and Colon Cancer. Boston, Kluwer Academic Publishers. 2002;1:9-38
51. Leong SP, Donegan E, Heffernon W, et al. Adverse reactions to isosulfan blue during selective sentinel lymph node dissection in melanoma. Annals of Surgical Oncology 2000;7(5):361-6
52. Smidt ML, Janssen CM, Barandregt WB, et al. "Sentinel lymph node biopsy performed under local anesthesia is feasible." American Journal of Surgery 2004; 187(6): 684-7
53. Leong SP, Steinmetz I, Habib FA, et al. Optimal selective sentinel lymph node dissection in primary malignant melanoma. Archives of Surgery 1997;132(6):666-72, discussion 673
54. McMasters KM, Reintgen DS, Ross MI, et al. Sentinel lymph node biopsy for melanoma: How many radioactive nodes should be removed? Annals of Surgical Oncology 2001;8(3):192-7
55. Treseler PA, Tauchi PS. Pathologic analysis of the sentinel lymph node. Leong SP, Wong JH, editors. The Surgical Clinics of North America. Philadelphia, WB Saunders. 2000;80:1695-1719
56. Tanis PJ, Boom RP, Koops HS, et al. Frozen section investigation of the sentinel node in malignant melanoma and breast cancer. Annals of Surgical Oncology 2001;8(3):222-6
57. Gershenwald JE, Tseng CH, Thompson W, et al. Improved sentinel lymph node localization in patients with primary melanoma with the use of radiolabeled colloid. Surgery 1998;124(2):203-10
58. Ross MI, Reintgen DS, Balch CM. Selective lymphadenectomy: Emerging role for lymphatic mapping and sentinel node biopsy in the management of early stage melanoma. Seminars in Surgical Oncology 1993;9(3):219-23
59. Eshima D, Fauconnier T, Eshima L, et al. Radiopharmaceuticals for lymphoscintigraphy: Including dosimetry and radiation considerations. Seminars in Nuclear Medicine 2000;30(1):25-32
60. White DC, Schuler FR, Pruitt SK, et al. Timing of sentinel lymph node mapping after lymphoscintigraphy. Surgery 1999;126(2):156-61
61. Glass FL, Cottam JA, Reintgen DS, et al. Lymphatic mapping and sentinel node biopsy in the management of high-risk melanoma. Journal of the American Academy of Dermatology 1998;39(4 Pt 1):603-10
62. Martin RC, Fey J, Yeung H, et al. Highest isotope count does not predict sentinel node positivity in all breast cancer patients. Annals of Surgical Oncology 2001;8(7):592-7
63. McMasters KM, Wong SL, Chao C. Letter to the Editor: Comment on the article 'Highest isotope count does not predict sentinel node positivity in all breast cancer patients,' by Martin et al., August 2001, Annals of Surgical Oncology 2002;9(3):317-18
64. Wong SL, Edwards MJ, Chao C, et al. Sentinel lymph node biopsy for breast cancer: impact of the number of sentinel nodes removed on the false-negative rate. Journal of the American College of Surgeons 2001;192(6):684-91
65. McMasters KM, Tuttle TM, Carlson DJ, et al. Sentinel lymph node biopsy for breast cancer: a suitable alternative to routine axillary dissection in multi-institutional practice when optimal technique is used. Journal of Clinical Oncology 2000;18:2560-66

66. Martin RC 2nd, Edwards MJ, Wong SL, et al. Practical guidelines for optimal gamma probe detection of sentinel lymph nodes in breast cancer: results of a multi-institutional study. For the University of Louisville Breast Cancer Study Group. Surgery 2000;128(2):139-44
67. McMasters KM, Reintgen DS, Ross MI, et al. Sentinel lymph node biopsy for melanoma: how many radioactive nodes should be removed? Annals of Surgical Oncology 2001;8(3):192-7
68. Leong SP, Morita ET, Lee W, et al. In Melanoma Patients, the Most Radioactive Node is Not Always the Sentinel Node. Annual Meeting, Society of Nuclear Medicine. Sacramento, California; 2001
69. Kapteijn BA, Nieweg OE, Liem I, et al. Localizing the sentinel node in cutaneous melanoma: gamma probe detection versus blue dye. Annals of Surgical Oncology 1997;4(2):156-60
70. Ariyan S, Ariyan C, Farber LR, et al. Reliability of identification of 655 sentinel lymph nodes in 263 consecutive patients with malignant melanoma. Journal of the American College of Surgeons 2004;198(6):924-32
71. Leong SP. Selective sentinel lymphadenectomy for malignant melanoma. Leong SP, editor. Malignant Melanoma. The Surgical Clinics of North America 2003;83(1):157-85, vii
72. Oliveira Filho RS, Santos ID, Ferreira LM, et al. Is intra-operative gamma probe detection really necessary for inguinal sentinel lymph node biopsy? Sao Paulo Medical Journal 2000;118(6):165-8
73. Leong SP, Achtem TA, Habib FA. Discordancy between clinical predictions vs. lymphoscintigraphic and intraoperative mapping of sentinel lymph node drainage of primary melanoma. Archives of Dermatology 1999;135(12):1472-6
74. Reintgen D, Balch CM, Kirkwood J, et al. Recent advances in the care of the patient with malignant melanoma. Annals of Surgery 1997;225(1):1-14
75. Chung MA, Cady B. New lessons from the sentinel node. Surgical Oncology Clinics of North America 2001;10(2):461-73, xi-xii
76. Bonenkamp JJ, Logan DR, Suemnig AA, Thompson JF. The cost of sentinel node biopsy (SNB) for melanoma. Melanoma Research 2001;11:S107
77. Hettiaratchy SP, Kang N, O'Toole G, et al. Sentinel lymph node biopsy in malignant melanoma: a series of 100 consecutive patients. British Journal of Plastic Surgery 2000;53(7):559-662
78. Temple WJ, Baron R, Fey J, et al. Sensory morbidity after sentinel node biopsy (SLNB): A significant and persistent sequela. 55th Annual Cancer Symposium. Denver, Colorado, Lippincott Williams & Wilkins; 2002
79. Albo D, Wayne JD, Hunt KK, et al. Anaphylactic reactions to isosulfan blue dye during sentinel lymph node biopsy for breast cancer. American Journal of Surgery 2001;182(4):393-8
80. Cimmino VM, Brown AC, Szocik JF, et al. Allergic reactions to isosulfan blue during sentinel node biopsy — a common event. Surgery 2001;130(3):439-42
81. Montgomery AM, Reisfeld RA, Cheresh DA. Integrin alpha v beta 3 rescues melanoma cells from apoptosis in three-dimensional dermal collagen. Proceedings of the National Academy of Sciences of the USA 1994;91(19):8856-60
82. Krouse RS, Schwarz RE. Blue dye for sentinel lymph node mapping: not too sensitive, but too hypersensitive? [Letter] Annals of Surgical Oncology. In Press, 2000
83. Leong SP. Blue dye for sentinel lymph node mapping: not too sensitive, but too hypersensitive? [Letter, Reply]. Annals of Surgical Oncology. In Press, 2000
84. Leong SP, Kim RP, Rhee JY. Incidence of blue dye adverse reactions for melanoma and breast cancer selective sentinel lymphadenectomy based on a large multi-institutional survey. 3rd International SLN Conference. Yokohama, Japan; 2002

85. Leong SP, Kashani-Sabet M, Desmond RA, et al. Clinical significance of melanoma: Micrometastasis to sentinel lymph nodes and other high-risk factors based on long-term follow-up. World Journal of Surgery. In Press
86. Gershenwald JE, Thompson W, Mansfield PF, et al. Multi-institutional melanoma lymphatic mapping experience: the prognostic value of sentinel lymph node status in 612 stage I or II melanoma patients. Journal of Clinical Oncology 1999;17(3):976-83
87. McMasters KM, Wong SL, Edwards MJ, et al. Factors that predict the presence of sentinel lymph node metastasis in patients with melanoma. Surgery 2001;130(2):151-6
88. Ross M. Lymphatic mapping and sentinel node biopsy for early-stage melanoma: How we do it at the MD Anderson Cancer Center. Journal of Surgical Oncology 1997;66(4):273-6
89. Cherpelis BS, Haddad F, Messina J, et al. Sentinel lymph node micrometastasis and other histologic factors that predict outcome in patients with thicker melanomas. Journal of the American Academy of Dermatology 2001;44(5):762-6
90. Statius Muller MG, van Leeuwen PA, de Lange-De Klerk ES, et al. The sentinel lymph node status is an important factor for predicting clinical outcome in patients with Stage I or II cutaneous melanoma. Cancer 2001;91(12):2401-8
91. Clary BM, Mann B, Brady MS, et al. Early recurrence after lymphatic mapping and sentinel node biopsy in patients with primary extremity melanoma: a comparison with elective lymph node dissection. Annals of Surgical Oncology 2001;8(4):328-37
92. Essner R, Conforti A, Kelley MC, et al. Efficacy of lymphatic mapping, sentinel lymphadenectomy, and selective complete lymph node dissection as a therapeutic procedure for early-stage melanoma. Annals of Surgical Oncology 1999;6(5):442-9
93. Gadd MA, Cosimi AB, Yu J, et al. Outcome of patients with melanoma and histologically negative sentinel lymph nodes. Archives of Surgery 1999;134(4):381-7
94. Starz H, Balda BR, Kramer KU, et al. A micromorphometry-based concept for routine classification of sentinel lymph node metastases and its clinical relevance for patients with melanoma. Cancer 2001;91(11):2110-21
95. Starz H, De Donno A, Balda BR. The Augsburg experience: histological aspects and patient outcomes. Annals of Surgical Oncology 2001;8(9 Suppl):48S-51S
96. Morton D, Essner R, Hoon DS, et al. Long-term results of lymphatic mapping and sentinel lymphadenectomy for early-stage melanoma: Implications of nodal microanatomy and molecular staging on detection of nodal micrometastasis. American Surgical Association 123rd Annual Meeting, Washington, DC, American Surgical Association; 2003
97. Wang X, Heller R, VanVoorhis N, et al. Detection of submicroscopic lymph node metastases with polymerase chain reaction in patients with malignant melanoma. Annals of Surgery 1994;220(6):768-74
98. Bostick P, Morton D, Turner R, et al. Prognostic significance of occult metastases detected by sentinel lymphadenectomy and reverse transcriptase-polymerase chain reaction in early-stage melanoma patients. Journal of Clinical Oncology 1999;17(10):3238-44
99. Davis EG, Chao C, McMasters KM, et al. Polymerase chain reaction in the staging of solid tumors. Cancer Journal 2002;8(2):135-43
100. McMasters K, Reintgen D, Ross MI, et al. Sunbelt melanoma trials: sensitivity and specificity of reverse transcriptase polymerase chain reaction (RT-PCR) markers for sentinel lymph nodes (SLN). Proceedings of the American Society of Clinical Oncology 1999;18:537a
101. Leong SP. Paradigm of metastasis for melanoma and breast cancer based on the sentinel lymph node experience. Annals of Surgical Oncology 2004;11(3 Suppl):192S-7S
102. Zettersten E, Shaikh L, Ramirez R, et al. Prognostic factors in primary cutaneous melanoma. Leong SP, editor. Malignant Melanoma. The Surgical Clinics of North America 2003;83(1):61-75

103. Clark WH Jr, Elder DE, Guerry D 4th, et al. Model predicting survival in stage I melanoma based on tumor progression. Journal of the National Cancer Institute 1989;81(24):1893-904
104. Liu V, Mihm MC. Pathology of malignant melanoma. Leong SP, editor. Malignant Melanoma. The Surgical Clinics of North America 2003;83(1):31-60, v
105. Balch CM, Buzaid AC, Soong SJ, et al. Final version of the American Joint Committee on Cancer Staging System for Cutaneous Melanoma. Journal of Clinical Oncology 2001;19(16):3535-648
106. Reintgen DS, Cruse CW, Wells K, et al. The orderly progression of melanoma nodal metastases. Annals of Surgery 1994;220(6):759-67
107. AJCC. Cancer Staging Manual. 6th ed. Page DL, Fleming ID, Fritz AG, Balch CM, Haller DG, Morrow M. New York: Springer, 2003
108. Wang E, Miller LD, Ohnmacht GA, et al. Prospective molecular profiling of melanoma metastases suggests classifiers of immune responsiveness. Cancer Research 2002;62(13):3581-6
109. Leong SP. Future perspectives on malignant melanoma. Leong SP, editor. Malignant Melanoma. The Surgical Clinics of North America 2003;83(2):453-6, x
110. Farmer ER, Gonin R, Hanna MP. Discordance in the histopathologic diagnosis of melanoma and melanocytic nevi between expert pathologists. Human Pathology 1996;27(6):528-31
111. Kelley SW, Cockerell CJ. Sentinel lymph node biopsy as an adjunct to management of histologically difficult to diagnose melanocytic lesions: a proposal. Journal of the American Academy of Dermatology 2000;42(3):527-30
112. Leong SP. The role of sentinel lymph nodes in human solid cancer. Devita, Hellman, Rosenberg, editors. PPO Updates. Vol 12. Philadelphia, Lippincott-Raven;1998:1-12
113. Cochran AJ, Balda BR, Starz H, et al. The Augsburg Consensus. Techniques of lymphatic mapping, sentinel lymphadenectomy, and completion lymphadenectomy in cutaneous malignancies. Cancer 2000;89(2):236-41
114. Balch CM, Lange JR. Lymphatic mapping and sentinel node lymphadenectomy for cancer: an overview. Annals of Surgical Oncology 2001;8(9 Suppl):1S-4S
115. Nieweg OE, Tanis PJ, Rutgers EJ. Summary of the Second International Sentinel Node Conference. European Journal of Nuclear Medicine 2001;28(5):646-9
116. Essner R, Cochran AJ. Sentinel node biopsy: not only a staging tool? Recent Results in Cancer Research 2002;160:133-48
117. Shen J, Wallace AM, Bouvet M. The role of sentinel lymph node biopsy for melanoma. Seminars in Oncology 2002;29(4):341-52
118. Zervos EE, Burak WE Jr. Lymphatic mapping in solid neoplasms: state of the art. Cancer Control 2002;9(3):189-202
119. Kapteijn BA. Biopsy of the Sentinel Node in Melanoma, Penile Carcinoma and Breast Carcinoma: The Case for Lymphatic Mapping. Amsterdam, PrintPartners Ipskamp; 1997
120. Keshtgar MRS, Waddington WA, Lakhani SR, et al. The Sentinel Node in Surgical Oncology. New York, Springer; 1999
121. Uren RF, Thompson JF, Howman-Giles RB. Lymphatic Drainage of the Skin and Breast: Locating the Sentinel Nodes. Singapore, Harwood Academic Publishers; 1999
122. Whitman ED, Reintgen D. Radioguided Surgery. Austin, Landes Bioscience; 1999
123. Nieweg OE, Essner R, et al., editors. Lymphatic Mapping and Probe Applications in Oncology. New York, Marcel Dekker; 2000
124. Schlag PM, Veronesi U, editors. Recent Results in Cancer Research: Lymphatic Metastasis and Sentinel Lymphonodectomy. Berlin, Springer-Verlag; 2000
125. Robert ME, Wen DR, Cochran AJ. Pathological evaluation of the regional lymph nodes in malignant melanoma. Seminars in Diagnostic Pathology 1993;10(1):102-15
126. Rivers JK, Roof MI. Sentinel lymph-node biopsy in melanoma: is less surgery better? Lancet 1997;350(9088):1336-7

127. Kirkwood JM, Strawderman MH, Ernstoff MS, et al. Interferon alpha-2b adjuvant therapy of high-risk resected cutaneous melanoma: the Eastern Cooperative Oncology Group Trial EST 1684. Journal of Clinical Oncology 1996;14(1):7-17
128. Wagner
129. Reintgen DS. Changing standards of surgical care for the melanoma patient. Annals of Surgical Oncology 1996;3(4):327-8
130. Coit D, Wallack M, Balch C. Society of Surgical Oncology practice guidelines. Melanoma surgical practice guidelines. Oncology 1997;11(9):1317-23
131. Emilia JC, Lawrence W Jr. Sentinel lymph node biopsy in malignant melanoma: the standard of care? Journal of Surgical Oncology 1997;65(3):153-4
132. Houghton A, Coit D, Bloomer W, et al. NCCN melanoma practice guidelines. National Comprehensive Cancer Network. Oncology 1998;12(7A):153-77
133. Leong SP. Sentinel lymph node mapping and selective lymphadenectomy: The standard of care for melanoma. Current Treatment Options in Oncology 2004;5(3):185-94
134. Balch CM, Buzaid AC, Atkins MB, et al. A new American Joint Committee on Cancer staging system for cutaneous melanoma. Cancer 2000;88(6):1484-91
135. Carpenter R. Sentinel node biopsy should be introduced into routine practice before results of randomized trials are available. The Breast 2001;10:281-4
136. Merkel FS. Tastzellen und Taskorperchen bei den Haustieren und biem Menschen. Archiv fuer Mikroskopische Anatomie 1875;11:636-52
137. De Wolff-Peeters C, Marien K, Mebis J, et al. A cutaneous APUDoma or Merkel cell tumor? A morphologically recognizable tumor with a biological and histological malignant aspect in contrast with its clinical behavior. Cancer 1980;46(8):1810-6
138. Pollack SV, Goslen JB. Small-cell neuroepithelial tumor of skin: a Merkel-cell neoplasm? The Journal of Dermatologic Surgery and Oncology 1982;8(2):116-22
139. Toker C. Trabecular carcinoma of the skin. Archives of Dermatology 1972;105(1): 107-10.
140. Stephens JS, Gibbs JF, Huang PP, Kraybill WG. Merkel cell carcinoma: a review of the literature and an unusual case of metastasis to in-transit epitrochlear lymph nodes. Contemporary Surgery 1999;54(6):344-7
141. Freeman MS, Tillman LA. Merkel cell carcinoma. Surgical Rounds. January 2003, pp 31-6
142. Koljonen V, Bohling T, Granhroth G, Tukiainen E. Merkel cell carcinoma: a clinicopathological study of 34 patients. European Journal of Surgical Oncology 2003;29:607-10
143. Lehrer MS, Hershock D, Ming ME. Merkel cell carcinoma. Current Treatment Options in Oncology 2004;5(3):195-1999
144. Goessling W, McKee PH, Mayer RJ. Merkel cell carcinoma. Journal of Clinical Oncology 2002;20(2):588-98
145. Tai PT, Yu E, Winquist E, et al. Chemotherapy in neuroendocrine/Merkel cell carcinoma of the case series and review of 204 cases. Journal of Clinical Oncology 2000;18(12):2493-9
146. Pfeifer T, Weinberg H, Brady MS. Lymphatic mapping for Merkel cell carcinoma. Journal of the American Academy of Dermatology 1997;37(4):650-1
147. Cherpelis BS, Marcusen C, Lang PG. Prognostic factors for metastasis in squamous cell carcinoma of the skin. Dermatologic Surgery 2002; 28(3):268-73
148. Tanis PJ, Nieweg OE, Hart AA, et al. The illusion of the learning phase for lymphatic mapping. Annals of Surgical Oncology 2002;9(2):142-7
149. Simmons RM. Review of sentinel lymph node credentialing: how many cases are enough? Journal of the American College of Surgeons 2001;193(2):206-9
150. Wells KE, Joseph E, Ross M, et al. Lymphatic mapping for melanoma before and after wide local excision. 4th World Conference on Melanoma, Sydney, Australia. Melanoma Research. 1997;7:S105

151. Kelemen PR, Essner R, Foshag LJ, et al. Lymphatic mapping and sentinel lymphadenectomy after wide local excision of primary melanoma. Journal of the American College of Surgeons 1999;189(3):247-52
152. Whitman ED, Yardi P, Boatman A, et al. Sentinel node mapping after wide local excision in melanoma patients at a regional referral center. 2nd International Sentinel Node Congress. Santa Monica, California; 2000
153. Evans HL, Krag DN, Teates JW, et al. Lymphoscintigraphy and sentinel node biopsy accurately stages melanoma in patients presenting after wide excision. Society of Surgical Oncology's Cancer Symposium. Denver, Colorado; 2002
154. Leong SP, Thelmo MC, Kim RP, et al. Delayed harvesting of sentinel lymph nodes after previous wide local excision of extremity melanoma. Annals of Surgical Oncology 2003;10(2):196-200
155. Thelmo MC, Sagebiel RW, Treseler PA, et al. Evaluation of sentinel lymph node status in spindle cell melanomas. Journal of the American Academy of Dermatology; 44(3):451-5
156. Jaroszewski DE, Pockaj BA, DiCaudo DJ, et al. The clinical behavior of desmoplastic melanoma. American Journal of Surgery 2001;182(6):590-5
157. Payne WG, Kearney R, Wells K, et al. Desmoplastic melanoma. American Surgeon 2001;67(10):1004-6
158. Gyorki DE, Busam K, Panageas K, et al. Sentinel lymph node biopsy for patients with cutaneous desmoplastic melanoma. Annals of Surgical Oncology 2003;10(4):403-7
159. Tanabe KK. Lymphatic mapping and epitrochlear lymph node dissection for melanoma. Surgery 1997;121(1):102-4
160. Hunt JA, Thompson JF, Uren RF, Howman-Giles R, Harman CR. Epitrochlear lymph nodes as a site of melanoma metastasis. Annals of Surgical Oncology 1997;5(3):248-52
161. Thelmo MC, Morita ET, Treseler PA, et al. Micrometastasis to in-transit lymph nodes from extremity and truncal malignant melanoma. Annals of Surgical Oncology 2001;8(5):444-8

Chapter 4

SELECTIVE SENTINEL LYMPHADENECTOMY FOR BREAST CANCER

Charles E. Cox, Elizabeth S. Weinberg, Ben Furman, Laura B. White, Jayesh Patel, Daniel C. Dickson, Jeff King
Department of Surgery, H. Lee Moffitt Cancer Center and Research Institute at the University of South Florida, Tampa, Florida

HISTORICAL BACKGROUND

In 1960 Gould first coined the term "sentinel node" implying the first node in the drainage pathway from the malignant tumor.[1] In 1977 Cabanas described a "sentinel node" for staging penile carcinoma.[2] Seminal work reported by Norman and Reintgen demonstrated the ambiguity of dermal drainage patterns in melanoma and redefined the concept of Sappy's line in terms of physiologic lymphatic drainage.[3,4] This work pointed out the necessity of lymphoscintigraphy as a mainstay in all cases of truncal or head and neck melanomas with the exception that extremity melanomas demonstrated well-defined areas of drainage except for in transit nodal drainage. Another seminal work, which antedated lymphatic mapping, led to the discovery that submicroscopic nodal metastases could be diagnosed in patients. Lymph nodes of the primary basin were placed in tissue culture from which viable melanoma cells could be grown from 30% of these otherwise histological negative nodes. Subsequent technological advances with PCR (polymerase chain reaction) technology for the evaluation of tyrosinase enzyme developed by Reintgen have proven the power of nodal prognosis at the submicroscopic level for melanoma.[5] These observations, along with the simple observation by Morton and colleagues that in every case of preoperative lymphoscintigraphy a singular node received direct drainage from the primary tumor, have paved the way for sentinel lymph node mapping.[6,7] Using a surgical marker of Lymphazurin blue dye, Morton was able to intraoperatively localize the node and identify the metastatic disease early in its spread. Concurrent technology that developed hand-held gamma detection probes for detection of radiolabeled antitumor antibodies, was transferred by Alex and Krag and allowed for the direct identification of the sentinel node following injection of the lymphoscintigraphic agent in breast cancer.[6-9] Guiliano followed, soon thereafter, from Morton's group demonstrating the capacity of lymphazurin to accurately identify the sentinel node in breast cancer.[10-13] Albertini, Cox, and Reintgen described the combination technique of radiocolloid and blue dye with a significant improvement in detection of the sentinel nodes in carcinoma of the breast.[10, 11]

These applications of new technology brought with them the promise of improved detection and prognosis by submicroscopic markers. Finding the sentinel node and applying PCR to its evaluation for submicroscopic disease would and indeed has revolutionized the surgical management of solid tumors. Serial sectioning, IHC staining, or growing of the nodal tissues in tissue culture to increase the detection rate of metastasis to the lymph nodes was a daunting, expensive, and labor-intensive proposition to be used on all the lymph nodes collected from a complete lymph node dissection and thus the fact that all these events came together at the same time led to great hope and great discovery. The basins were mapped, the sentinel node was harvested, and each single node could then be exhaustively evaluated for metastatic disease. The only thing that remained was the testing of the hypothesis that the sentinel node seen on mapping was indeed representative of the remainder of the basin. Herein lies a pivotal observation in the whole evolution of sentinel node mapping. Gershenwald, Reintgen, and Morton published the initial work on melanoma mapping with blue dye alone and standard histologic evaluation of nodes by H&E staining. Of 243 patients enrolled in the initial study of blue dye mapping for melanoma, 10 went on to develop metastatic recurrence in the mapped basin, within an 18-month period of observation, when the node was histologically negative by H&E. Eight of these ten patients on repeat sectioning of the initial sentinel node and stains with IHC techniques for S-100 revealed the presence of micrometastatic disease. Since Moffitt Cancer Center and the John Wayne Cancer Institute were part of this study, the significance of performing IHC stains on nodes to avoid false-negative assessments of the nodal basin became paramount for breast cancer nodal evaluation. Divergence in evaluation of nodal disease with IHC stains for breast cancer came from Krag and the NSABP group that previously reported in breast cancer that micrometastatic disease was of little consequence to clinical outcome and thus the added expense and trouble to do IHC stains on the nodes by them was deemed superfluous, extremely costly, pedantic, and irrelevant. There was a rush to review to literature and demonstrate that micrometastatic disease had prognostic significance for breast cancer. The Ludwig trial and others that had retrospectively studied the nodes for micromets indeed demonstrated a therapeutic and prognostic significance in breast cancer, as with melanoma. In this flurry to equate breast cancer with melanoma outcomes, the entire point of reducing false-negative assessments of the nodal basin in breast cancer was all but overlooked.

The use of sentinel node mapping in breast cancer was indeed going to be a significant change in the therapy with the potential of leaving some patients worse than if all the nodes had been removed. Therefore, it became critical in the minds of those promulgating sentinel node removal only that all that could be done to certify the accuracy of the sentinel node evaluation to assure that it did indeed reflect with accuracy the remaining status of the basin should be done.[14] Since the data on mapping with melanoma required IHC techniques to validate and improve the accuracy of the evaluation, the groups who understood its significance employed routine IHC stains for cytokeratins for all breast cancer patients. Furthermore, the work of Turner et al. clearly demonstrated the efficacy of the method. 1/2100 was found to have disease when the SLN was removed and evaluated with IHC methodology.[15]

The previous decade has demonstrated that the sentinel lymph node mapping is a more sensitive and accurate technique for nodal evaluation and may supplant the complete removal of nodes in the node-negative population for breast cancer. These facts have been clearly accepted for melanoma and have defined lymphatic mapping as the standard of care for the assessment of nodal spread for melanoma.

GROWING NEED FOR MORE EFFECTIVE STRATEGIES FOR BREAST CANCER CARE

In the United States the epidemiology of breast cancer demonstrates that from 1970 forward 10 million women entered the ages where breast cancer became a risk. As a woman's age increases, the probability of breast cancer also mounts. As of 1995 approximately 185,000 women were being detected with breast cancer; based on the population increase and the predictions of probability in the next 10 years approximately 296,000 women would present with a new diagnosis of breast cancer and the next 20 years would see over 419,000 new breast cancer cases per year. Current data are on track with these predictions with the number of new breast cancers diagnosed in 2003 at a level of 212,000 cases in the United States (Figure 1).

Figure 1. The epidemiology of breast cancer.

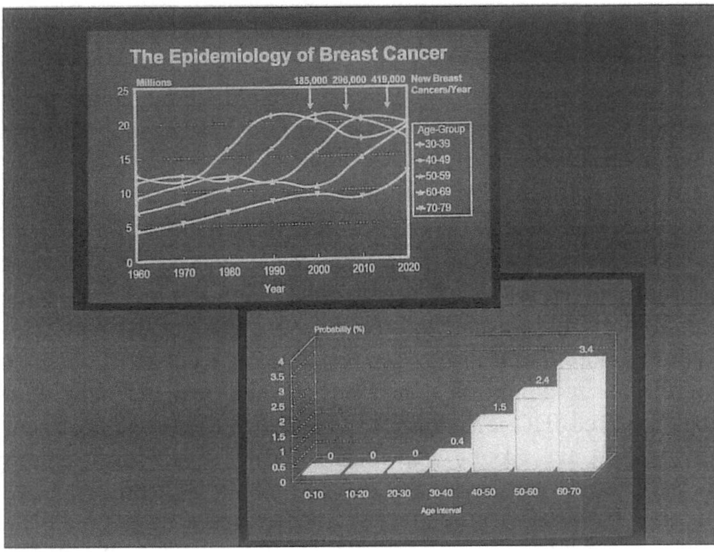

With this rapid rise in the number of breast cancer patients, new and improved techniques for the treatment of breast cancer have been met with acceptance. The advantages of sentinel lymphadenectomy are that it provides staging information with reduced surgical morbidity, reserve axillary lymph node dissection for patients with proven axillary nodal metastases, and ultimately should reduce overall cost. In addition, consumer-driven demand for less invasive procedures, applied high technology, a press with a voracious appetite for the dissemination of new technologies, and a system intent on cost containment strategies, have each played a role in the rapid evolution of more efficient means to diagnose and treat breast cancer. Lymphatic mapping and subsequent SLN dissection has dramatically achieved these goals while reducing the morbid outcomes associated with CALND.

SLN AND BREAST CARCINOMA

An initial protocol utilizing approximately 450 uCi of technetium-labeled sulfur colloid combined with 5 cm^3 of Lymphazurin blue dye injected in an intraparenchymal location was performed. Following harvest of the SLN a complete axillary node dissection was performed on all patients. Gamma detectors of all makes and models were utilized, each providing excellent radio-guidance for the detection of the SLN. The identification of the SLN was determined as a node that contained a tenfold increase and counted over nonsentinel lymph node counts or any blue node or a dilated blue lymphatic channel that went to a node which was blue or any hot and blue lymph node.

This initial study included 186 patients of whom 13 failed to map. 173 patients mapped successfully resulting in 120 who had negative SLNs and 53 patients who had positive SLNs. Of the 120 negative cases, only one patient was found to have a positive node in the complete axillary lymph node dissection. The sensitivity, specificity, and accuracy values for this group are listed below:

Sensitivity:53/54= 98.2%
Specificity:119/119=100%
Accuracy:172/173=99.4%

The SLN evaluation has proved to be a very reliable and sensitive technique. The false-negative rate as reported in the literature is an important concern. The false-negatives, as recorded for SLN mapping, is calculated as the number of false-negative exams divided by the number of true positives plus false-negatives. Of importance in all series of lymphatic mapping, approximately 30% of patients will have positive lymph nodes. Therefore, a 10% false-negative rate for 100 patients would translate into a total of 3 patients for the entire series. This represents a 1.85% (1/54) false-negative rate for the above-reported series.

Perhaps a better way of representing these data is shown in Figure 2.

Figure 2. The negative predictive value of sentinel lymph node mapping in breast cancer.

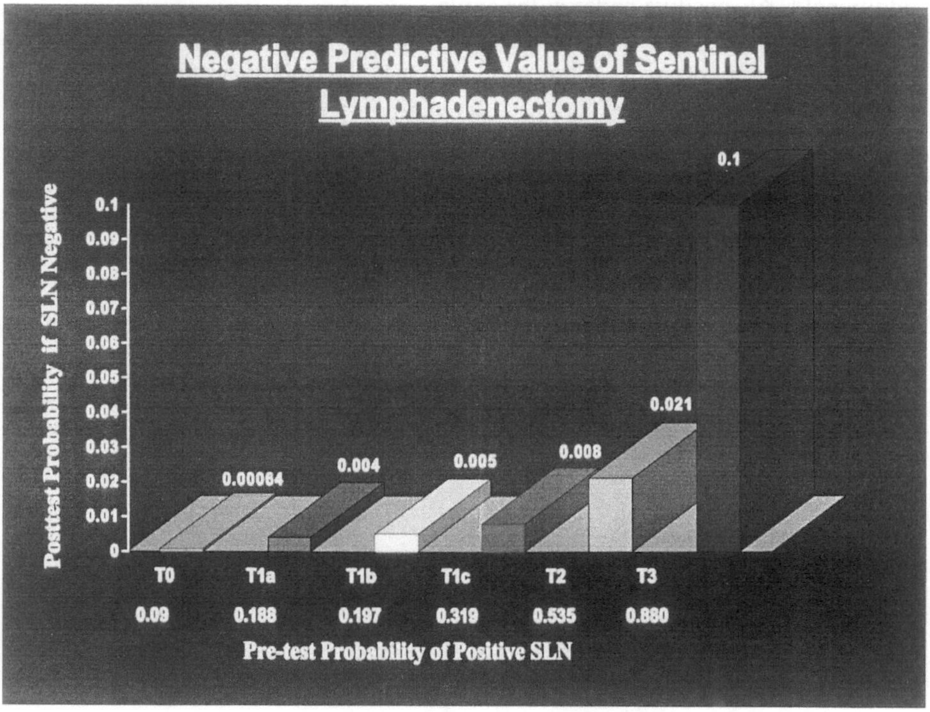

Those patients with early breast cancer T0 would have a 0.06% chance of missing a positive node. For T1A lesions the percentage would be 0.4%, for T1B, 0.5%, for T1C, 0.8%, for T2, 2.1% with patients in the T3 category potentially having a 10% probability of missing a positive node when the SLN was negative.

SLN mapping has proven to be extremely accurate with a false-negative rate of below 2%. To date no patient has had clinical recurrence in the axilla after negative sentinel lymphadenectomy. This currently represents approximately 2526 patients with negative mappings over a period of approximately 9 years with over 10,375 patient-years of follow-up.

The sentinel lymphadenectomy generally has an accuracy rate of 95%[16] and has a false-negative rate that ranges from 0 to 11%[11,17-25]. The false-negative rate of the sentinel lymphadenectomy is equal to or better than the false-negative rate of the complete axillary node dissection. The similar false-negative rate is attributable to the method of evaluation of the lymph nodes. As previously mentioned, when mapping began in melanoma, 243 patients were mapped with blue dye and 10 patients recurred in a period of approximately 18 months. In these 10 patients evaluated by H&E stains alone, the SLNs were stained with S-100 stains and immunohistochemical techniques, which showed that 8 out of the 10 had S-100-positive cells in the node. This study demonstrated that long-term false negatives, which recur, could have been detected earlier by more thorough evaluation of the lymph nodes. Therefore, the importance of cytokeratin staining in breast cancer patients is to avoid false negatives. Six to twenty-six percent of patients with IHC-positive SLNs will have additional H&E-positive nodes in the axilla.

Table 1. Incidence of positive axillary nodes when an SLN is positive only for micrometastasis.

Author	Institute	Year	Patients	Non-SLNs +
Turner	JWCI	2000	93	26%
Kamath	Moffitt	2001	101	15.2%
Jakub	Moffitt	2002	971	14.5%
Nos[b]	Inst. Curie	2003	83	6.0%

* 25% of SLN mets detected by CK-IHC Median SLN metastasis = 2.0 mm.

[b] 31% of SLN mets detected by CK-IHC stains.

Table 1 demonstrates the incidence of additional positive nonsentinel lymph nodes when micrometastatic disease is detected in the SLN.[26-29]

The photomicrograph in Figure 3 demonstrates the difficulty of identifying malignant cells within a lymph node using H&E. However, with immunohistochemical staining, the cells can be readily and easily detected (Figure 4).

Figure 3. Lymph node with micrometastases stained with hematoxylin and eosin (H&E) (high power 100X).

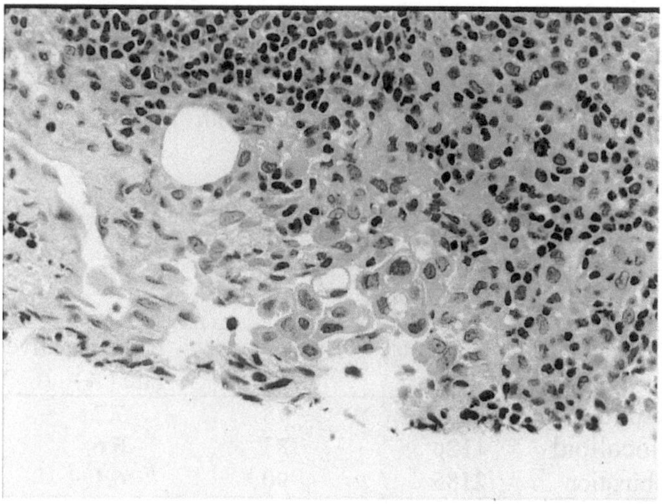

Figure 4. Lymph node stained with CK-IHC stains (low power 10X).

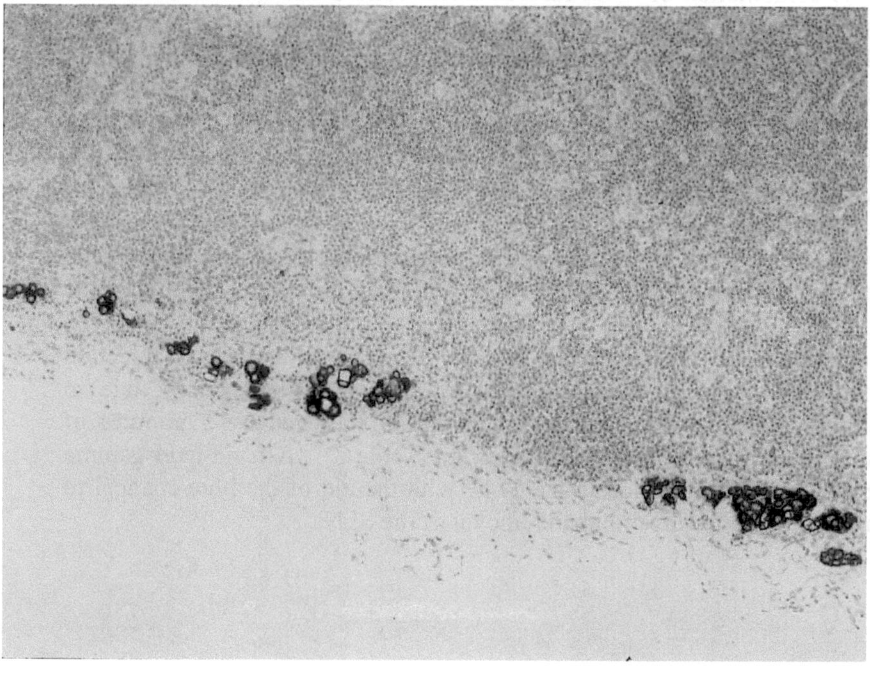

TECHNICAL CONSIDERATIONS OF LYMPHATIC MAPPING

Ability to perform lymphatic mapping and sentinel lymphadenectomy requires coordinated efforts from surgeons, radiologists, pathologists, and operating room staff. Dr. Giuliano described his method of dye localization as five species of Lymphazurin dye injected into the axillary side along the biopsy site. Five minutes of manual compression to the breast is utilized to aid in lymphatic flow. An incision is made approximately 1 cm below the axillary hairline; one proceeds to the depth of the clavipectoral fascia and begins to look carefully for a blue dye channel leading to the SLN. Table 2 shows the average results of many authors[11-13,17,18,30-49] in their experience with sentinel lymphadenectomy using blue dye only, radiocolloid only, or both as the localization technique.

Table 2. Worldwide experience with sentinel lymphadenectomy: Blue dye versus radiocolloid SLN detection

(See CD Rom for full meta-analyis)

Technique	No. patients	Success rate (%)	False negative rate (%)
Blue dye	1435	78	7.2
Radiocolloid	1126	83	6.6
Combination	2185	90	6.1

A combination of ^{99m}Tc-labeled sulfur colloid and Lymphazurin blue dye has been shown to be most effective for identification of the SLN.[50] The radiocolloid injection, usually performed by nuclear medicine, should be done 1 to 8 hours prior to axillary exploration, with the optimal injection time 2–3 hours before operation. Approximately 200–2000 uCi of radiolabeled sulfur colloid is diluted to 6 ml as the injectant, and given in 1-ml aliquots, intraparenchymally at the tumor margin, periareolar, or intradermal locations. Lymphoscintigraphy may be helpful for medial lesions, but is not necessary, and is not routinely done at many cancer centers. Lymphazurin blue dye is injected prior to beginning the operation. The blue dye can be injected intraparenchymally or given subdermally in the subareolar region. However, intradermal injection should be avoided, unless the injected area is to be excised, due to tattooing, which will occur. Again, this is followed by 5 minutes of intermittent manual breast massage (See Table 3). A hand-held gamma probe is then used to locate the SLN, with the aid of the blue channel to direct surgical localization and removal of the SLN.

The pathologist examines the SLN intraoperatively, using either imprint cytology methods or frozen section. If either of these modalities reveals cancer within the SLN, a complete axillary lymph node dissection is performed. The pathologist later examines the removed negative SLNs using H&E staining. If positive, no further exam is required. When initial H&E screen is negative, cytokeratin staining is performed routinely. A complete axillary node dissection is conducted if either of these modalities reveals the presence of tumor cells within the SLN.

Table 3. Success rates and false-negative rates associated with various injection techniques for sentinel lymphadenectomy. (See CD Rom for full meta-analyis[11, 36, 39, 45, 46, 51-57])

Injection site	No. patients	Success rate (%)	False negative rate (%)
Subareolar	76	99	0
Peritumoral	1055	89	8.6
Dermal/intradermal	775	98	6.5
Subdermal	510	96	7.2

PROCEDURE

The following procedural protocol is based on a breast SLN task-specific checklist provided by the American College of Surgeons Oncology Group for surgeons being trained, mentored, and evaluated in sentinel lymphadenectomy. This checklist is employed for surgeons learning how to perform SLN biopsies. Figures 5 and 6 offer anatomical landmarks considered during the mapping procedure. (See CD Rom for full color photos of each step, narrated video method, downloadable intraoperative checklist for scoring performance, and web link for recording personal mapping data).

The procedure is as follows:

1. Patient selected has disease appropriate for mapping (based on review of exam, imaging studies, and past history).
2. Timing of operation appropriate for radionucleotide injection (>30 minutes for same day or next day).
3. Patient must be clinically node negative .
4. Surgeon must have an intraoperative pathology plan.
5. Surgeon must review radionucleotide injection procedure.
6. Patient should then be positioned correctly on operating room table.
7. Surgeon injects blue dye correctly (peritumoral or subareolar).

8. Massage breast for 5 minutes.
9. "Hot spot" must then be marked on axilla prior to incision.
10. Incision is selected beneath axillary hair line.
11. Clavipectoral fascia is identified.
12. Dissection is directed to blue and/or hot lymph nodes.*
    * A properly excised node is any blue node or any hot node with an ex vivo radioactivity count ratio of SLN to non-SLN of 10:1, an in vivo radioactivity count ratio of SLN to background of 3:1, or both (JACS).
13. Probe must be used appropriately to assess potential sentinel nodes.
14. Sentinel nodes are then removed with ligature/clip of lymphatic channels as appropriate for size of lymphatics/vessels.
15. Ten-second ex-vivo count or peak instantaneous count must be obtained on each removed node.
16. Lymph nodes are labeled appropriately for pathologist.
17. Reevaluation on axilla for hot and/or blue nodes.
18. Removal of all nodes with counts greater than 10% of hottest SLNs.
    A properly excised node is any blue node or any hot node with an ex vivo radioactivity count ratio of SLN to non-SLN of 10:1, an in vivo radioactivity count ratio of SLN to background of 3:1, or both (JACS).
19. Surgeon then palpates axilla prior to closing incision.

Extras

1. Surgeon should preoperatively review lymphoscintogram if it was done and develop an operative plan based on these findings.
2. A careful examination is conducted near lateral thoracic vein if no SLNs are identified.
3. A full axillary node dissection is performed if no SLNS are identified or an SLN is positive.

Figure 5. The external anatomy used to locate the sentinel lymph node.

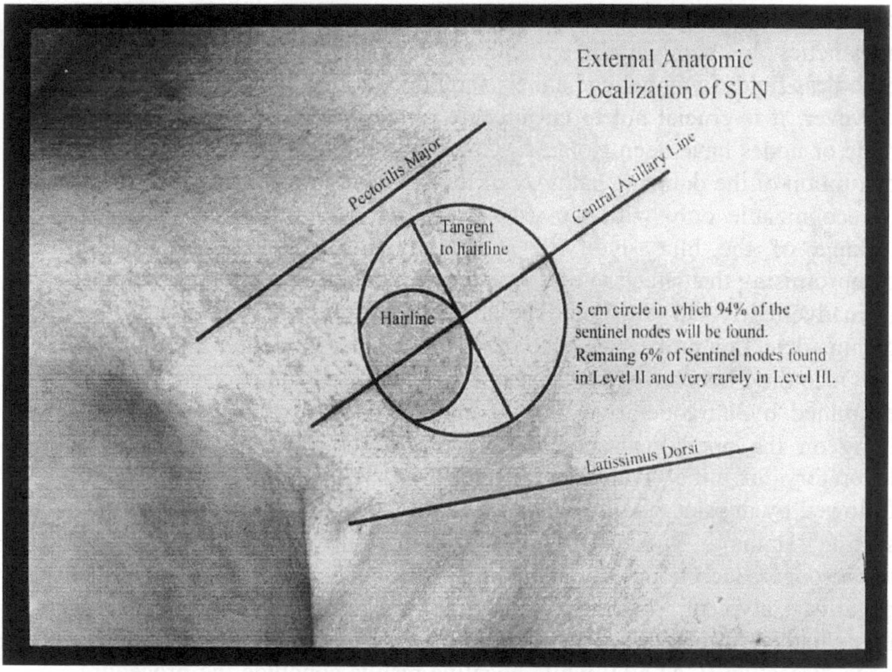

Figure 6. The internal anatomy used to locate the sentinel lymph node.

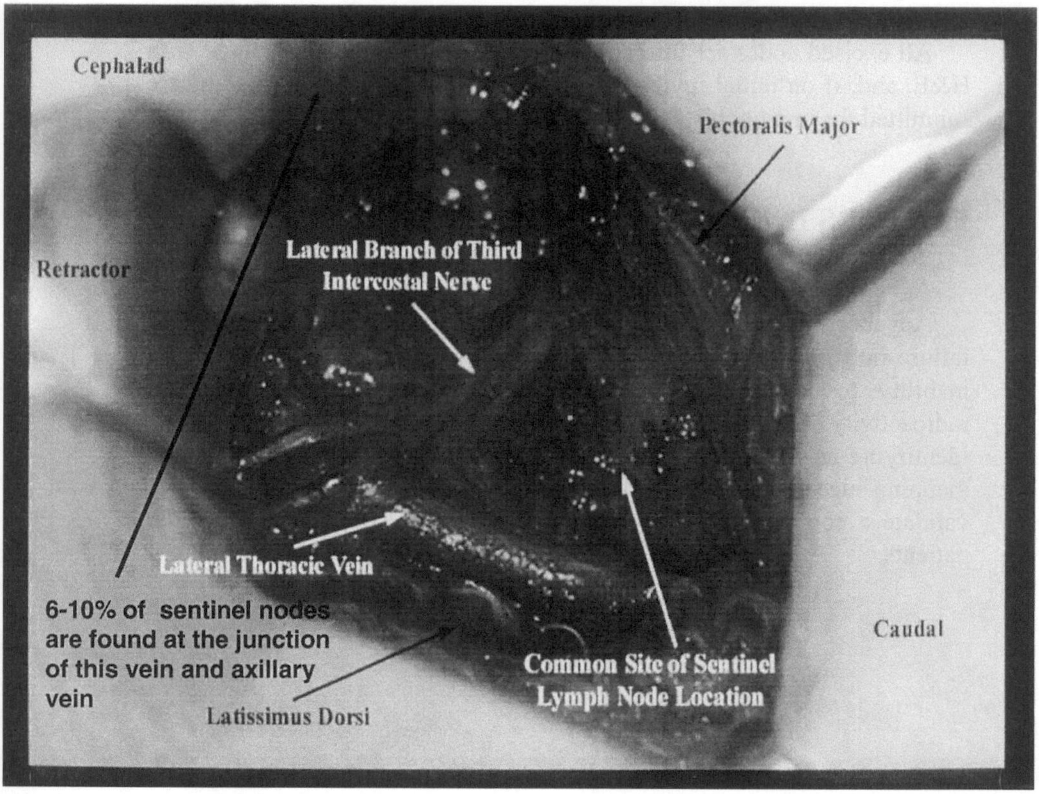

Visualization of the lymphatic channels requires good exposure and a bloodless field. Electrocautery should be used for dissection. If local anesthetics are being used, epinephrine may be added to enhance the bloodless field. Lymphatic channels should be clipped when encountered, however, it is crucial not to cut or clip a blue lymphatic channel until a node or nodes have been isolated. Cutting a blue channel will result in a disruption of the drainage pathway of the blue dye into the SLN rendering it recognizable only with the use of the gamma probe. Furthermore, leakage of the blue dye will stain the surrounding tissues further compromising the detection of a blue lymph node. If the blue dye channel is inadvertently cut, it should be located and clipped; the use of the gamma detection probe then becomes critical in locating the SLN.

Once the SLNs have been successfully identified and excised, they are examined by intraoperative imprint cytology: While the patient is still lying on the operating table, the SLNs are submitted to a pathology laboratory for initial evaluation. There, they are examined by sectioning followed by imprint cytology. The cytologist touches a slide to each nodal section, stains it with Diff-Quick solution, and observes it under a microscope. Each node is assigned to a diagnostic category of positive, negative, atypical, or suspicious and reported to the OR team immediately. A positive diagnosis results in a complete axillary lymph node dissection (CALND) while negative results conclude the procedure. A diagnosis of suspicious or atypical usually results in further analysis with either frozen section or rapid intraoperative cytokeratin staining.

All excised nodes are further sectioned in 2 mm intervals, stained with H&E, and, if on initial review are found to be negative, step sections are submitted for immunohistochemical stains for cytokeratin (CK).

FACTORS INFLUENCING SLN DETECTION

Age and Body Mass Index

Advanced age and marked obesity have been linked to an increased failure rate in SLN biopsies. An SLN mapping failure is defined as an inability to identify the SLNs by blue dye or invivo counts of radioactivity. Age has been shown to negatively impact the success rate of identifying an SLN at the rate of 0.75%/year of age over 40.[58] Although mapping success decreases with increasing age, age alone is not enough to validate a complete axillary dissection without an SLN biopsy in older patients.

Body mass index (BMI) has been explored as a potential cause for mapping failure. A study of 1600 mapping patients showed that of a random sample of 26 patients whose mapping failed, the mean BMI was 29.54 lb/in.^{2} Conversely, the BMI for a random sample of patients whose mapping was a success was 26.42 lb/in.^{2} Statistical analysis revealed that BMI (lb/in^2) is a significant factor in mapping failure (p=0.042).[58] Surgeons should keep in mind that they are less likely to successfully detect an SLN in individuals with a higher BMI. Factors such as the mapping agent, injection method, and surgical technique will all impact the success or failure of a mapping procedure. It is important to keep all of these factors in mind when assessing the cause of mapping failure. Figure 7 shows the correlation between age and BMI and mapping failure.

Several studies have demonstrated that the only patient-related factors for mapping failures are age and BMI. Among many other factors, these two factors have remained the only ones that cannot be modified to reduce the failure rate. Therefore, the other factors such as surgical skill, injection techniques, massage, appropriate dyes, colloidal particle size, adequate well-calibrated instrumentation, careful pathologic analysis, and experience may be the only factors that *can* be altered to affect mapping failures.

Figure 7. Nomogram depicting the probability of successful mapping. It shows the patient's body mass index and their age: there is a higher degree of mapping failure as the body mass index increases and the age increases. See CD Rom for personal probability calculations. (Courtesy of Cox et al. Age and body mass index may increase the chance of failure in sentinel lymphadenectomy. *The Breast Journal.* Blackwell Publishing.)

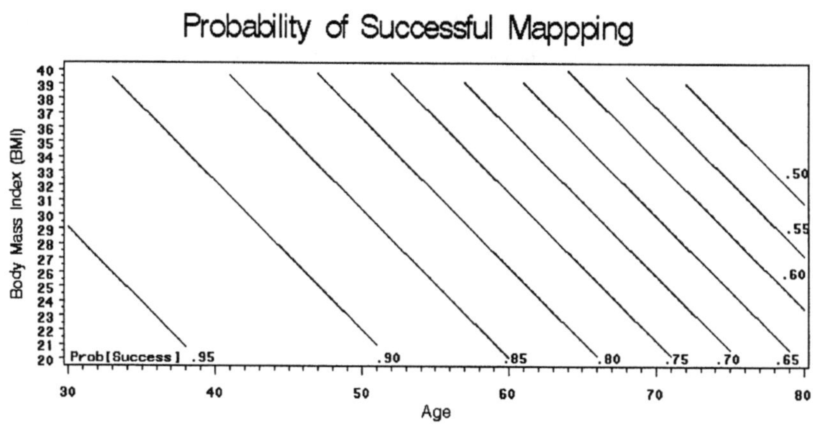

Learning Curves, Operative Experience and Volume of Practice

As one can clearly see in Figure 8, the more mapping procedures a physician conducts, the more successful he or she is. A study conducted at Moffitt Cancer center created lymphatic learning curves for a series of physicians who were mentored in lymphatic mapping. Most of the physician's failure rate declined after just a small number of mapping cases[59]. However, Moffitt physician E had a high failure rate after compiling the learning curves and was therefore asked to retake the lymphatic mapping course offered at Moffitt Cancer Center with subsequent improvement. On the other hand, physician F had a low failure rate early on in their experience, probably due to the fact that physician F was mentored by physician A.

Upon compilation of a number of physician learning curves much disparity was noted in the various experiences with the caveat that despite poor results by some surgeons the false negative rates were low when strict adherence to the guidelines of the mapping procedure were followed. Inability to locate the SLN resulted in 2 false negative cases out of 350 cases performed by 9 surgeons using a combined blue dye radioactive dye approach following a defined course in lymphatic mapping. In an effort to evaluate the reasons for failure to find the SLN, the surgical volume performed over a 30 day period (Surgical Volume Index, SVI) was plotted against rate of failure to find the SLN. The calculated logistic regression curve for successful breast cancer lymphatic mapping based on surgical volume demonstrates the intuitive results that the more cases a surgeon performs in a given time period the better he or she will perform. (Figure 9)

Figure 8. Learning curves for physicians A-F at the Moffitt Cancer Center. (next page)

Figure 8

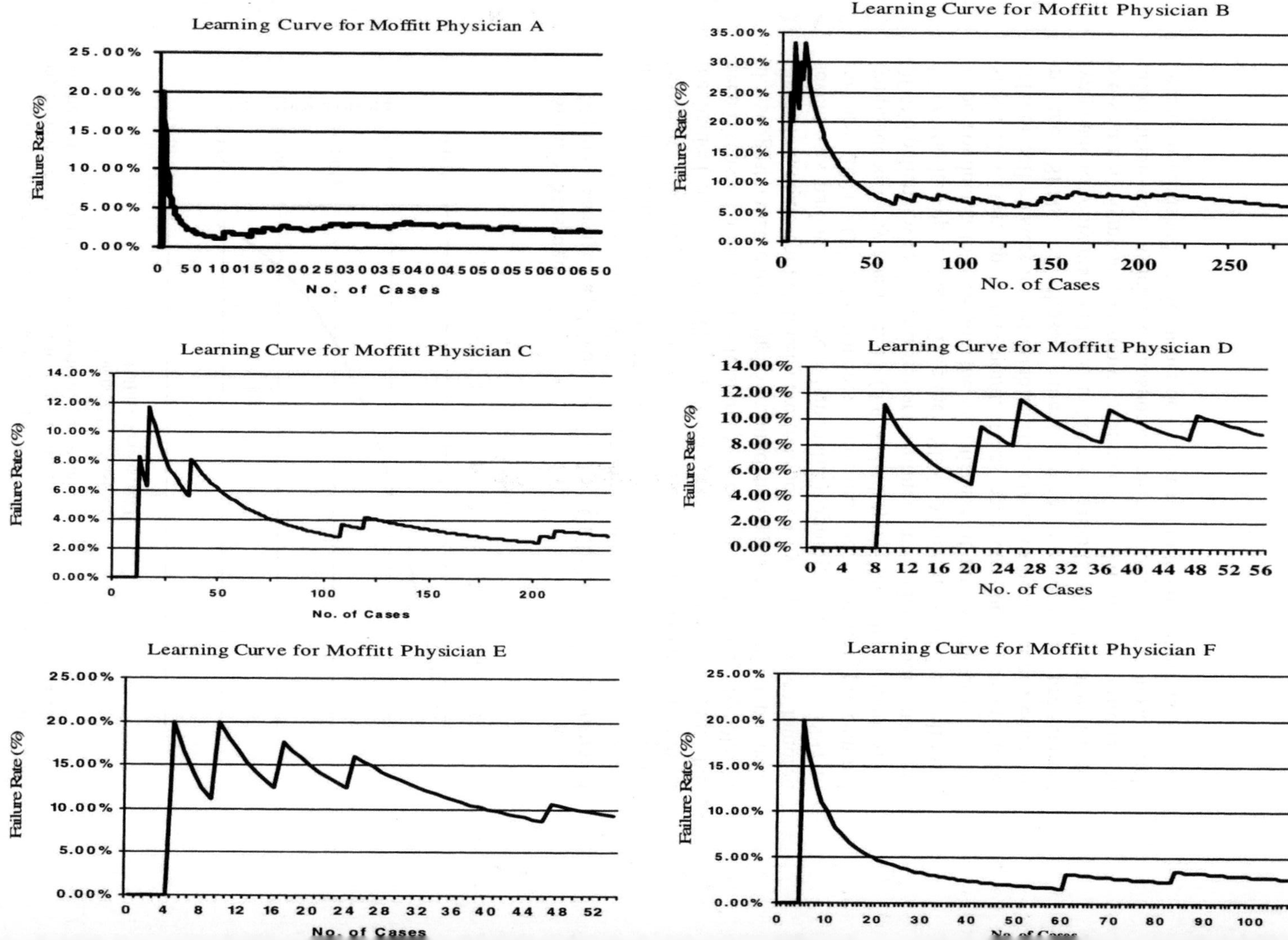
Learning Curve for Moffitt Physician A
Failure Rate (%)
25.00%
20.00%
15.00%
10.00%
5.00%
0.00%
0 50 100 150 200 250 300 350 400 450 500 550 600 650
No. of Cases
Learning Curve for Moffitt Physician B
Failure Rate (%)
35.00%
30.00%
25.00%
20.00%
15.00%
10.00%
5.00%
0.00%
0 50 100 150 200 250
No. of Cases
Learning Curve for Moffitt Physician C
Failure Rate (%)
14.00%
12.00%
10.00%
8.00%
6.00%
4.00%
2.00%
0.00%
0 50 100 150 200
No. of Cases
Learning Curve for Moffitt Physician D
Failure Rate (%)
14.00%
12.00%
10.00%
8.00%
6.00%
4.00%
2.00%
0.00%
0 4 8 12 16 20 24 28 32 36 40 44 48 52 56
No. of Cases
Learning Curve for Moffitt Physician E
Failure Rate (%)
25.00%
20.00%
15.00%
10.00%
5.00%
0.00%
0 4 8 12 16 20 24 28 32 36 40 44 48 52
No. of Cases
Learning Curve for Moffitt Physician F
Failure Rate (%)
25.00%
20.00%
15.00%
10.00%
5.00%
0.00%
0 10 20 30 40 50 60 70 80 90 100

Figure 9. Logistic regression demonstrates that for the number of cases performed in a 30 day cycle the calculated failure rate for a given surgeon would be inversely related to the numbers of cases that the surgeon performs per month.

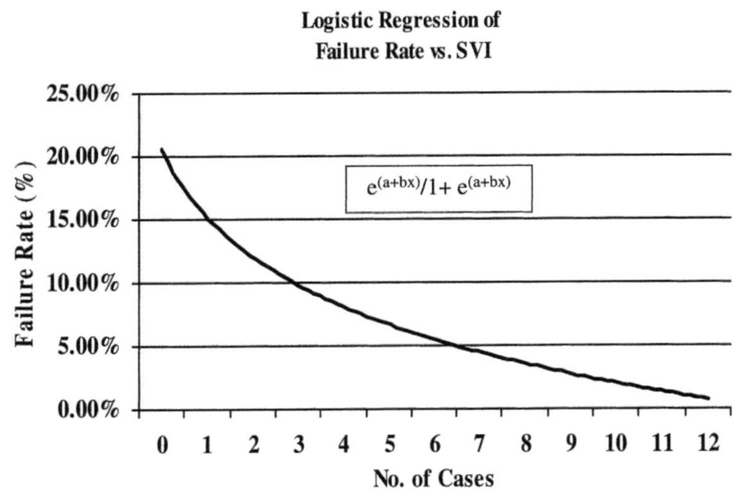

Manual Massage

Manual massage, as advocated by Dr. Guiliano, has demonstrated improved mapping success[25,47,60]. However, with massage it has been implicated that dislodged cells may worsen prognostic outcome by "seeding" the tumor throughout the body. The concept of benign mechanical transport (BMT), or tumor spread caused by massage, has been discussed often in the literature. However, a recent study, by Diaz et al., suggests that during the 5 minute massage prior to lymph node dissection, some epithelial cells are transported by BMT. Seven hundred seventy-six patients underwent lymphatic mapping from March 1997 to January 2001. Of 320 patients who did not undergo pre-sentinel lymphadenectomy massage, 11 (3.4%) had epithelial cells in their SLN. Of 456 patients who did undergo pre-sentinel lymphadenectomy massage, 45 (9.9%) had epithelial cells in their SLN. Many more studies will need to be conducted to ascertain the significance of micrometastases in the SLNs. However, up to this point, it has been concluded that epithelial cells or cell clusters *not* of established metastases occur more frequently in the SLNs of those patients who undergo a pre-sentinel lymphadenectomy massage than in those of patients who do not undergo a pre-sentinel lymphadenectomy massage.[61] Histologic criteria to differentiate cells which are transported into the nodes versus those which became established await further definition and outcomes analysis.

SPECIAL SITUATIONS IN LYMPHATIC MAPPING

Internal Mammary Nodes

According to recent studies, 2% to 29% of all patients who receive a sentinel lymphadenectomy will map to at least one internal mammary node (IMN) and 10% to 14% of those patients who map to the IM area will have at least 1 IMN positive.[62] In all lymphatic mapping cases, the internal mammary locations should be thoroughly evaluated especially in the second and third parasternal interspaces.[63] By separating the fibers of the pectoralis major muscle and dividing the intercostal muscles at the parasternal location, radioguided excision may be accomplished. Careful localization and delicate dissection will result in the uneventful removal of the IMN(s). Following removal, marking the location with a small surgical clip will allow radiographic localization should the node return positive on final pathology.

Impeccable care must be taken during the dissection to avoid entering the pleural space, which could result in a pneumothorax. If this occurrs the patient is treated with intraoperative pleural aspiration and postoperative observation until the resolution of the pneumothorax.

If an IMN cannot be safely removed, an intraoperative clip at the site of the node can be placed, the patient can be scanned or X-rayed postoperatively,[63] and the location of the IMN can be tattooed for later radiation. If the IMN is positive on final pathological evaluation, then radiation is given to the IMN chain. In contrast, a negative IMN would obviate the need for radiation in at least 865 of the cases. Figure 10 shows the disease-free survival for patients who have any number of positive IMNs alone. A patient with a positive IMN has a disease-free survival equivalent to that of patients with only axillary node involvement.[64]

Figure 10. Overall survival curves for axillary and internal mammary nodes involvement. Node Negative (AN-) & Node Positive (AN+) Node Negative (IMN-) & Node Positive (IMN+) (Veronesi et al.)

Survival Curves For Axillary & Internal Mammary Node Involvement

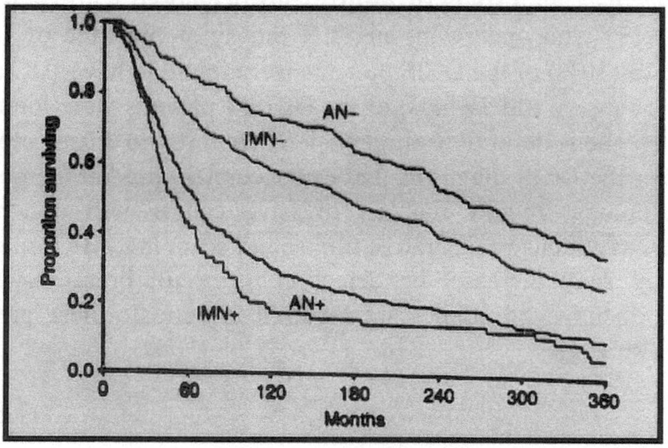

As mentioned previously, intradermal, subareolar, and intra-parenchymal injection techniques have been used with much success, but deep intraparenchymal injection is the technique that allows identification of the IMN chain.

Ductal Carcinoma in Situ

Ductal carcinoma in situ (DCIS) has been described as proliferating malignant ductal cells, which are contained by the basement membrane, which occasionally reach the lobular units without invasion into the surrounding stroma.[65] DCIS with microinvasion (DCISM), on the other hand, is defined in the same manner except that cancer cells have begun to invade through the myoepithelial layer of the mammary ducts or lobules. Due to the major advances in high-quality mammography, DCIS was the most rapidly growing subtype of breast cancer from 1983 to1992, with a growth rate in detection of 500 percent. DCIS currently represents approximately 15–25% of all newly reported breast cancer patients. Furthermore, only 2 % of these 27,000 to 46,000 new patients diagnosed with DCIS each year are expected to die of the disease over their lifetime and less than 5% of DCISM patients are expected to die of their disease.

Due to the low incidence of nodal metastases in DCIS (<2%) and DCISM (<5%) patients,[65] the validity of SLN analysis for these patients has been under scrutiny for some time. For patients with invasive cancer, sentinel node evaluation has been shown to increase detection of metastases in the axilla by 9 % to 31 % [65] and has therefore become standard of care for these patients at many cancer treatment centers. This technique has been found to be useful for patients with even the smallest risk of lymph node involvement.[66] Therefore, it has been proposed by a few institutions[65,67-70] that mapping DCIS patients can be of great value. The primary reason to map DCIS patients is the fact that 13% to 29% will have unsuspected invasive cancer at the time of their definitive operation. *Patients requiring or requesting mastectomy for DCIS must undergo lymphatic mapping at the time of the definitive procedure or lose forever the ability to be mapped if they are found to have an occult breast cancer in the specimen.* In a study of 240 patients diagnosed with DCIS (224) or DCISM (16) who underwent an SLN biopsy at the time of definitive surgery, 23 (10%) of the DCIS patients were found to have IDC after their definitive surgery and 7 (44%) of the DCISM patients were found to have IDC after their definitive surgery.[65] There are no clear preoperative criteria for the DCIS diagnosis that can accurately predict the outcome on final pathologic review that an invasive cancer will not be found. However, assiduous preoperative ultrasound scanning, MRI imaging, and PET scans may increase the detection of occult breast cancers; cost effective documented studies are required to validate these preoperative detection strategies.

Prophylactic Mastectomy

A prophylactic mastectomy (PM) is an operation that removes the entire breast, the nipple areolar complex, and the tail of Spence in the absence of a diagnosed cancer in that breast. The sole purpose is to prevent the occurrence of breast cancer and has become a widely accepted alternative, in selected patients, to routine close surveillance. Reasons for a PM may include one or more of the following: histologic risk factors such as LCIS, a positive family history, BRCA 1 and 2 positive diagnoses, cosmesis, symmetry with a contralateral mastectomy for carcinoma, and/or cancer phobia. The main indication is genetic mutations linked to breast cancer.[71]

Premenopausal patients with a strong family history of breast cancer will most likely require genetic counseling to determine their personal risk, recurrence risk, and risk to family or offspring. Gene-positive patients of young patients with a recent diagnosis of breast cancer may opt for childbearing preservation by harvesting eggs and/or utilizing embryo cryopreservation. However, these patients need counseling regarding the risk of hormonal stimulation with breast cancer associated with ovulatory stimulation by clomiphene citrate and tamoxifen.[72] Other patients may choose to preserve ovarian function by utilizing hormonal blocking of ovaries during chemotherapy. The primary drug used for this purpose is gonadotropin releasing hormone (GnRH) for 4–6 weeks during chemotherapy.

Patients with a strong history of breast cancer, who have a lesion treatable with lumpectomy may receive a lumpectomy with SLN biopsy and subsequent genetic screening. If diagnosed as BRCA 1/2 positive following the lumpectomy and SLN biopsy, the patient will not receive radiation, but will get a bilateral mastectomy and reconstruction with oophorectomy while the negative patient may receive radiation to the breast alone. Prophylactic oophorectomy should be offered to all women with BRCA1 or 2 mutations, especially those beyond the childbearing years .[73]

The Moffitt series by Dupont et al. demonstrates that up to 5% of prophylactic mastectomies harbor occult cancer and many patients with a history of carcinoma have an increased risk, 0.5–1.0% per year, of developing a contralateral breast cancer.[74]

Mapping PM patients is built on a few basic premises.[71] First, the incidence of inadvertent axillary node removal in prophylactic mastectomy is approximately 15%, mapping may help avoid this problem. Second, lymph node mapping may eliminate the need for total axillary dissection if cancer is detected in the prophylactic breast when the SLN is negative. Third, SLN mapping may detect occult nodal disease prior to the detection of disease in the breast. As a result of lymphatic mapping and sentinel lymphadenectomy, most patients can be spared the potential risks and long-term morbidity of a complete axillary node dissection. If mapping is not performed at the time of prophylactic mastectomy and a breast cancer is detected, a second operative procedure would be required. Still, with studies showing that the absence of known disease in the breast does not preclude the presence of occult disease in the axilla,[71,74] the routine practice of mapping prophylactic patients is a logical extension of the mapping procedure.

Implants and Reduction Mammoplasty

The ever-increasing popularity of plastic surgery breast augmentation and reduction mammoplasty raises the question of whether or not patients can be mapped following these procedures. Lymphatic mapping conducted at the H. Lee Moffitt Cancer Center on over 50 patients with prior breast augmentation proved to be 100% successful. However, despite these favorable results, good clinical judgment by the attending surgeon is imperative.

When a patient undergoes a breast reduction, the inferior pedicle technique causes the least disruption of lymphatic flow to the axillary basin. However, difficulty in mapping can arise when the tumor is located within the pedicle flap region (5 to 7 o'clock).

A review included 12 patients with previous reduction mammoplasty who underwent surgery at the H. Lee Moffitt Cancer Center for breast cancer. Five patients were mapped for nodal evaluation, four tumors were located outside of the pedicle flap, and all four mapped successfully. Conversely, the other patient with the tumor located inside the pedicle flap region failed to map successfully. One may conclude that cosmetic breast surgery does not completely eliminate the ability to undergo successful mapping. However, depending on the location of the tumor, cosmetic surgery can possibly jeopardize the mapping success rate.

Neoadjuvant Chemotherapy

Treatment of locally advanced breast cancer (LABC) or any Stage III cancer with neoadjuvant chemotherapy offers advantages such as assessing tumor response, reduction in tumor size with possible breast conservation and possible axillary clearance of nodal disease. Kuerer et al. report that neoadjuvant chemotherapy clears axillary metastasis in 23% of all breast cancer patients with LABC and 10% will have occult nodal disease on negative findings with H&E.[75] The more important observation is that these patients with negative findings on CALND following neoadjuvant therapy with known nodal disease assessed by H&E exam have a 5-year survival rate of 80–90% while patients with residual nodal disease have survival rates of 50–60%. However, the patients recruited to neoadjuvant chemotherapy treatment are usually those LABC patients with clinically palpable nodes or enlarged nodes noted on imaging studies. Many studies report that the overall success rate in SLN mapping after neoadjuvant chemotherapy ranges from 84 to 90% and the false-negative rate can range from 0 to 33%[75-77] depending on the patient's reaction to the chemotherapy and the initial tumor stage and size. The great debate still remains whether to map before or after neoadjuvant chemotherapy. Lymph node mapping post neoadjuvant treatment would *ideally* predict the pathological clearance of nodal disease and help avoid a CALND in 23% of patients. However, does mapping post neoadjuvant therapy accurately access the entire nodal basin when reports of up to 33% false negatives exist?

When mapping was be conducted on patients with tumors > 4.5 cm without clinically palpable lymph nodes to determine the true axillary status, accrual due to pathological positivity of nodes was increased by 87%.

Clinical Outcome Based on Follow-up

Figure 11 presents an algorithm that is currently used at the Moffitt Cancer Center in the management of patients with Lymphatic mapping.

Figure 11. Axillary dissection algorithm and sentinel lymphadenectomy as an established procedure.

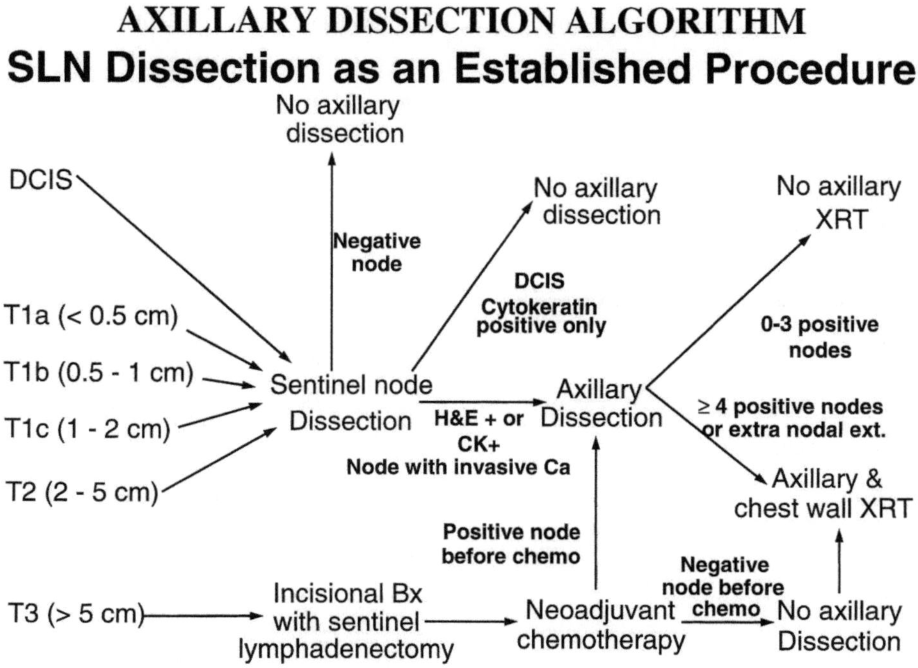

Continuous follow-up is required for all SLN mapping patients not only to evaluate potential axillary nodal recurrence, but also to accurately assess failure rates and occult metastasis. Typically, the largest complaint made by patients who undergo CALND is morbidity caused by lymphedema. Approximately 40% of all patients who undergo CALND have lymphedema in the shortterm and approximately 5% will suffer with chronic lymphedema for the rest of their lives.[25] Numerous studies have reported that SLN mapping reduces morbidity for those who avoid a CALND.[20, 22, 39, 78] In 2003, Veronesi et al. reported on the side effects of 100 patients who received a CALND vs. 100 patients who avoided a CALND because their sentinel nodes were found to be negative for metastasis.[20] Table 4 exhibits their findings regarding the benefits of avoiding a CALND: those who avoid a CALND have more arm mobility, less swelling, less pain, less numbness in the upperarm, and better aesthetic appearance in the longrun.

Table 4. Side effects in SLN-only dissection patients vs. CALND patients (Courtesy of Massachusetts Medical Society. Copyright 2003)

Side effect	Axillary-dissection group (n = 100)		Sentinel-node group (n = 100)	
	No. of patients			
	6 mo	24 mo	6 mo	24 mo
Axillary pain [a]				
No	9	61	84	92
Yes, sporadic	72	34	14	7
Yes, continuous	19	5	2	1
Numbness or paresthesias on operated side [b]				
No	15	32	98	99
Yes	85	68	2	1
Arm Mobility [c]				
80–100%	73	79	100	100
60–79%	22	18	0	0
40–59%	5	2	0	0
20-39%	0	1	0	0
< 20%	0	0	0	0

Aesthetic appearance of axillary scar [d]				
Good	91	85	98	100
Bad	9	15	2	0
Arm swelling (difference in circumference) [e]				
No difference	31	25	89	93
< 1 cm	44	38	11	6
1–2 cm	17	25	0	1
> 2 cm	8	12	0	0

[a] Postoperative axillary pain was evaluated as continuous (lasting > 50% of the day), sporadic, or absent.

[b] Numbness and paresthesias were assessed by comparing skin sensitivity on the inner and outer upper arms, axillae, and chest wall on the operated side with that on the untreated side. Sensitivity was recorded as either the presence or absence of numbness.

[c] Arm mobility was judged by asking the patient to assign the restriction in motion in the operated arm a value on a scale of 0% (severe restriction) to 100% (no restriction).

[d] The appearance of the axillary scar was judged by asking the patient simply to say whether the result was good or bad.

[e] Arm swelling and edema were assessed by comparing the circumference (in centimeters) of the treated arm 15 cm above the lateral epicondyle with that of the untreated arm.

FUTURE PERSPECTIVES

Lymphatic mapping from its inception has allowed for directed pathologic evaluation utilizing methodologies such as immunohistochemistry, RT-PCR, and now gene microarray technology in the analysis of lymph nodes.[79] SLN biopsy has become the standard of care for breast cancer at many facilities and will continue to become the primary tool for early cancer treatment around the world. Due to the fact that the patient's outcome and treatment is chiefly based on the analysis of the lymphatics, these advances will continue to drive the need for more accurate evaluation and pathologic staging as evidenced by the changes in the AJCC staging system. Selective sentinel lymphadenectomy will also continue to drive the need for clarification in the significance of micrometastatic disease whether it is in the SLN or other sites that are accessible for analysis such as bone marrow and the blood.[80] This capacity should drive the next wave of therapeutic intervention, defining which group will benefit from chemotherapy and which will not. New diagnostics of gene microarray and proteomics promise to make these goals a reality.

Many new, innovative tools and procedures are being developed for better management of breast cancer. Lymphatic mapping for breast cancer diagnosis is a quick, accurate technique that provides increased precision in detection of lymphatic metastasis. The risk/benefit analysis of lymphatic mapping provides an improvement in staging with reduced morbidity, elimination of general anesthesia, elimination of a surgical drain, and elimination of a hospital stay for a large portion of the population treated. Many facilities around the world are integrating the SLN biopsy procedure into their routine care for breast cancer patients by training their surgeons through advanced education and certification programs. Significant advantages and improvements like these manifest that lymphatic mapping will soon become the standard of care for all breast cancer staging at all major cancer treatment facilities worldwide.

REFERENCES

1. Gould EA, Winship T, Philbin PH, Kerr HH. Observations on a "sentinel node" in cancer of the parotid. *Cancer* Jan-Feb 1960;13:77-78.
2. Cabanas RM. An approach for the treatment of penile carcinoma. *Cancer* Feb 1977;39(2):456-466.
3. Norman J, Cruse CW, Espinosa C, et al. Redefinition of cutaneous lymphatic drainage with the use of lymphoscintigraphy for malignant melanoma. *Am J Surg* Nov 1991;162(5):432-437.
4. Norman J Jr., Cruse W, Ruas E, et al. The expanding role of lymphoscintigraphy in the management of cutaneous melanoma. First Place Winner: Conrad Jobst award. *Am Surg* Dec 1989;55(12):689-694.
5. Reintgen DS, Conrad AJ. Detection of occult melanoma cells in sentinel lymph nodes and blood. *Semin Oncol* Feb 1997;24(1 Suppl 4):S11-15.
6. Morton DL, Wen DR, Foshag LJ, Essner R, Cochran A. Intraoperative lymphatic mapping and selective cervical lymphadenectomy for early-stage melanomas of the head and neck. *J Clin Onco.* Sep 1993;11(9):1751-1756.
7. Morton DL, Wen DR, Wong JH, et al. Technical details of intraoperative lymphatic mapping for early stage melanoma. *Arch Surg* Apr 1992;127(4):392-399.
8. Alex JC, Weaver DL, Fairbank JT, Rankin BS, Krag DN. Gamma-probe-guided lymph node localization in malignant melanoma. *Surg Onco.* Oct 1993;2(5):303-308.
9. Alex JC, Krag DN. Gamma-probe guided localization of lymph nodes. *Surg Oncol* 1993;2(3):137-143.
10. Albertini JJ, Cruse CW, Rapaport D, et al. Intraoperative radio-lympho-scintigraphy improves sentinel lymph node identification for patients with melanoma. *Ann Surg* Feb 1996;223(2):217-224.
11. Albertini JJ, Lyman GH, Cox C, et al. Lymphatic mapping and sentinel node biopsy in the patient with breast cancer. *JAMA.* Dec 11 1996;276(22):1818-1822.
12. Giuliano AE, Kirgan DM, Guenther JM, Morton DL. Lymphatic mapping and sentinel lymphadenectomy for breast cancer. *Ann Surg* Sep 1994;220(3):391-398; discussion 398-401.
13. Giuliano AE. Sentinel lymphadenectomy in primary breast carcinoma: an alternative to routine axillary dissection. *J Surg Oncol* 1996;62(2):75-77.

14. Bilchik AJ, Giuliano A, Essner R, et al. Universal application of intraoperative lymphatic mapping and sentinel lymphadenectomy in solid neoplasms. *Cancer J Sci Am* Nov-Dec 1998;4(6):351-358.
15. Turner RR, Ollila DW, Krasne DL, Giuliano AE. Histopathologic validation of the sentinel lymph node hypothesis for breast carcinoma. *Ann Surg* Sep 1997;226(3):271-276; discussion 276-278.
16. Schwartz GF, Giuliano AE, Veronesi U. Proceedings of the consensus conference on the role of sentinel lymph node biopsy in carcinoma of the breast, April 19-22, 2001, Philadelphia, Pennsylvania. *Cancer* May 15 2002;94(10):2542-2551.
17. Borgstein PJ, Pijpers R, Comans EF, van Diest PJ, Boom RP, Meijer S. Sentinel lymph node biopsy in breast cancer: guidelines and pitfalls of lymphoscintigraphy and gamma probe detection. *J Am Coll Surg* Mar 1998;186(3):275-283.
18. Krag DN. Minimal access surgery for staging regional lymph nodes: the sentinel-node concept. *Curr Probl Surg* 1998;35(11):951-1016.
19. Hill AD, Tran KN, Akhurst T, Yeung H, Yeh SD. Lessons learned from 500 cases of lymphatic mapping for breast cancer. *Ann Surg* 1999;229(4):528-535.
20. Veronesi U, Paganelli G, Viale G, et al. A randomized comparison of sentinel-node biopsy with routine axillary dissection in breast cancer. *N Engl J Med* Aug 7 2003;349(6):546-553.
21. Weerts JM, Maweja S, Tamigneaux I, Dallemagne B, Jourdan JL. The sentinel lymph node biopsy in breast cancer. *Acta Chir Belg* 2002;102(2):110-113.
22. Giuliano AE, Jones RC, Brennan M, Statman R. Sentinel lymphadenectomy in breast cancer. *J Clin Oncol* Jun 1997;15(6):2345-2350.
23. Cody HS 3rd, Borgen PI. State-of-the-art approaches to sentinel node biopsy for breast cancer: study design, patient selection, technique, and quality control at Memorial Sloan-Kettering Cancer Center. *Surg Oncol* Aug 1999;8(2):85-91.
24. Jakub JW, Pendas S, Reintgen DS. Current status of sentinel lymph node mapping and biopsy: facts and controversies. *Oncologist* 2003;8(1):59-68.
25. Cox CE, Haddad F, Bass S, et al. Lymphatic mapping in the treatment of breast cancer. *Oncology (Huntingt)* Sep 1998;12(9):1283-1292; discussion 1293-1284, 1297-1288.
26. Giuliano AE, Haigh PI, Brennan MB, et al. Prospective observational study of sentinel lymphadenectomy without further axillary dissection in patients with sentinel node-negative breast cancer. *J Clin Oncol* 2000;18(13):2553-2559.
27. Kamath VJ, Giuliano R, Dauway EL, et al. Characteristics of the sentinel lymph node in breast cancer predict further involvement of higher-echelon nodes in the axilla: a study to evaluate the need for complete axillary lymph node dissection. *Arch Surg* 2001;136(6):688-692.
28. Jakub JW, Diaz NM, Ebert MD, et al. Completion axillary lymph node dissection minimizes the likelihood of false negatives for patients with invasive breast carcinoma and cytokeratin positive only sentinel lymph nodes. *Am J Surg.* Oct 2002;184(4):302-306.
29. Nos C, Harding-MacKean C, Freneaux P, et al. Prediction of tumour involvement in remaining axillary lymph nodes when the sentinel node in a woman with breast cancer contains metastases. *Br J Surg* 2003;90(11):1354-1360.
30. Guenther JM, Krishnamoorthy M, Tan LR. Sentinel lymphadenectomy for breast cancer in a community managed care setting. *Cancer J Sci Am* 1997;3(6):336-340.
31. Flett MM, Going JJ, Stanton PD, et al. Sentinel node localization in patients with breast cancer. *Br J Surg* 1998;85(7):991-993.
32. Altinyollar H, Kapucuoglu N, Pak I, et al. Lymphatic mapping and sentinel lymphadenectomy in early stage breast carcinoma. *J Exp Clin Cancer Res* 2000;19(2):141-144.

33. Noguchi M, Motomura K, Imoto S, et al. A multicenter validation study of sentinel lymph node biopsy by the Japanese Breast Cancer Society. *Breast Cancer Res Treat* 2000;63(1):31-40.
34. Rodier JF, Routiot T, Mignotte H, et al. Lymphatic mapping and sentinel node biopsy of operable breast cancer. *World J Surg* 2000;24(10):1220-1225.
35. Su F, Jia W, Li H, et al. Sentinel lymph node biopsy in breast cancer: value for predicting the status of axillary node. *Zhonghua Wai Ke Za Zhi* 2000;38(10):784-786.
36. McMasters KM, Wong SL, Martin RC 2nd, et al. Dermal injection of radioactive colloid is superior to peritumoral injection for breast cancer sentinel lymph node biopsy: results of a multiinstitutional study. *Ann Surg* May 2001;233(5):676-687.
37. Krag DN, Weaver DL, Alex JC, Fairbank JT. Surgical resection and radiolocalization of the sentinel lymph node in breast cancer using a gamma probe. *Surg Oncol* Dec 1993;2(6):335-339; discussion 340.
38. Pijpers R, Meijer S, Hoekstra OS, et al. Impact of lymphoscintigraphy on sentinel node identification with technetium-99m-colloidal albumin in breast cancer. *J Nucl Med* Mar 1997;38(3):366-368.
39. Veronesi U, Paganelli G, Galimberti V, et al. Sentinel-node biopsy to avoid axillary dissection in breast cancer with clinically negative lymph-nodes. *Lancet* Jun 28 1997;349(9069):1864-1867.
40. Krag D, Weaver D, Ashikaga T, et al. The sentinel node in breast cancer—a multicenter validation study. *N Engl J Med* Oct 1 1998;339(14):941-946.
41. Snider H, Dowlatshahi K, Fan M, Bridger WM, Rayudu G, Oleske D. Sentinel node biopsy in the staging of breast cancer. *Am J Surg* Oct 1998;176(4):305-310.
42. Delaloye JF, Antonescu C, Besseghir N, Genton CY, Bischof-Delaloye A, De Grandi P. [Sentinel lymph node biopsy in breast cancer: the Lausanne experience]. *Rev Med Suisse Romande* Jun 2000;120(6):491-494.
43. Cserni G, Boross G, Baltas B. Value of axillary sentinel nodal status in breast cancer. *World J Surg* 2000;24(3):341-344.
44. Borgstein PJ, Meijer S, Pijpers R. Intradermal blue dye to identify sentinel lymph-node in breast cancer. *Lancet* Jun 7 1997;349(9066):1668-1669.
45. Barnwell JM, Arredondo MA, Kollmorgen D, et al. Sentinel node biopsy in breast cancer. *Ann Surg Oncol* Mar 1998;5(2):126-130.
46. Nwariaku FE, Euhus DM, Beitsch PD, et al. Sentinel lymph node biopsy, an alternative to elective axillary dissection for breast cancer. *Am J Surg* Dec 1998;176(6):529-531.
47. Bass SS, Lyman GH, McCann CR, et al. Lymphatic mapping and sentinel lymph node biopsy. *Breast J* Sep 1999;5(5):288-295.
48. Peley G, Farkas E, Teglas M, Orosz Z, Andocs G. [Feasibility and accuracy of the combined radioisotope and blue-dye guided sentinel lymph node biopsy in breast cancer]. *Magy Seb* Dec 2000;53(6):241-246.
49. Zervos EE, Burak WE Jr. Lymphatic mapping for breast cancer: experience at The Ohio State University. *Breast Cancer* 2000;7(3):195-200.
50. Edwards MJ, Whitworth P, Tafra L, et al. The details of successful sentinel lymph node staging for breast cancer. *Am J Surg* 2000;180(4):257-261.
51. O'Hea BJ, Hill AD, El-Shirbiny AM, et al. Sentinel lymph node biopsy in breast cancer: initial experience at Memorial Sloan-Kettering Cancer Center. *J Am Coll Surg* Apr 1998;186(4):423-427.
52. Mertz L, Mathelin C, Marin C, et al. [Subareolar injection of 99m-Tc sulfur colloid for sentinel nodes identification in multifocal invasive breast cancer]. *Bull Cancer* Nov 1999;86(11):939-945.
53. Bass SS, Cox CE, Ku NN, Berman C, Reintgen DS. The role of sentinel lymph node biopsy in breast cancer. *J Am Coll Surg* Aug 1999;189(2):183-194.

54. Smith LF, Cross MJ, Klimberg VS. Subareolar injection is a better technique for sentinel lymph node biopsy. *Am J Surg* Dec 2000;180(6):434-437; discussion 437-438.
55. Tafra L, Lannin DR, Swanson MS, et al. Multicenter trial of sentinel node biopsy for breast cancer using both technetium sulfur colloid and isosulfan blue dye. *Ann Surg* Jan 2001;233(1):51-59.
56. Kern KA. Sentinel lymph node mapping in breast cancer using subareolar injection of blue dye. *J Am Coll Surg* Dec 1999;189(6):539-545.
57. Boolbol SK, Fey JV, Borgen PI, et al. Intradermal isotope injection: a highly accurate method of lymphatic mapping in breast carcinoma. *Ann Surg Oncol* Jan-Feb 2001;8(1):20-24.
58. Cox CE, Dupont E, Whitehead GF, et al. Age and body mass index may increase the chance of failure in sentinel lymph node biopsy for women with breast cancer. *Breast J* Mar-Apr 2002;8(2):88-91.
59. Cox CE, Salud CJ, Cantor A, et al. Learning curves for breast cancer sentinel lymph node mapping based on surgical volume analysis. *J Am Coll Surg* Dec 2001;193(6):593-600.
60. Bass SS, Cox CE, Salud CJ, et al. The effects of postinjection massage on the sensitivity of lymphatic mapping in breast cancer. *J Am Coll Surg* Jan 2001;192(1):9-16.
61. Diaz N, Vrcel V, Ebert MD, et al. Epithelial cells in sentinel lymph nodes associated with breast massage prior to SLN biopsy: a mode of benign mechanical transport. *Mod Pathol* 2003;16:28A.
62. Dupont EL, Salud CJ, Peltz ES, et al. Clinical relevance of internal mammary node mapping as a guide to radiation therapy. *Am J Surg* Oct 2001;182(4):321-324.
63. Cox CE, Salud CJ, Harrinton MA. The role of selective sentinel lymph node dissection in breast cancer. *Surg Clin North Am* Dec 2000;80(6):1759-1777.
64. Veronesi U, Marubini E, Mariani L, et al. The dissection of internal mammary nodes does not improve the survival of breast cancer patients. 30-year results of a randomised trial. *Eur J Cancer* 1999;35:1320-1325.
65. Cox CE, Nguyen K, Gray RJ, et al. Importance of lymphatic mapping in ductal carcinoma in situ (DCIS): why map DCIS? *Am Surg* Jun 2001;67(6):513-519; discussion 519-521.
66. Jakub JW, Ebert MD, Diaz NM, et al. Effect of lymphatic mapping on diagnosis and treatment of patients with T1a, T1b favorable breast cancer. *Ann Surg* Jun 2003;237(6):838-841; discussion 841-833.
67. Cody HS, Van Zee KJ. Point: Sentinel lymph node biopsy is indicated for patients with DCIS. *NCCN* 2003;1(2):199204.
68. Jakub JW, Cox CE, Pippas AW, et al. Controversial topics in breast lymphatic mapping. *Semin Surg Oncol* 2004;In press.
69. Klauber-DeMore N, Tan LK, Liberman L, et al. Sentinel lymph node biopsy: is it indicated in patients with high-risk ductal carcinoma-in-situ and ductal carcinoma-in-situ with microinvasion? *Ann Surg Oncol* Oct 2000;7(9):636-642.
70. Pendas S, Dauway E, Giuliano R, Ku N, Cox CE, Reintgen DS. Sentinel node biopsy in ductal carcinoma in situ patients. *Ann Surg Oncol* Jan-Feb 2000;7(1):15-20.
71. Dupont EL, Kuhn MA, McCann C, Salud C, Spanton JL, Cox CE. The role of sentinel lymph node biopsy in women undergoing prophylactic mastectomy. *Am J Surg* Oct 2000;180(4):274-277.
72. Oktay K, Buyuk E, Davis O, Yermakova I, Veeck L, Rosenwaks Z. Fertility preservation in breast cancer patients: IVF and embryo cryopreservation after ovarian stimulation with tamoxifen. *Hum Reprod* Jan 2003;18(1):90-95.
73. Abrams JD, Cody HS, Appleton A, et al. *Sentinel Lymph Node Biopsy*. London: Martin Dunitz Ltd.; 2002.

74. Lopez MJ, Porter KA. The current role of prophylactic mastectomy. *Surg Clin North Am* Apr 1996;76(2):231-242.
75. Kuerer HM, Sahin AA, Hunt KK, et al. Incidence and impact of documented eradication of breast cancer axillary lymph node metastases before surgery in patients treated with neoadjuvant chemotherapy. *Ann Surg* Jul 1999;230(1):72-78.
76. Miller AR, Thomason VE, Yeh IT, et al. Analysis of sentinel lymph node mapping with immediate pathologic review in patients receiving preoperative chemotherapy for breast carcinoma. *Ann Surg Oncol* Apr 2002;9(3):243-247.
77. Haid A, Tausch C, Lang A, et al. Is sentinel lymph node biopsy reliable and indicated after preoperative chemotherapy in patients with breast carcinoma? *Cancer* Sep 1 2001;92(5):1080-1084.
78. Miguel R, Kuhn AM, Shons AR, et al. The effect of sentinel node selective axillary lymphadenectomy on the incidence of postmastectomy pain syndrome. *Cancer Control* Sep-Oct 2001;8(5):427-430.
79. Cox CE, Yeatman T, Salud CJ, Bass SS. Significance of sentinel node micrometastasis. *Cancer Control* Nov 1999;6(6):601-605.
80. Yeatman TJ, Cox CE. The significance of breast cancer lymph node micrometastases. *Surg Oncol Clin N Am* Jul 1999;8(3):481-496, ix.

Chapter 5

SENTINEL LYMPH NODE MAPPING IN COLON AND RECTAL CANCER:
ITS IMPACT ON STAGING, LIMITATIONS, AND PITFALLS

Sukamal Saha[1], Adrian G. Dan[1], Carsten T. Viehl[2], Markus Zuber[3], David Wiese[1]
[1]Michigan State University, Flint, Michigan, [2]University of Basel, Switzerland,
[3]Kantonsspital Olten, Olten, Switzerland

Abstract: Sentinel lymph node (SLN) mapping has been widely applied in the staging of solid neoplasms including colon and rectal cancer. Since the first reported feasibility study in 1997, there have been numerous publications validating SLN mapping as a highly accurate and powerful upstaging technique for colon and rectal cancer. In addition to refining the technical aspects of this procedure, these studies have investigated the use of other tracers and operative techniques, while determining the indications, limitations, and pitfalls of SLN mapping in patients with colorectal cancers. This chapter reviews the rationale for performing SLN mapping for the accurate staging of colon and rectal cancers, and provides a brief review of the historical background of the development of the procedure. Landmark publications, which have contributed to the current status of the technique, are discussed. We will focus on the technical details of the procedure, and on the pathological evaluation of the specimen and the SLNs. The various tracers and techniques of SLN mapping in colon and rectal cancer will be discussed. We have performed SLN mapping in more than 240 consecutive patients over the past 7 years. The success rates for identifying at least one SLN for colon and rectal cancer were 100% and 90.6%, respectively. The accuracy rates were 95.8% and 100%, respectively. In terms of upstaging, 32.3% of colon cancer patients with nodal metastases and 16.7% of rectal patients with nodal metastases were upstaged by the detection of micrometastases found in the SLNs only. Finally, we will also discuss the current role as well as the future research directions for SLN mapping in colon and rectal cancer.

INTRODUCTION

Colorectal cancer remains one of the major causes of morbidity and mortality from gastrointestinal malignancies, with the last published account of 783,000 new cases and approximately 437,000 deaths globally in 1990.[31] It is the third most common malignancy in the United States with an estimated 147,500 new cases and is the third leading cause of cancer-related deaths with approximately 57,100 deaths in the year 2003.[17] As with most other solid malignancies, the stage of the tumor at the time of initial diagnosis remains the most important prognostic factor for predicting survival in colorectal cancer. Although surgery alone is considered curative in patients in whom the disease is confined within the bowel wall (AJCC stages I and II), the survival decreases dramatically by about 25–35% once the disease has spread beyond the bowel wall and into the draining lymph nodes (AJCC stage III). The addition of adjuvant chemotherapy following surgical resection has been shown to be curative in more than one third of patients with nodal metastasis.[6,45] Therefore, the diagnostic accuracy of nodal metastasis remains essential and critical for the proper prediction of survival as well as for appropriate therapeutic planning. About 10–25% of patients with presumed localized disease (AJCC stage I and II) will develop progression of their disease and will ultimately succumb to distant metastases within 5 years of having potentially "curative surgery." Although the causes of such systemic failure may be multifactorial, it is reasonable to assume that many of these patients indeed had occult nodal micrometastases, which remained undetected by conventional pathological examination of the lymph nodes. This subset of patients is the basis of our estimation of the 10–20% rate of understaging found in colorectal cancer patients when conventional surgery without SLN mapping and conventional pathological methods are employed. Various pathological methods have been developed to enhance the detection rates of such nodal micrometastases. These include serial sectioning,[32,41] immunohistochemistry (IHC) using cytokeratin,[15,16] and most recently, reverse transcriptase polymerase chain reaction (RT-PCR).[28,34] These technical advances have indeed increased the rate of detection of nodal metastases in colorectal cancer but with an enormous burden to the pathologist in terms of time, cost, and labor intensity. It is therefore impractical to apply such advanced techniques arbitrarily to just any or all lymph nodes within a specimen.

The identification of an adequate number of lymph nodes within a specimen by the pathologist also remains a major obstacle in the accurate staging of colon and rectal cancer. This problem is augmented by the fact that most histologically positive lymph nodes are less than 5 mm in size and are therefore difficult to identify.[16,33] While pathological methods such as fat clearance techniques[39] and pinning and stretching techniques[8] have been developed to increase the yield of lymph nodes per specimen, they also remain highly time and labor intensive. The SLN mapping technique therefore provides an ideal avenue for improved staging accuracy in patients with colorectal cancer.

While Gould and colleagues coined the term "sentinel node" in 1960,[14] the physiologic concept of SLN mapping was originally proposed and described by Cabanas in 1977 for the treatment of penile cancer.[5] In 1992, the work of Morton and colleagues[29] redefined and improved the technique of SLN mapping in patients with malignant melanoma. Since the 1990s, this technique has been used for the accurate staging of nodal metastasis in a multitude of solid tumors including breast cancer,[12,22] colon and rectal cancers,[35] gynecological malignancies,[2] thyroid cancer,[19] prostate cancer,[43] lung cancer,[26] gastric and esophageal cancers,[21] pancreatic and small bowel cancers,[40] and anal canal cancer.[20] By the late 1990s, studies of the efficacy of SLN mapping for breast cancer, melanoma, and colorectal cancer had firmly established the reliability and high accuracy rates with which the technique can be performed. Multiple studies[12,29,36] have shown the status of the SLN(s) to reflect the histological status of the particular lymph node basin with more than a 90% accuracy. In melanoma and breast cancer, this accurate staging may help avoid the unnecessary morbidity associated with the dissection of the regional lymph nodes in patients with negative SLNs. The occurrence of aberrant drainage in colorectal tumors, for which the operation should be changed to extend the margins of resection, has been shown to be a very relevant yet infrequent finding.[3] In colon and rectal cancer, however, SLN mapping has emerged as a proven and powerful upstaging technique as has been shown in numerous studies.[1,4,11,30,37] Studies were also conducted to evaluate the usefulness of various tracers such as fluorescein or technetium sulfur colloid (TSC) as enhancers or alternates, and to explore new techniques such as laparoscopic, ex vivo, and minimally invasive approaches to SLN mapping for colon and rectal tumors.

The SLN is defined as the first through fourth node(s) to receive direct drainage from the primary tumor site and which have the highest potential of harboring metastatic disease. Therefore, if the SLNs can be identified during colorectal cancer surgery, these nodes can be meticulously examined by the pathologists with detailed analysis by multilevel microsections, IHC, or RT-PCR methods. This may lead to the detection of occult nodal micrometastatic disease, which may have otherwise remained undetected by conventional pathological examination of a single section of the lymph node. In turn, this may upstage a significant number of patients with early colon and rectal cancer to whom potentially curative systemic chemotherapy can then be offered, leading to improved survival.

Over the past 7 years, our group has undertaken a prospective study regarding the use of the SLN mapping technique for staging of colon and rectal cancer. The objectives of our research are as follows:

- To determine the feasibility of the SLN mapping technique in colon and rectal cancer by utilizing isosulfan blue dye as the gold standard tracer (Lymphazurin; U.S. Surgical Corp.,Norwalk, CT).

- To assess the accuracy of the technique for determining the correct status of the regional lymph node basin.

- To identify any aberrant mesenteric lymphatic drainage patterns requiring any extension of the planned resection margins.

- To determine the indications/contraindications, limitations, and pitfalls of the technique.

- To evaluate the efficacy of other tracers that may be used as enhancers such as TSC or alternates such as fluorescein 10% (Fluorescein; Alcon Laboratories Inc., Fort Worth, TX) to the blue dye.

SENTINEL LYMPH NODE MAPPING FOR COLON CANCER—HOW WE DO IT

From October 1996 through August 2003, 189 consecutive patients with the diagnosis of colon cancer were prospectively entered under an Institutional Review Committee approved protocol after informed consent was obtained. Preoperative evaluation for all patients included a complete history and physical examination, routine laboratory studies including liver function studies and carcinoembryonic antigen (CEA), colonoscopy, and computed tomography of the abdomen and pelvis. Prior to surgery all patients were given standard bowel preparation along with prophylactic oral and intravenous antibiotics.

At the time of laparotomy, the location of the tumor is identified either by manual palpation or visually by recognizing the endoscopic tattooing in patients who underwent polypectomy during colonoscopy. Initially, the extent of the primary tumor and the presence of any distant metastases are evaluated. The tumor-bearing portion of the colon is mobilized by dividing the lateral peritoneal attachments and any adhesions present. Utmost precautions are taken to avoid cutting through the peritoneum covering the mesentery in order to avoid any disruption of the mesenteric lymphatic pathways that lead to the lymph nodes.

Injection of Lymphazurin

Once the tumor-bearing area of the colon is isolated, 1–2 ml of Lymphazurin 1% is injected using a tuberculin syringe and a 30-gauge needle (Figure 1). The dye is injected subserosally in a circumferential manner around the primary tumor. Great care is taken to avoid any spillage of the dye onto the surface of the mesentery or any injection into the bowel lumen. Intraluminal injection of the dye can lead to its absorption away from the primary tumor and may highlight lymph nodes that are not the "true" SLNs. This may lead to higher "skip metastases" rates and lower accuracy rates, as was seen in the study by Joosten et al.[18]

Identification of the Sentinel Lymph Nodes

Usually within 5–10 minutes after the injection, the blue dye travels via the lymphatics to the nearby mesenteric lymph nodes, which turn pale to deep blue. The first to fourth blue-staining lymph nodes, with the most direct drainage from the primary tumor, are marked with suture as "SLN(s)" (Figure 2). The SLNs are most often seen on the retroperitoneal surface and marked accordingly for future identification by the pathologist. It should be noted that the blue dye often travels very quickly through the lymphatics and lymph nodes, and the "true" SLNs may lose their blue color after a short time. Hence, by the time the specimen reaches the hands of the pathologist, the dye may be found in lymph nodes farther down the lymphatic chain, while the "true" SLN may not be blue at all. This underscores the importance of the initial tagging of the SLNs with suture at the time of their identification intraoperatively. In the event that *in vivo* identification of one or more SLNs is not accomplished during the operation, an additional 1–2 ml of Lymphazurin 1% can be injected *ex vivo*. This might allow the pathologist to identify an SLN during the pathologic dissection of the mesentery. Once the SLNs are identified, a standard oncologic resection is performed to include adequate proximal and distal margins, along with the regional lymph nodes in the attached mesentery. Occasionally a blue node is identified outside of the usual lymphatic bearing area and should be considered an SLN and included within the margins of the resection. In patients with unusually thick or fatty mesentery, limited surgical dissection of the mesenteric fat may be required to identify the blue-stained lymph nodes.

SENTINEL LYMPH NODE MAPPING FOR RECTAL CANCER — HOW WE DO IT

For patients with tumors at the rectosigmoid junction and of the rectum above the peritoneal reflection, the dye is injected in a similar manner as for colon cancer. For low to mid rectal tumors, located below the retroperitoneal reflection, the blue dye is injected with a 25-gauge spinal needle from below through a proctoscope, into the submucosal and muscular layers underneath the tumor. If any blue nodes are seen during the initial mobilization of the rectum, they are immediately marked with suture as SLNs. In many patients, especially those with low rectal tumors, no blue nodes outside of the mesorectum are found during total mesorectal excision (TME). In these cases, an oncologic resection was done first by TME, followed by the *ex vivo* submucosal injection of an additional 1-2 ml of the blue dye. Any blue nodes near the tumor within the mesorectum found *ex vivo* either by the surgeon or by the pathologist may be regarded as an SLN.

OTHER TRACERS

Lymphazurin 1% has been the most frequently utilized dye for lymphatic mapping in colon and rectal cancer. With the advent of SLN mapping in colorectal and other cancers, the widespread use of the dye has led to reports of rare anaphylactic reactions,[23,25,27] as well as interference with pulse oxymetry monitoring.[7,24] In some countries, Lymphazurin is not easily available and its use may be cost prohibitive. We have therefore attempted to validate the use of fluorescein 10% as an alternative dye for SLN mapping.[9] Fluorescein 10% is commonly available throughout the world, comparatively inexpensive, and not associated with any known allergic reactions. We have used fluorescein 10% in the last 120 patients with results comparable to Lymphazurin. Fluorescein dye can be injected in a similar manner to Lymphazurin, using a tuberculin syringe and 1-2 ml of the dye. The dye travels quickly via the lymphatics and turns the SLNs fluorescent. These can be visually identified in a dark room under Wood's light illumination as bright yellow nodes (Figure 3). No allergic reaction has been observed during the use of either Lymphazurin or fluorescein dye in our series.

As has been shown in SLN mapping for melanoma[10] and breast cancer,[22] TSC can also be used for lymphatic mapping in colorectal cancer. We have used 0.5–1 mCi of TSC in 57 patients using a guarded syringe for injection in a similar manner to Lymphazurin and fluorescein.[38] SLN designation using TSC was based on increased radioactivity in "hot nodes" detected with the use of a gamma probe. Kitagawa et al. in Japan have also used technetium tin colloid for successful lymphatic mapping in colon cancer.[21] We have found that TSC is a useful adjunct to Lymphazurin. Although the identification of many "hot" nodes is facilitated by their blue coloration when Lymphazurin is also used, TSC radioactive nodes have a comparable accuracy in correctly predicting the status of the nodal basin. As a matter of fact, those SLNs that are both "blue" and "hot" are about twice as likely to yield histologic positivity, and may represent SLNs that should receive particularly special attention from the pathologist.

EX VIVO MAPPING

An alternative approach to *in vivo* SLN mapping has been described by Wong et al.[46] After a standard oncologic resection, the specimen is dissected by the pathologist along the antimesenteric border, regardless of whether the tumor is along that line. Lymphazurin 1% is injected at four quadrants submucosally, with 0.25 ml of dye injected at each location. The specimen is then gently massaged for 5 minutes. All identified blue nodes are then designated as SLNs. Wong and colleagues reported a 92.3% (24/26) success rate of identifying at least one SLN, with an average of 3.0 SLNs per patient. Advanced pathological methods were employed only in those patients in whom nodal metastases were not detected by standard pathological methods. Of 14 such patients, 29% (4/14) were upstaged by the identification of nodal micrometastases. Of these, 14% (2/14) were only identified by IHC means.

LAPAROSCOPIC EXPERIENCE

Lymphatic mapping has also been described in colon tumors by some authors using laparoscopic techniques.[47] The dye may be injected into the submucosa by endoscopy or into the subserosal layer under laparoscopic visualization. Kitagawa et al.[21] have described the technique for successfully locating the SLNs using a laparoscopic gamma probe while others have used Lymphazurin 1%. Wood and colleagues[47] reported a success rate of 100% as well as an accuracy rate of 100% in a series of nine patients who underwent laparoscopic SLN mapping with an average of two SLNs identified per patient. As laparoscopic colectomy for early colon cancer becomes more common, these techniques will become increasingly more important, especially in cases where the root of the mesentery is difficult to resect laparoscopically (i.e., morbid obesity).

PATHOLOGICAL EXAMINATION

The surgical specimens were sent to the pathology department in fresh state. The SLNs were dissected free from the specimen, sectioned grossly at 2- to 3-mm intervals and blocked separately in individual cassettes. The remainder of the specimen was formalin-fixed and dissected according to standard pathologic protocols for evaluation of the tumor and margins, and for harvesting of the non-SLNs. For some cases, postfixation of the pericolic adipose tissues for 2 to 18 hours in Carnoy's fluid aided in the identification and retrieval of non-SLNs, which appeared white against the pale yellow background of fat.[44] For each SLN, five sections were prepared at 20- to 40-micron intervals; the first four were stained routinely with hematoxylin and eosin (H&E), while the last section was labeled for cytokeratins by IHC (AE-1/AE-3 cocktail; Ventana Medical Systems, Tucson, AZ) (Figure 4). Other sections of the tumor and non-SLNs were routinely stained with H&E. For some studies, frozen sections of representative SLNs, non-SLNs, and tumor were obtained for RT-PCR analysis.

From the pathologist's perspective, the principal goal of evaluating colorectal cancer resection specimens is to provide accurate and relevant data regarding the staging and prognosis of disease. To this end, it is incumbent on the pathologist to precisely sample and assess sections of the tumor, appropriate margins, and regional lymph nodes. Meaningful assessment of the nodes in turn requires that a sufficient number be harvested. Indeed, for standard pathological examination, the proportion of nodes involved by tumor in patients with regional metastases depends purely on the number of nodes harvested; in fact, the predictive probability of detecting disease continues to rise with the number of nodes obtained.[13] There is no absolute minimum number of nodes that will guarantee identification of all nodal metastases. Furthermore, even very small nodes are capable of harboring metastatic tumor. Because of this, pathologists have become more aware of the need to harvest as many nodes as reasonably possible, a time-consuming effort. Methods have been developed to help increase node yields, such as stretching and pinning out the mesentery for fixation, or using clearing agents to render the nodes visible within the mesenteric fat. All of these methods require added time and effort.

Use of the SLN mapping technique in colorectal cancer, however, is quick and to the point. It has been shown to improve the accuracy of staging by directing the pathologist's attention to the one to four nodes most likely to harbor metastasis. Focused attention on these specific nodes, together with routine lymph node dissection, improves the detection of metastatic disease, thus improving staging accuracy. Because some of these nodes represent micrometastasis, detected on occasion only by IHC, the focus must now turn toward the issue of relevance. That is, does this upstaging truly affect patient outcome with or without neoadjuvant therapy? To this point, early studies have shown mixed results. But without the foundation of accurate pathologic assessment, i.e., demonstration of detectable tumor within the nodes, such studies will necessarily suffer the bias of potential pathologic understaging.

TECHNICAL CHALLENGES

The true benefit of SLN mapping in colorectal cancer lies in its ability to identify the SLNs with micrometastatic disease, which would remain undetected if the nodes were examined by conventional techniques. Hence, such nodal micrometastases are more likely to be detected in early T1, T2, or T3 tumors, rather than in more bulky T4 lesions or tumors invading adjacent structures. In such large tumors, however, the amount of dye injected circumferentially would be higher than the usual 2ml. A Swiss group,[42] as described below, first tested the amount of dye needed in relation to the size of the tumor.

Swiss Trial

Two factors were tested in this trial for lymphatic mapping in colorectal cancer: the amount of the injected dye in relation to the diameter of the primary tumor and the relationship of SLN status with bone marrow micrometastases. In this trial,[42] at least 0.5 ml of the blue dye per centimeter of tumor diameter was found to be highly successful in identifying at least one SLN. Hence, some of the higher failure rates seen in some published series may indeed be due to the inadequate amount of dye for the relative size of the tumor. We agree with the authors that at least 0.5 ml of the dye for each centimeter of tumor diameter is reasonable for lymphatic mapping, especially for larger tumors. The addition of radio-colloid did not increase the success rate of SLN mapping in identifying the true SLNs.

Although bone marrow micrometastases have been found to be of prognostic significance in breast cancer, such a correlation was lacking for colorectal cancer. In this trial, a higher incidence of positive bone marrow micrometastases was detected in patients with positive SLNs than in patients with negative SLNs (50% vs. 27%), although no statistical significance could be reached.

CLINICAL OUTCOME FOR COLON CANCER

Of the 242 consecutive patients in this study, 189 patients had colon cancer. The number and locations of the primary tumors were as follows: appendix 1; cecum 40; right colon 66; hepatic flexure 6; transverse colon 23; left colon 7; and sigmoid colon 46. Ages ranged from 40 to 97 years (median 73 years). The SLN mapping technique successfully identified 1–4 SLNs in 189 out of 189 patients (100%). A total of 2703 lymph nodes were examined (mean 14.3 per patient), of which 440 (16.3%) lymph nodes were identified as SLNs. Of these, one SLN was identified in 26% of patients, two SLNs in 32%, three SLNs in 29%, and four SLNs in 13% of patients. In 124 (65.6%) patients the SLNs were negative for metastasis. Of these 124 patients, in 116 (93.5%) patients the SLNs as well as all the non-SLNs were negative for metastasis. In the other 8 (6.5%) patients, the SLNs were negative but 11 of the non SLNs were positive for metastasis (skip metastasis). In 65 patients, the SLNs were positive for metastasis. In 30 (46.2%) of the 65 patients, the SLNs were the only site of metastasis with all other non-SLNs being negative. In 21 (32.3)% of the 65 patients with histologically positive SLNs, micrometastasis was identified only in 1–2 of 10 microsections of a single SLN. Of these 21, 8 (12.3% of the 65 patients with histologically positive SLNs) were confirmed by IHC only; thus representing truly occult micrometastasis. The extent of surgery was altered by evidence of an aberrant lymphatic drainage detected by the SLN mapping technique in four colon cancer patients. Overall, the sensitivity of SLN mapping for colon cancer in our series was 89.0%, the specificity was 100%, and the negative predictive value was 93.5%. The accuracy of correctly predicting the status of the nodal basin was 95.6%. Solitary micrometastasis in the SLNs, as was found in 32.3% of the 65 patients with histologically positive SLNs, may have upstaged these patients from AJCC stage I/II to stage III, allowing them to possibly benefit from adjuvant chemotherapy.

Of the 242 consecutive patients, 53 had rectal lesions. Of these, 37 were in the rectum and 16 were in the rectosigmoid. Ages for this group ranged from 32 to 85 years (median 71 years). The SLN mapping technique successfully identified 1–4 SLNs in 48 out of 53 patients (90.6%). In 5 patients, the SLN mapping technique failed to identify any blue node (all 5 patients were treated with neoadjuvant chemoradiation therapy). The following analysis is based on the remaining 48 patients with rectal cancer in whom at least one SLN was identified. A total of 685 lymph nodes were examined (mean 12.9 per patient), of which 91 (13.3%) were designated as SLNs. Of these, one SLN was identified in 48% of patients, two SLNs in 27%, three SLNs in 21%, and four SLNs in 4% of patients. In 36 (75%) patients the SLNs were negative for metastasis. In all of these 36 patients

(100%), the SLNs as well as all the non-SLNs were negative for metastasis. There were no cases of skip metastases for rectal cancer. In 12 (25%) patients, the SLNs were positive for metastasis. In 4 of these 12 patients, the SLNs were the exclusive site of metastasis with all other non-SLNs being negative. In 2 (16.7% of the 12 patients with nodal metastases) of these patients, micrometastasis was identified only in 1–2 of 10 microsections of a single SLN. In one patient (8.3% of the 12 patients with nodal metastases), micrometastasis was identified by IHC only; thus representing truly occult micrometastasis. The extent of surgery was altered by evidence of an aberrant lymphatic pathway detected by the SLN mapping technique in three patients. Overall, the sensitivity, specificity, negative predictive value, and accuracy of SLN mapping for rectal cancer in our series were all 100%. Solitary micrometastasis in the SLNs, as was found in 16.7% of the 12 patients with nodal metastases, may have upstaged these patients from AJCC stage I/II to stage III, allowing them to benefit from adjuvant chemotherapy.

The incidence of metastasis in SLNs vs. non-SLNs was 22.5% vs. 6.7% for colon cancer and 18.7% vs. 8.4% for rectal cancer. In the presence of negative SLNs, metastases were found in 11 out of 1724 (0.6%) of non-SLNs only (skip metastasis) for colon cancer and 0 out of 401 (0%) of non-SLNs for rectal cancer. To evaluate the effect of multilevel micro sectioning of the SLNs only as opposed to the non SLNs, for the first 25 consecutive patients all SLNs as well as the non-SLNs were sectioned at 10 levels in identical manner. Of the 390 lymph nodes examined (average 15.6 per patient), 13 (36%) of the 36 SLNs were positive for metastasis, while only 24 (7%) of the 354 non-SLNs had metastasis. When all the initially negative non-SLNs were sectioned at 10 levels and reexamined, only 0.6% (2 of 330 lymph nodes) revealed previously undetected micrometastasis. These results further confirm the unique distribution of metastasis via the lymphatics to the SLNs with minimal chance of skip metastasis. Thus, there may be no further benefit in performing multilevel sections of the non-SLNs as opposed to the SLNs.

OVERVIEW

Clinical oncologists have long known the decrease in overall survival associated with nodal metastases of most solid tumors. Adjuvant chemotherapy is considered standard of care for patients with nodal metastases in colorectal cancer and has been shown to reduce cancer-related mortality by about one-third.[6,45] The ability to cure a significant number of patients with metastatic disease underscores the importance of identifying those patients who would benefit from chemotherapy. Technological and pathological advances over the past decade have made it possible to upstage patients from AJCC stages I and II to AJCC stage III by identifying nodal micrometastases using various techniques i.e., serial sectioning, IHC, and RT-PCR. The SLN mapping technique allows the pathologists to focus their attention on the few nodes with the highest probability of harboring metastatic disease. The arbitrary use of these advanced and costly methods for all the resected nodes within a specimen would be highly inefficient and cost prohibitive. Our series along with a review of the literature has shown that the SLN mapping technique can be performed with a success rate and accuracy rate of more than 90% in patients with early stage colorectal cancer.

The failure of the technique to identify an SLN is often a result of pre-operative chemoradiation therapy for mid- to low-rectal cancers and may be due to fibrosis of the submucosal lymphatics. In the face of intense peritoneal inflammation, as may be encountered with fecal contamination in perforated carcinoma, the dye may not be able to penetrate the large inflamed lymph nodes. In instances where the primary tumor is large and invades adjacent structures (i.e., T4), the lymphatic pathway may be altered. This may lead to failure to identify an SLN or to skip metastasis. Often in such advanced cases some lymph nodes may become completely replaced by tumor, hence the dye may not penetrate those nodes (Figure 5). However, the blue lymphatics may lead the surgeon to those nodes and they should still be marked as SLNs. If the clinically positive nodes are detectable at laparotomy, then the mapping is not of any benefit, as metastatic nodal disease is already evident. The relative limitations and contraindications of the procedures are listed in Table 1.

Table 1. Limitations and contraindications of SLN mapping

Limitations	Contraindications
• Previous colon surgery	• Distant metastasis
• Neoadjuvant chemo/radiation therapy	• Clinically positive lymph nodes
• Large tumor invading adjacent organs	
• Perforate carcinoma	
• Multiple primary tumors	

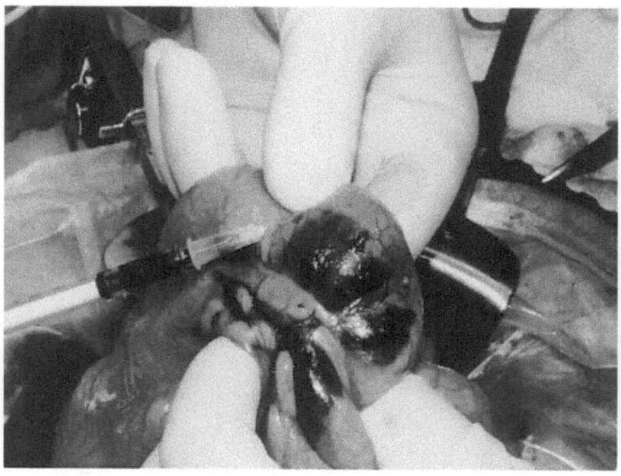

1.

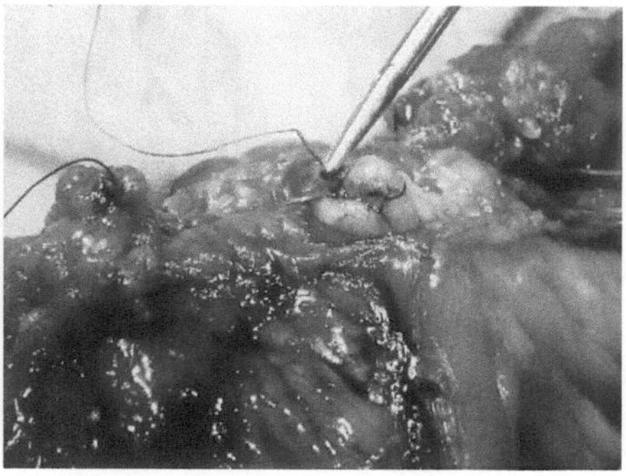

2.

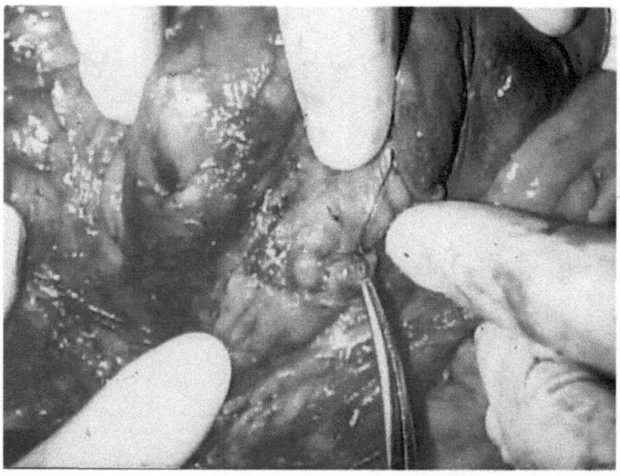

3.

Figure 1. Lymphazurin 1% is being injected subserosally around a tumor in the sigmoid colon of a 70-year-old female.

Figure 2. The sentinel lymph node is marked with suture as it appears soon after the dye injection.

Figure 3. Fluorescein 10% is also being injected subserosally showing greenish-yellow stained sentinel lymph node near the primary tumor.

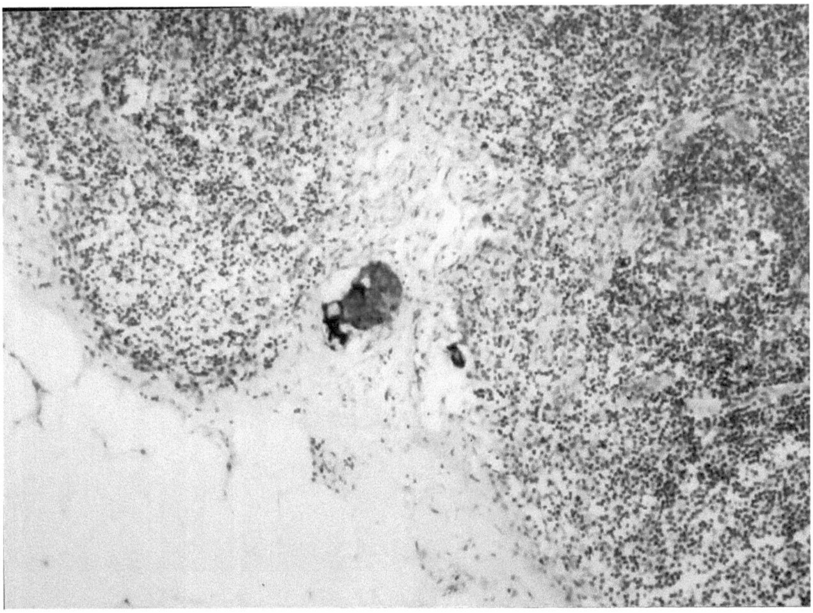

4.

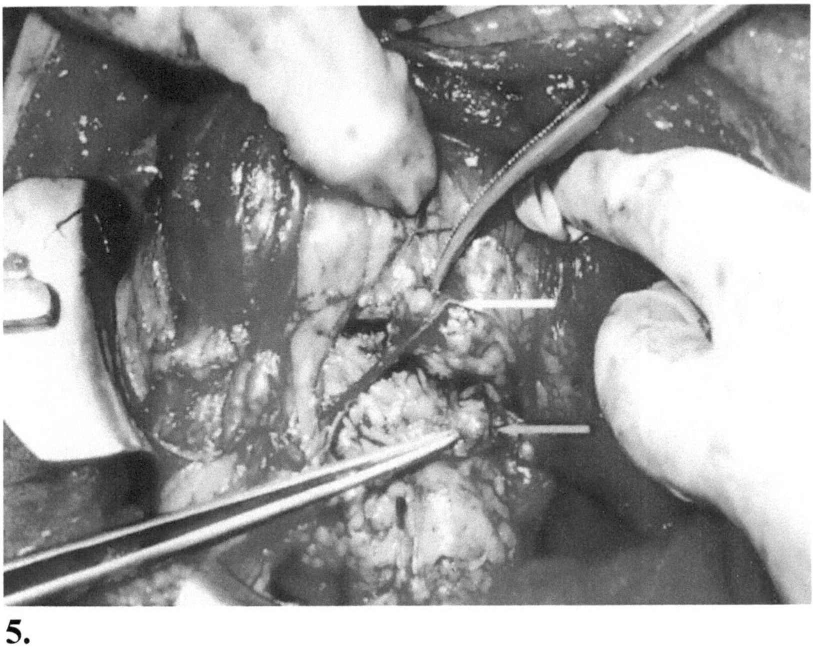

5.

Figure 4. Occult micrometastasis seen in small 9-mm sentinel lymph node detected only by immunohistochemistry.

Figure 5. In some advanced cases lymph nodes may become completely replaced by tumor and the dye may not penetrate the nodes.

As previously stated, the SLN mapping technique can be performed with feasibility rates and accuracy rates for predicting the status of the nodal basin of well over 90%. Unlike in melanoma and breast cancer, the primary purpose of SLN mapping in colorectal cancer is not to change the extent of the operation, but to upstage patients. As the technical aspects of the mapping are relatively simple, the overall learning curve of the SLN mapping technique in colorectal cancer is shorter. Adhering to the details of the intraoperative technique and the pathological evaluation are critical to lowering the incidence of skip metastasis. The fine-tuning of the technique over the past few years has included studies with alternative tracers and studies to determine the appropriate amounts of dye in relation to the size of the mass. The use of fluorescein over the past few years has further validated the utility of this tracer with results comparable to those of Lymphazurin, at a substantially lower cost ($99 per vial of Lymhazurin vs. ~$2 per vial of fluorescein) and without the associated risks of allergic reactions or interference with patient oxygen saturation monitoring. TSC has also been successfully used for SLN mapping and has been found to be a helpful adjunct to Lymphazurin. Those nodes that are identified by both Lymphazurin and TSC have been shown to have a much higher yield for metastatic disease and deserve the special attention of the pathologist.[38] However, due to the simplicity of its use without the need of additional equipment and its widespread availability in the United States, lymphazurin remains the gold standard for SLN mapping in colorectal cancer.

Plans are under way for a large, multi-institutional study by the American College of Surgeons Oncology Group (ACOSOG – Z0170) to evaluate and to verify the efficacy of this technique and to assess its impact on the survival of patients with colorectal cancer. If verified in such trials, the application of the SLN mapping technique in colorectal cancer may become part of the standard practice of general surgeons given its simplicity, high accuracy, low cost, and especially its ability to aid the pathologists to focus their attention on 1-4 SLNs for detailed analysis. Upstaged patients can be offered neo-adjuvant chemotherapy, which may increase their survival.

REFERENCES

1. Bendavid Y, Latulippe J, Younan R, et al. Phase I study on sentinel lymph node mapping in colon cancer: A preliminary report. J Surg Oncol 2002;79:81-84.
2. Bilchik A, Giuliano A, Essner R, et al. Universal application of intraoperative lymphatic mapping and sentinel lymphadenectomy in solid neoplasms. Cancer J 1998;4(6): 351-358.

3. Bilchik A, Saha S, Tsioulias G, et al. Aberrant drainage of missed micrometastases: The value of lymphatic mapping and focused analysis of sentinel lymph nodes in gastrointestinal neoplasms. Ann Surg Oncol 2001;8(9S):82-85.
4. Bilchik A, Nora D, Tollenaar R, et al. Ultrastaging of early colon cancer using lymphatic mapping and molecular analysis. Euro J Cancer 2002;38(7):977-985.
5. Cabanas RM. An approach for treatment of pe1nile carcinoma. Cancer 1977;39(2):456-6.
6. Cohen AM, Kelsen D, Saltz L, et al. Adjuvant therapy for colorectal cancer. Curr Probl Cancer 1998;22:5-65.
7. Coleman RL, Whitten CW, O'Boyle J, Sidhu B. Unexplained decrease in measured oxygen saturation by pulse oxymetry following injection of lymphazurin 1% (isosulfan blue) during a lymphatic mapping procedure. J Surgi Oncol 1999; 70(2):126-129.
8. Crucitti F, Doglietto GB, Bellantone R, et al. Accurate specimen preparation and examination is mandatory to detect lymph nodes and avoid understaging in colorectal cancer. J Surg Oncol 1992; 51:153-158.
9. Dan A, Saha S, Wiese D, et al. Comparative analysis of Lymphazurin 1% vs. fluorescein 10% in sentinel lymph node (SLN) mapping for colorectal (CR) tumors. Archi Surg 2004 (in press)
10. Essner R, Bostick P, Glass E, Foshag L, Haigh P, Wang H, Morton D. Standardized probe-directed sentinel node dissection in melanoma. Surgery 2000; 127: 26-31.
11. Fitzgerald T, Khalifa M, Zahrani M, et al. Ex vivo sentinel lymph node biopsy in colorectal cancer: A feasibility study. J Surg Oncol 2002;80:27-32.
12. Giuliano AE, Kirgan DM, Guenther JM, Morton DL. Lymphatic mapping and sentinel lymphadenectomy for breast cancer. Ann Surg 1994;220(3):391-401.
13. Goldstein NS. Lymph node recoveries from 2427 pT3 colorectal resection specimens spanning 45 years: recommendations for a minimum number of recovered lymph nodes based on predictive probabilities. Am J Surg Pathol 2002;26(2):179–89.
14. Gould EA, Winship T, Philbin PH, Hyland, et al. Observations on a "sentinel node" in cancer of the parotid. Cancer 1960;13:77-8.
15. Greenson JK, Isenhart CE, Rice R, et al. Identification of occult micrometastases in pericolic lymph nodes of Dukes' B colorectal cancer patients using monoclonal antibodies against cytokeratin and CC49; correlation with long-term survival. Cancer 1994;73(3):563-569.
16. Haboubi NY, Abdalla SA, Amini S, et al. The novel combination of fat clearance and immunohistochemistry improvise prediction of the outcome of patients with colorectal carcinomas: A preliminary study. Int J Colorectal Dis 1998;13(2):99-102.
17. Jemal A, Murray T, Samuels A, et al. Cancer statistic, 2003. CA – A Cancer Journal for Clinicians 2003; 53(1): 5-26, 2003.
18. Joosten J, Strobbe L, Wauters C, et al. Intraoperative lymphatic mapping and the sentinel node concept in colorectal carcinoma. Br J Surg 1999;86:482-486.
19. Keleman PR, van Herle AJ, Giuliano AE. Sentinel lymphadenectomy in thyroid malignant neoplasms. Arch Surg 1998;133(3):288-292.
20. Keshtgar MR, Amin A, Taylor I, et al. The sentinel node in anal carcinoma. Eur J Surg Oncol 2001;27(1):113-4.
21. Kitagawa Y, Fugii H, Mukai M, et al. The role of the sentinel lymph node in gastrointestinal cancer. Surg Clin North Am 2000;80(6):1799-1809.

22. Krag DN, Weaver DL, Alex JC, et al. Surgical resection and radiolocalization of the sentinel node in breast cancer using a gamma probe. Surg Oncol 1993; 2(6):335-39.
23. Kuerer HM, Wayne JD, Ross MI. Anaphylaxis during breast cancer lymphatic mapping. Surgery 2001; 129(1): 119-120.
24. Larsen VH, Freudendal A, Fogh-Andersen N. The influence of patent blue V on pulse oxymetry and haemoximetry. Acta Anaesthesiol Scand Suppl 1995; 107: 53-55.
25. Leong SP, Donegan E, Hefferson W, Dean S, Katz JA. Adverse reactions to isosulfan blue during selective sentinel lymph node dissection in melanoma. Ann Surgl Oncol 2000; 7(5): 361-366.
26. Little AG, DeHoyos, Kirgan DM, et al. Intraoperative lymphatic mapping for non-small cell lung cancer: The sentinel node technique. J Thorac Cardiovasc Surg 1999;117(2):220-34.
27. Longnecker SM, Guzzardo MM, Van Voris LP. Life-threatening anaphylaxis following subcutaneous administration of isosulfan blue 1%. Clin Pharmacol 1985; 4(2): 219-221.
28. Mori M, Mimori K, Inoue H, et al. Detection of cancer micrometastases in lymph nodes by reverse transcriptase polymerase chain reaction. Cancer Res 1995;55(25):3417-20.
29. Morton DL, Wen DR, Wong HH, et al. Technical details of intraoperative lymphatic mapping for early stage melanoma. Archi Surg 1992;127(4):392-399.
30. Paramo J, Summerall J, Poppiti R, et al. Validation of sentinel node mapping in patients with colon cancer. Ann Surg Oncol 2002;9(6):550-554.
31. Parkin DM, Pisani P, Ferlay J. Global cancer statistics. CA: A Cancer Journal for Clinicians 1999;49(1)33-64.
32. Pickreen JW. Significance of occult metastases, a study of breast cancer. Cancer 1961;14:1261-1271.
33. Rodriguez-Bigas MA, Maamoun S, Weber TK, et al. Clinical significance of colorectal cancer: metastases in lymph nodes <5 mm in size. Ann Surg Oncol 1996:3:124-130.
34. Rosenberg R, Hoos A, Mueller J, et al. Prognostic significance of cytokeratin-20 RT-PCR reaction in lymph nodes of node-negative colorectal cancer patients. J Clin Oncol 2002:;0(4):1049-1055.
35. Saha S, Ganatra BK, Gauthier J, et al. Localization of sentinel lymph node in colon cancer. A feasibility study. Society of Surgical Oncology 50th Annual Cancer Symposium. 1997, Chicago, IL. Abstract P-80, page 54.
36. Saha S, Wiese D, Badin J, et al. Technical details of sentinel lymph node mapping in colorectal cancer and its impact on staging. Ann Surg Oncol 2000;7(2):120-124.
37. Saha S, Bilchik A, Wiese D, et al. Ultrastaging of colorectal cancer by sentinel lymph node mapping technique – A multicenter trial. Ann Surg Oncol 2001;8(9S):94-98.
38. Saha S, Dan A, Berman B, et al. Lymphazurin 1% vs. TSC for lymphatic mapping in colorectal tumors – A comparative analysis. Ann Surg Oncol 2004; 11(1): in press.
39. Scott KWM, Grace RH. Detection of lymph node metastases in colorectal carcinoma before and after fat clearance. Br J Surg 1989; 76:1165-1167.
40. Tsioulias GJ, Wood TF, Morton DL, et al. Lymphatic mapping and focused analysis of sentinel lymph nodes upstage gastrointestinal neoplasms. Arch Surg 2000; 135: 926-931.

41. Turner RR, Ollila DW, Stern S, Giuliano AE. Optimal histopathologic examination of the sentinel lymph node for breast carcinoma staging . Am J Surg Pathol 1999;23(3):263-267.
42. Viehl CT, Hamel CT, Marti WR, et al. Identification of sentinel lymph nodes in colon cancer depends on the amount of dye injected relative to tumour size. World J Surg 2003; 27(12): in print.
43. Wawroschek F, Vogt H, Weckermann D, et al. The sentinel lymph node concept in prostate cancer— first results of gamma probe-guided sentinel lymph node identification. Eur Urol 1999;36(6):595-600.
44. Wiese D, Saha S, Badin J. Pathologic evaluation of sentinel lymph nodes in colorectal carcinoma. Arch Pathol Lab Med 2000;124:1759-1763.
45. Wolmark N, Rockette H, Fisher B, et al. The benefit of leucovorin-modulated fluorouracil as postoperative adjuvant therapy for primary colon cancer: Results from National Surgical Adjuvant Breast and Bowel protocol C-03. J Clin Oncol 1993;11(10):1879-1887.
46. Wong JH, Steineman S, Calderia C, et al. Ex vivo sentinel node mapping in carcinoma of the colon and rectum. Ann Surg 2001;233(4):515-521.
47. Wood T, Saha S, Morton D, et al. Validation of lymphatic mapping in colorectal cancer: In vivo, ex vivo, and laparoscopic techniques. Dis Colon Rectum 2001;8(2):150-157.

Chapter 6

SENTINEL LYMPH NODE MAPPING IN ESOPHAGEAL AND GASTRIC CANCER

Yuko Kitagawa, Hirofumi Fujii, Makio Mukai, Atsushi Kubo, Masaki Kitajima
Keio University School of Medicine, Tokyo, Japan

Abstract In recent years, the sentinel lymph node (SLN) concept has been widely investigated in a variety of solid tumors including gastrointestinal (GI) cancer. This chapter reviews the rationale and refined technical aspects for SLN mapping in upper GI cancer for the intraoperative accurate diagnosis of nodal status to perform individualized minimally invasive surgical approaches. We have described the technical details of the procedure as we have performed it in over 350 consecutive patients with esophageal and gastric cancer and introduced pitfalls and issues remaining.

The technical details and clinical applications of SLN mapping differfor patients with esophageal cancer and gastric cancer. Radio-guided method with lymphoscintigraphy using radioisotope-labeled colloid (RI) is essential for SLN mapping for esophageal cancer. Selective lymphadenectomy and SLN-targeted chemoradiotherapy would be feasible and beneficial for the patients with esophageal cancer. For gastric cancer, combined method with dye and RI is recommended for stable and accurate sampling of SLN in the laparoscopic setting. Laparoscopic local resection for superficial gastric cancer with negative SN status would be a reasonable and less-invasive novel procedure based on the SLN concept. We can utilize this procedure not only for an accurate staging but also as a great tool to change the patient care of upper GI cancer by individualized minimally invasive treatments.

INTRODUCTION

The term "orderly progression" can hardly be employed to describe the pattern of spread of upper gastrointestinal (GI) cancer, unlike melanoma and breast cancer. Anatomical skip metastases were found in 50–60% of esophageal cancer and in 20–30% of gastric cancer in a retrospective analysis of the location of solitary metastases.[14,16] Sano et al. reported that the perigastric nodal area close to the primary tumor is the first site of metastasis in only 62% of gastric cancers, based on a retrospective analysis of cases of solitary metastasis.[18] From these clinical observations, extended radical procedures such as esophagectomy with three-field lymph node dissection and gastrectomy with D2 lymphadenectomy have become recognized as standard procedures in Japan even for clinically node negative cases.[1,15] However, a significant increase of morbidity and mortality after these invasive procedures was reported in randomized trials.[4,6] To eliminate the necessity of uniform application of highly invasive surgery, sentinel lymph node (SLN) mapping may play a role in obtaining individual information to allow modification of the surgical procedure and other multidisciplinal approaches.

Several studies supporting the validity of the SN concept in upper GI cancers have been reported in the past few years.[5,8-10,17] The increasing prominence of endoscopic surgery since the early 1990s has changed surgical thinking in the field of GI surgery. Now the application of SN mapping in the management of GI malignancies is a riveting topic in surgical oncology. Here we review the current status and optimized procedures with some of the remaining issues in SLN mapping of esophageal and gastric cancer.

SENTINEL LYMPH NODE MAPPING FOR GASTRIC CANCER

Current status of SLN mapping for gastric cancer

As in other solid tumors, there are two major procedures to detect SLN in gastric cancer: The radio-guided procedure using radioisotope-labeled colloid and the dye-guided method.

We have performed a validation study for radio-guided SLN mapping for gastric cancer. From 1999 through 2003, 270 consecutive patients with the clinical diagnosis of T1 or T2N0 gastric cancer were prospectively entered under an Institutional Review Committee approved protocol of radio-guided SLN mapping for gastric cancer after informed consent was obtained. An updated result in our institute is summarized in Table 1.

Table 1. Updated data of SLN mapping for gastric cancer (Keio University Hospital, Tokyo, Japan, Jan. 1999– Dec. 2003)

Indication	cT1or T2 N0
Detection rate	97% (262 / 270)
SLN number	4.1
Sensitivity	92% (34 / 37)
Accuracy	99% (259 / 262)

SLNs in gastric cancer are usually multiple and show multidirectional distributions. The radio-guided method is a reliable and stable technique for detecting multiple SLNs in gastric cancer using a gamma probe. However, there are practical limitations such as the requirement of radiation safety regulations and special equipment in community hospitals to employ the radio-guided method as a routine clinical procedure.

The dye-directed method is also applicable to gastric cancer particularly in open surgery, in which mobilization of the stomach and real-time observation of lymphatic flow are feasible. Although there are several limitations to the dye-directed method such as fast transit and blind sites in dense fat, blue dye is useful for visualizing lymphatic vessels. There are several options in performing actual procedures, such as types of dye, injection routes (submucosal and subserosal), volume of tracer, and observation timing. In general, technical factors affect the results of SLN mapping for gastric cancer by the dye-guided method.

Technical errors using the single mapping agent approach are reduced by adding a different approach for lymphatic mapping. The radio-guided method allows us to confirm the complete harvest of SLNs with multidirectional and widespread distribution by gamma probing while the dye procedure enables us to perform real-time observation of the visualized lymphatic vessels. Therefore, at this moment, we recommend a combination of dye- and radio-guided methods for systematic SLN mapping of gastric cancer. Almost acceptable results for SLN mapping for gastric cancer have been reported from several institutes as single institutional studies using various methodologies as shown in Table 2.[13]

Table 2. SLN mapping for gastric cancer

Investigators	Published	Tracer[a]	Number of cases	Detection rate (%)	Sensitivity (%)
Kitagawa et al.	2000	RI	36	97	100 (5/5)
Hiratsuka et al.	2001	Dye (ICG)	74	99	90 (9/10)
Kitagawa et al.	2002	RI	121	96	92 (22/24)
Ichikura et al.	2002	Dye (ICG)	62	100	85 (11/13)
Miwa et al.	2003	Dye (PB)	211	96	89 (31/35)

[a]RI,colloid labeled with radioisotope;
PB, patent blue;
ICG; indocyanine green

A multicenter prospective validation study for SLN mapping for gastric cancer has been started in Japan in 2004.

Indication of SLN mapping for gastric cancer

Clinical T1 or T2N0 gastric cancer is a suitable target of this procedure. Because the main purpose of introducing this technology into gastric cancer surgery is to extend the indication of minimally invasive surgery for pathologically node negative cases, there is no advantage to include advanced cases for which modified less-invasive surgical approaches are not applicable. The size of the primary lesion is also an important factor to consider regarding this technique. It is difficult to cover a whole lymphatic drainage route from a larger tumor. We enroll patients with single primary lesions having diameters not exceeding 4 cm.

Choice of radioactive tracer

There are several types of radioactive tracers for SN mapping. Technetium-99m tin colloid and technetium-99m phytate are commonly used in Japan. In initial pilot studies, we have chosen technetium –99m tin colloid, which has a relatively large particle size. In our experience, tin colloid migrates into the SLNs within 2 hours and remains there for more than 20 hours through phagocytosis by macrophages. This characteristic of the tracer particle allows us to perform stable detection of SLN regardless of the timing. Technetium-99m phytate has a smaller particle size and there is a risk of migration into the secondary nodes beyond the actual SLN. At this moment, technetium-99m tin colloid is recommended as an optimal tracer for SLN mapping for gastric cancer.[8]

Administration of radioactive tracer

The day before surgery, technetium-99m tin colloid solution in a volume of 2.0 ml (150 MBq) was injected in four quadrants into the submucosal layer of the primary lesion using an endoscopic puncture needle (Figure 1). Technetium-99m Sn colloid solution was labeled by adding 1.5 ml of tin(II) chloride [Sn(II) Cl2] solution (Nihon Medi-Physics Co., Ltd., Nishinomiya, Japan) to 1.5 ml of -99m technetium pertechnetate solution with 111 MBq of radioactivity. Submucosal injection of the tracer is easy to perform by the endoscopic approach and accurate injection of an adequate amount of tracer is crucial for the precise SLN mapping for gastric cancer.

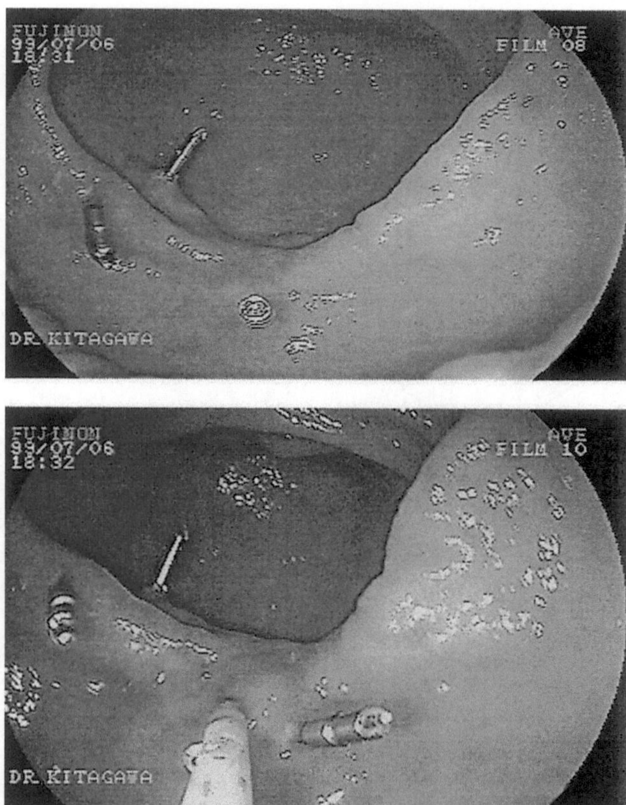

Figure 1. Endoscopic injection of radioactive tracer for gastric cancer. **(A)** Primary lesion of superficial slightly depressed type gastric cancer; **(B)** Endoscopic injection of tracer. Technetium–99m tin colloid solution in a volume of 2.0 ml (150 MBq) was injected in four quadrants into the submucosal layer of the primary lesion using an endoscopic puncture needle.

Intraoperative detection of SLN by a combination of dye and radio-guided methods

Real-time observation of lymphatic vessels and drainage routes from the primary lesion by the dye-guided method is helpful in addition to the radio-guided detection of SLNs using gamma probe. We prefer to perform intraoperative endoscopic injection of blue dye (Lymphazurin; 1% isosulfan blue, Tyco Healthcare) rather than subserosal direct injection for several reasons: (1) Intraoperative subserosal identification of T1 lesions is not so easy. (2) An accurate injection of the blue dye is critically important for SLN mapping. (3) In laparoscopic setting, subserosal injection of the blue dye is not practical. Injection procedure itself is the same as that for the radioactive tracer. Lymphatic vessels are visualized very clearly immediately after the injection (Figure 2).

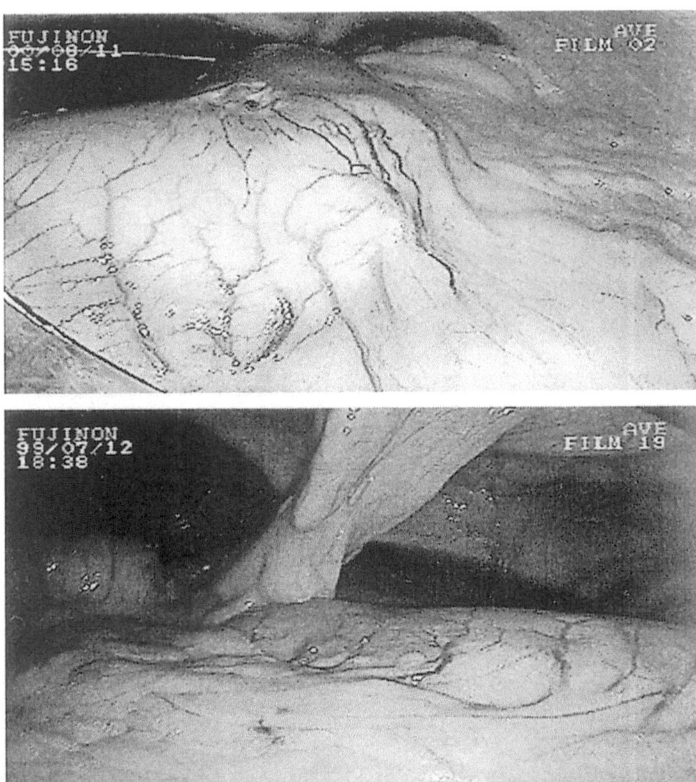

Figure 2. Laparoscopic view of lymphatic vessels from stomach stained by blue dye. Lymphatic vessels are visualized very clearly immediately after the injection of Lymphazurin.

Because of the rapid transit of blue dye, the best observation timing is 5 to 15 minutes after injection. Mobilization of stomach without destruction of lymphatic drainage routes before injection of the blue dye is also critical in detecting multidirectional SLNs properly.
Gamma probe with high collimation is essential for intraoperative final identification of SLNs (Figure 3). It is technically important to avoid shine-through from the primary lesion by handling of the gamma probe for the intraoperative detection of SLN.

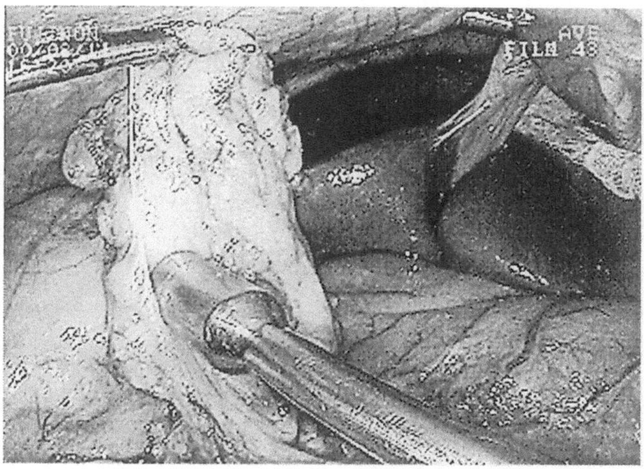

Figure 3. Laparoscopic detection of SLN in gastric cancer using Laparoprobe (Tyco Healthcare)

Intraoperative sampling of SLNs in gastric cancer-picking-up procedure or lymphatic basin dissection

A picking-up procedure of blue and/or hot nodes is feasible as a conventional SLN dissection. Miwa et al.[17] have proposed lymphatic basin dissection as a more reliable sampling procedure of SLNs of gastric cancer. Sentinel lymphatic basins can be identified by dye- and radio-guided methods and these basins should contain true SLNs. An identification of blue and/or hot nodes on the back table after lymphatic basin dissection is easier and more reliable than the picking-up method (Figure 4). Lymphatic basin dissection is considered a sort of selective lymphadenectomy containing SLNs and can be combined with modified resection of the stomach. Miwa et al.[17] recommend this procedure to avoid false-negative results by sampling error.

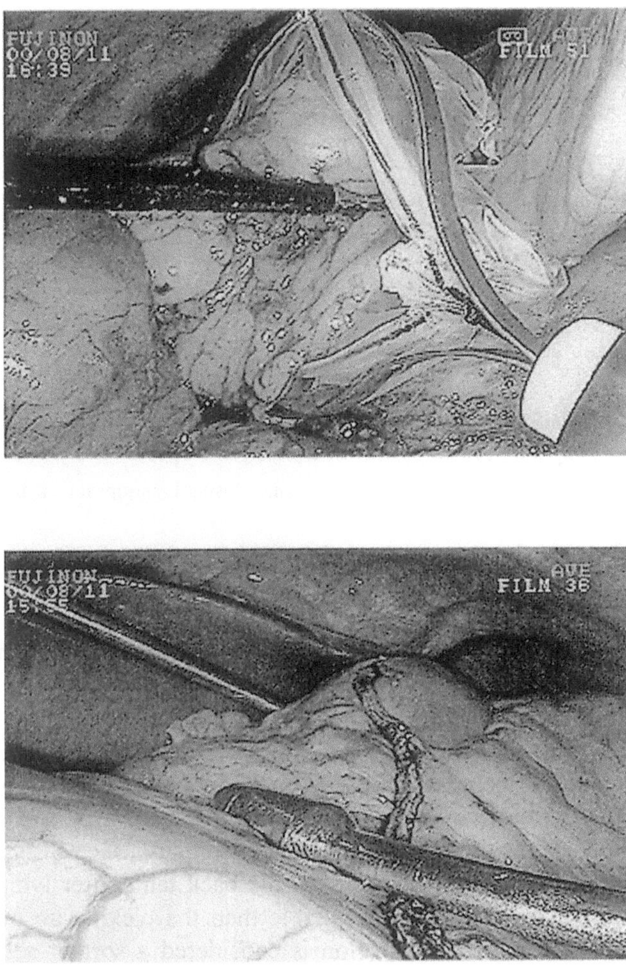

Figure 4. Laparoscopic sentinel basin dissection for gastric cancer. **(A)** Laparoscopic sampling of sentinel basin. Sentinel basin can be detected and retrieved by laparoscopic procedure. **(B)** Confirmation of no residual SLN by gamma probe after sentinel basin dissection.

Clinical impact of SLN mapping for gastric cancer

Gastric cancer is now one of the most suitable targets of an individualized less-invasive surgery based on the SLN concept. Despite the multidirectional and complicated lymphatic flow from gastric mucosa, the anatomical situation of the stomach is relatively suitable for SN mapping in comparison with organs embedded in closed spaces such as the esophagus and rectum. In particular, clinically T1N0 gastric cancer seems to be a good entity for which to try to modify the therapeutic approach. From the data reported in the literature, micrometastases tend to be limited within the sentinel basins in cT1N0 gastric cancer. Sentinel basins are therefore good targets of selective lymphadenectomy for cT1N0 gastric cancer with potential risk of micrometastasis. As indicated in Figure 5, cases with positive SLNs after selective dissection of sentinel basins can be treated by conventional radical surgery. Furthermore, laparoscopic local resection is theoretically feasible for curative treatment of SLN-negative early gastric cancer (Figure 6).[11] In Japan, clinical applications of this novel minimally invasive approach could have a great impact on patient care for gastric cancer because 60–70% of gastric cancer cases treated in major institutes belong to this category.

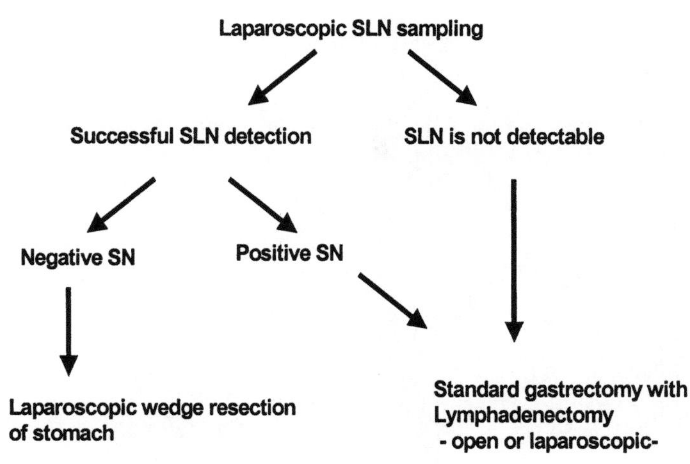

Figure 5. Therapeutic strategies of early gastric cancer with limited size of primary lesion based on SLN mapping.

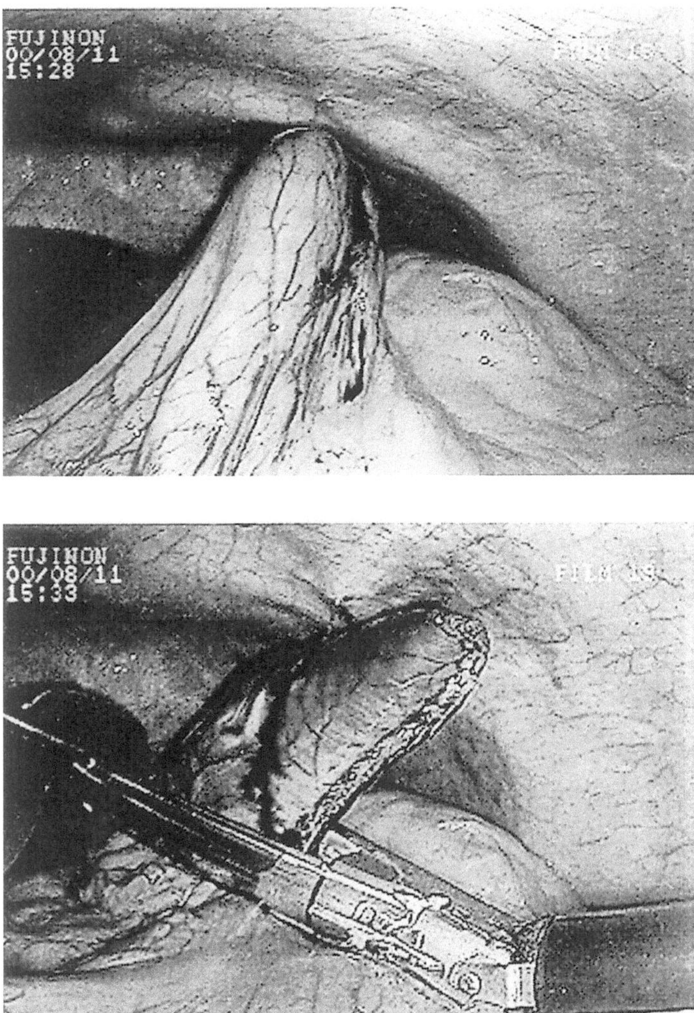

Figure 6. Laparoscopic wedge resection of stomach by lesion lifting method (Ohgami's method). **(A)** The primary lesion is lifted up by metal rod and wire. **(B)** The lesion is resected by endoscopic stapler.

SENTINEL LYMPH NODE MAPPING FOR ESOPHAGEAL CANCER

Current status of SLN mapping for esophageal cancer

SLN mapping for esophageal cancer is more complicated than that for gastric cancer. First of all, lymphatic mapping with the dye-guided method is not feasible for esophageal cancer. Regional lymph nodes of the thoracic esophagus are frequently pigmented by anthracosis and it is difficult to identify blue nodes. In organs such as the esophagus and rectum, real-time observation of the lymphatic route using dye is impossible without operative mobilization of the primary site. However, the mobilization itself destroys the active lymphatic flow from the primary lesion. For many of these reasons, the radio-guided method has been used for SLN mapping in esophageal cancer.[10,21] There are few studies demonstrating the feasibility and validity of the SN concept in esophageal cancer.[10,21] In Western countries, the number of earlystage esophageal cancers is very limited and it is difficult to perform clinical studies to investigate the lymphatic mapping in this entity. In esophageal cancer, SNs are multiple and widely spread from cervical to abdominal areas. In more than 80% of the cases, at least one SN is located in the second or third compartment of regional lymph nodes.[10] This characteristic distribution of SNs is attributed to the multidirectional lymphatic drainage routes from the esophagus. It is essential to plan and conduct a multicentric validation study of SLN mapping for esophageal cancer.

Significance of lymphoscintigraphy for SLN mapping for esophageal cancer

Preoperative endoscopic injection of radioactive tracer is basically the same as that described for gastric cancer. However, unlike gastric cancer, preoperative lymphoscintigraphy, taken 3 hours after tracer injection, has been found to be very useful in detecting SLNs in unexpected sites distant from the primary lesion of esophageal cancer (Figure 7). Distribution of SLNs in the esopageal cancer cases is widely spread from cervical to abdominal areas. Preoperative lymphoscintigraphy is essential for the SLN sampling for esophageal cancer.

Figure 7. Lymphoscintigraphy for esophageal cancer. Cervical and abdominal SLNs are visualized by lymphoscintigraphy.

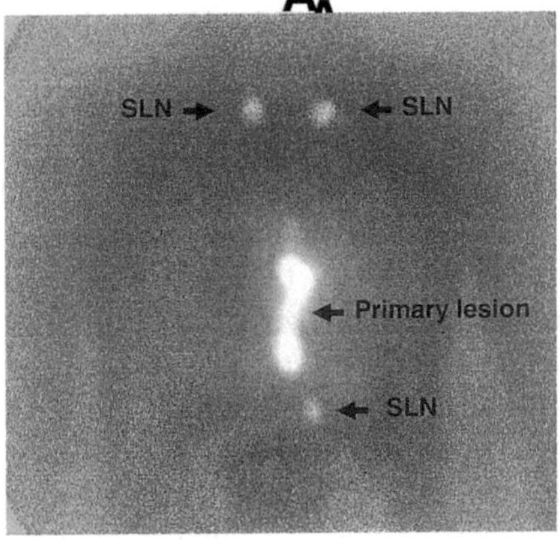

Intraoperative SLN sampling for esophageal cancer using gamma probe

SLNs located in the cervical area can be identified by percutaneous gamma probing. These SLNs in the cervical area can be resected by less invasive procedures as shown in Figure 8. Laparoscopic detection and sampling of abdominal SLNs is feasible, as described for gastric cancer. On the other hand, SLN sampling for mediastinal SLNs is relatively complicated and invasive because of the requirement of mobilization of thoracic esophagus. Shine-through from the primary lesion is also an obstacle for gamma probing for mediastinal SLNs.

Figure 8. Sampling of cervical SLN for esophageal cancer.

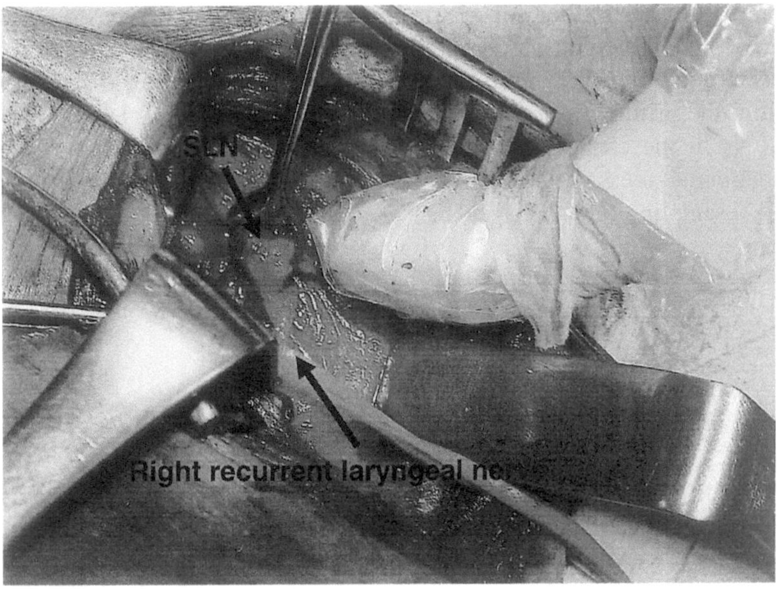

Clinical applications of SLN mapping in esophageal cancer
Selective lymphadenectomy based on SLN status

Transthoracic extended esophagectomy with three-field radical lymph node dissection has been recognized as a standard procedure for thoracic esophageal cancer in Japan because of widely spread and unpredictable metastatic patterns as previously described.[1] Indications of upper-mediastinal lymph node dissection for cervical esophageal cancer and lower-mediastinal lymph node dissection for abdominal esophageal cancer are then controversial. SLN mapping would provide significant information to perform an individualized selective lymphadenectomy based on SLN status.

A complete sampling of multiple and widespread SLNs in esophageal cancer is not a minimally invasive procedure unlike in melanoma and breast cancer. At present, local resection of the primary lesion of esophageal cancer with negative SN is not a practical procedure. However, selective and modified lymphadenectomy targeted on sentinel basins for clinically N0 esophageal cancer should become feasible and clinically useful. In our initial experience, clinically undetectable micrometastases in cT1N0 esophageal cancer tend to be limited within sentinel basins. Although three-field lymph node dissection is recognized as an extensive and curative procedure for thoracic esophageal cancer, its prognostic significance is still controversial. Uniform application of this highly invasive procedure could well increase the morbidity and reduce quality of life after surgery. Individualized selective lymphadenectomy for cN0 esophageal cancer based on SN status therefore seems to be a reasonable surgical approach.[12] The incidence of carcinoma of the esophagogastric junction, including Barrett's carcinoma, is increasing in Western countries, and more recently in Japan, and there are several surgical approaches for this clinical entity.[20] Individualized extent of resection and lymph node dissection for Barrett's carcinoma based on lymphatic mapping will become an important topic in surgical oncology for upper GI tract as shown in Figure 9.[19]

Figure 9. Individualized approach for Barrett's carcinoma based on lymphatic mapping. A case with negative SLN limited in abdominal area (A) can be treated by limited resection and jejunal interposition without extensive mediastinal lymph node resection (B).

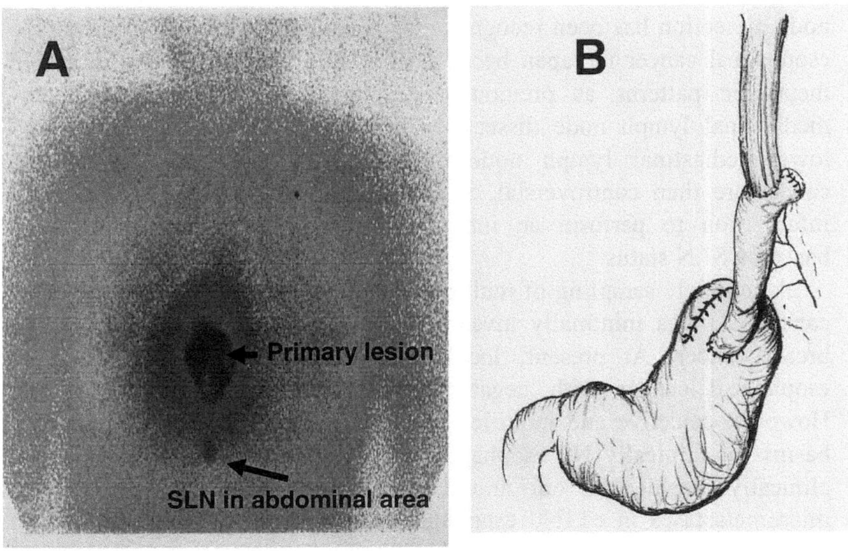

Accurate staging to determine the indication of adjuvant chemotherapy

Metastatic status of regional lymph nodes is an important prognostic factor regarding esophageal cancer. Ando et al.[2] reported that postoperative adjuvant chemotherapy with cisplatin and 5-FU has a preventive effect on relapse in patients with esophageal carcinoma when compared to surgery alone, on the basis of randomized trials. A benefit of the adjuvant chemotherapy was observed particularly in the patients with lymph node metastasis in this study. Therefore, accurate and sensitive detection of micrometastasis in lymph nodes in patients with esophageal cancer is clinically very important.

Although a number of reports demonstrate underestimation of micrometastasis in regional lymph nodes by conventional staging procedures employed for solid tumors, the application of intensive examinations such as step sectioning, immunohistochemistry and RT-PCR for all resected lymph nodes is not practical. A focused examination on SNs may help resolve this issue. Bilchik et al.[3] report that ultrasensitive assays by RT-PCR and electrochemiluminescent detection of multiple markers of SLNs from colorectal cancer patients can identify those who may be at high risk for recurrence and, therefore, are more likely to benefit from systemic adjuvant therapy.

Nonsurgical approaches for esophageal cancer targeted on SLN

Recently, chemoradiotherapy (CRT) has attracted attention as a multidisciplinary curative treatment for cT1N0 esophageal cancer. Although an acceptable effect on local control has been reported in this approach, distant node recurrence from the area out of the irradiation field is a serious problem to resolve in long-term observation. In this approach, control of invisible micrometastases is essential. Lymphoscintigrams revealing the distribution of SNs in each individual case are useful in designing the field of irradiation. Currently we are performing curative CRT for cT1N0 esophageal cancer with an individualized irradiation field instead of long T-type uniform irradiation fields.

Variables in Microarray Studies in Lymphoma

A comparison of the different studies of microarray analysis in lymphoma will demonstrate that there are variables in the type of platform used, the number of probe targets present, the control (if any) RNA source utilized, the number of cases studied, and the type of software used to analyze the data. Variables in tissue preservation, percent of tumor cells, and normalization of the data also likely exist, but will not be further detailed here as these data were variably reported. The two major platforms are cDNA microarrays, popularized by Pat Brown, and the oligoprobe microarray developed by Affymetrix. The number of targets in published studies in lymphoma have ranged from 588 to approximately 18,000. The source of control RNA included cell lines, reactive lymph nodes, isolated germinal centers, sorted cells from tonsils, or another subtype of lymphoma. Software analysis methods are characterized into two broad categories of unsupervised and supervised clustering, including ratio ranking, hierarchal clustering, self-organized mapping and others. The number of cases studied per subtype of lymphoma has ranged from 5 to 240.[1, 5, 7-13]

CONCLUSIONS

From recent single-institution reports performed on SLN mapping for gastric and esophageal cancer, the SLN concept seems to be valid even in the upper GI tract. Although further accumulation of the evidence based on multicenter clinical trials using standard protocol is required, SLN mapping would be a great tool to perform individualized surgical and nonsurgical treatment for upper GI cancer.

REFERENCES

1. Akiyama H, Tsurumaru M, Udagawa H, et al: Radical lymph node dissection for cancer of the thoracic esophagus. Ann Surg 220:364-373, 1994
2. Ando N, Iizuka T, Ide H et al: Surgery plus chemotherapy compared with surgery alone for localized squamous cell carcinoma of the thoracic esophagus: a Japan Clinical Oncology Group Study--JCOG9204. J Clin Oncol;21:4592-4596, 2003
3. Bilchik AJ, Saha S, Wiese D, et al: Molecular staging of early colon cancer on the basis of sentinel node analysis: a multicenter phase II trial. J Clin Oncol 19:1128-1136, 2001
4. Bonenkamp JJ, Hermans J, Sasako M, et al: Extended lymph-node dissection for gastric cancer. Dutch Gastric Cancer Group. N Engl J Med 340:908-914, 1999
5. Hiratsuka M, Miyashiro I, Ishikawa O, et al: Application of sentinel node biopsy to gastric cancer surgery. Surgery 129:335-340, 2001
6. Hulsher JBF, van Sandick JW, de Boer AGEM, et al: Extended transthoracic resection compared with limited transhiatal resection for adenocarcinoma of the esophagus. N Engl J Med 347:1662-1669, 2002
7. Ichikura T, Morita D, Uchida T, et al: Sentinel node concept in gastric carcinoma. World J Surg 26: 318-322, 2002
8. Kitagawa Y, Fujii H, Mukai M, et al: Radio-guided sentinel node detection for gastric cancer. Br J Surg 89:604-608, 2002a
9. Kitagawa Y, Fujii H, Mukai M, et al: Intraoperative lymphatic mapping and sentinel lymph node sampling in esophageal and gastric cancer. Surg Oncol Clin North Am 11:293-304, 2002b
10. Kitagawa Y, Fujii H, Mukai M, et al: The role of sentinel lymph node in gastrointestinal cancer. Surg Clin North Am 80:1799-1809, 2000
11. Kitagawa Y, Ohgami M, Fujii H, et al: Laparoscopic detection of sentinel lymph nodes in gastrointestinal cancer: A novel and minimally invasive approach. Ann Surg Oncol 8(9S):86-89, 2001
12. Kitajima M, Kitagawa Y: Surgical treatment of esophageal cancer—The advent of the era of individualization. N Engl J Med 21:1705-1709, 2002
13. Kitagawa Y, Kitajima M: Diagnostic validity of radio-guided sentinel node mapping for gastric cancer. Surgical Technology International (in press), 2004
14. Kosaka T, Ueshima N, Sugaya J, et al: Lymphatic route of the stomach demonstrated by gastric carcinomas with solitary lymph node metastasis. Surg Today 29: 695-700, 1999
15. Maruyama K, Gunven P, Okabayashi K, et al: Lymph node metastases of gastric cancer. General pattern in 1931 patients. Ann Surg 210:596-602, 1989
16. Matsubara T, Ueda M, Kaisaki S, et al: Localization of initial lymph node metastasis from carcinoma of the thoracic esophagus. Cancer 89: 1869-1873, 2000
17. Miwa K, Kinami S, Taniguchi K, et al: Mapping sentinel nodes in patients with early-stage gastric carcinoma. Br J Surg 90:178-182, 2003
18. Sano T, Katai H, Sasako M, et al: Gastric lymphadenectomy and detection of sentinel nodes. Recent Results Cancer Res 157:253-258, 2000
19. Stein HJ, Sendler A, Siewert JR: Site-dependent resection techniques for gastric cancer. Surg Oncol Clin North Am 11:405-414, 2002

20. Vizcaino AP, Moreno V, Lambert R, et al: Time trends incidence of both major histologic types of esophageal carcinomas in selected countries, 1973–1995. Int J Cancer 99:860-868, 2002
21. Yasuda S, Shimada H, Chino O, et al: Sentinel lymph node detection with Tc-99m tin colloids in patients with esophagogastric cancer. Jpn J Clin Oncol 33:68-72, 2003

Chapter 7

SENTINEL LYMPH NODE MAPPING IN LUNG CANCER

Michael J. Liptay
Evanston Northwestern Healthcare, Evanston, IL, USA

INTRODUCTION

Lung cancer remains the most common cause of cancer-related mortality in both sexes worldwide. Over 180,000 new cases will be diagnosed this year in the United States alone. Only 25–30% of these patients are considered candidates for potential curative resection. If pathologic lymph node involvement is recognized, the chances of a long-term survival are less than 50%. Improved staging techniques are the cornerstone of advancements in new therapeutic strategies allowing for homogeneous study group selection and balanced assessment of true effects.

Lymph node status is the single most important prognostic factor for localized potentially resectable non-small-cell lung cancer. Nodal involvement decreases the 5-year survival by nearly 40% compared to similar patients without nodal metastases. Nonetheless, up to 40% of completely resected "histologically node negative" patients relapse and die of their original cancers often recurring within 2 years. This is at least in part due to inaccurately staged nodal disease. Recent studies suggest that the presence of nodal micrometastatic disease in lung cancer may garner the same poor prognosis as metastases evident by conventional techniques. A powerful application of the sentinel node technique in lung cancer is the identification of specific nodes for further ultrastaging pathologic and molecular examination.

Sentinel node mapping has become the standard of care in both breast cancer and melanoma. The primary utility of these tumors is avoidance of nontherapeutic axillary or groin lymph node dissections and their incumbent morbidities. The morbidity of a complete mediastinal node dissection for lung cancer is not excessive and the procedure may be therapeutic.

Another important role is directing pathologic examination to specific sentinel nodes and applying more sensitive techniques on a limited amount of tissue to detect occult micrometastatic disease.

Sentinel node mapping in lung cancer is in the evaluation phase. Several techniques have been proposed as valid ways to identify the first site of nodal drainage. Radioisotopes injected both intraoperatively and preoperatively have been reported most frequently. This chapter will focus on our technique of intraoperative sentinel node mapping with technetium sulfur colloid.

TECHNIQUE

We have performed intraoperative sentinel node mapping in over 200 patients using the injection of technetium -99m suspensions directly into lung masses at the time of thoracotomy. Our original methods have been described in a previous publication detailing our experience with our first 52 patients.[1] Modification to the technique has included most importantly a decrease in the amount of radioactivity injected into the tumors from an original total dose of 2 mCi to our current dose of 0.25 mCi. This has allowed a significant decrease in background radiation from the tumor allowing improved identification of sentinel node stations *in vivo.*[2]

The tumor mass itself is injected in a four-outer-quadrant fashion with technetium sulfur colloid filtered once through a 20-micron filter. The filtering of the particles assures rapid passage of radioisotope through the lymphatics to allow for sentinel node identification without prolonging the planned resection.

The Radiation Safety regulations in Illinois require a licensed physician to dispense the radioisotope. Our protocol has a nuclear medicine physician prepare four tuberculin syringes under sterile technique with the 0.25 mCi dose divided. These are then passed on to the sterile operating field. The surgeon injects the radioisotope in a four-quadrant fashion directly into the tumor. The syringes are collected by the nuclear medicine personnel and the area surveyed with a Geiger counter to detect spillage and contamination. No other precautions are necessary such as special decontamination after the case or additional protection of OR personnel.

A standard dissection is then performed to complete an anatomic resection of the tumor. Readings are taken with the hand-held gamma probe counter (Navigator® system, United States Surgical Corporation) after calibration. The minimum necessary migration time from injection of the tumor with the technetium-99m sulfur colloid solution to the detection of radioactivity in the lymph nodes has been found to be 10 minutes.

During the time of migration, care is taken to avoid dissection of the bronchial structures and peribronchial tissues where the majority of lymphatics are located. The bronchial dissection and division are performed last in the majority of cases if the operation permits.

Successful studies utilizing preoperative injection of various radioisotopes within 24 hours of the planned surgery have been reported. Our technique is based on the intraoperative injection of the radioisotope with attention paid to: preparation, injection of the radioisotope into the tumor, anatomic dissection, *in vivo* and *ex vivo* readings, and re-surveillance for residual radioactivity.

PREPARATION

After the preoperative evaluation and informed consent, patients are taken to the operating room and the standard preparations made for mediastinoscopy (if indicated), thoracotomy, and resection. After thoracotomy, patients are injected with technetium-99 sulfur colloid (O.25 mCi) divided into four equal doses. The radioisotope is prepared according to the manufacturer's instructions and drawn through a 200-nm sterile filter once. For the injection preparation, the radioisotope is drawn into four tuberculin syringes (1 ml) and injected using 27 gauge needles.

Preparation of the radioisotope is performed under the direction of a nuclear medicine physician. After injection of the technetium the syringes are given back to nuclear medicine, the area is surveyed for residual radioactivity, and the materials are taken back for disposal.

INJECTION

Moist lap pads are positioned around the tumor in the chest to avoid spillage of radioisotope during injection into the tumor. The isotope is injected into the periphery of the lung tumor in a four-quadrant pattern. The injections are made into the tumor and not in the lung parenchyma surrounding the tumor to avoid the confounding incidence of aerosolization of the radioactivity into the parenchyma and airways. After injection the chest is irrigated with sterile water solution to wash out any stray radioisotope (Figure 1).

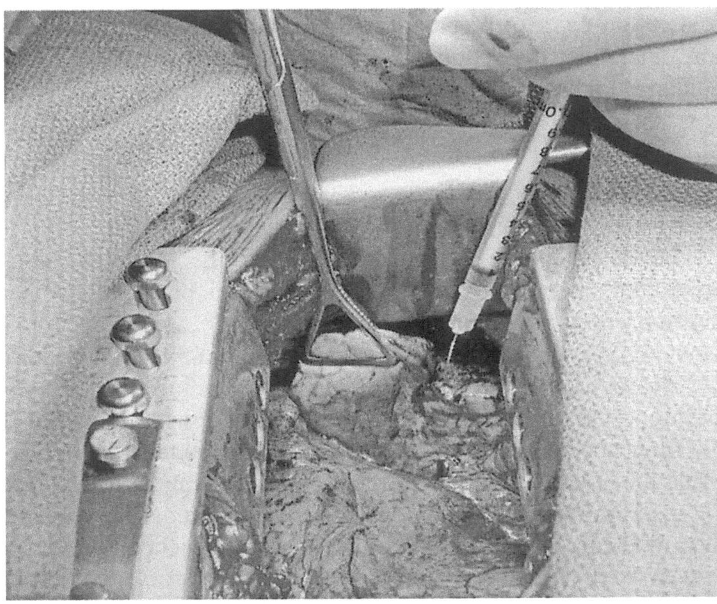

Figure 1. Radio-isotope injection. 0.25mCi of filtered Tc-99m was injected in four quadrants directly into tumor 10 minutes before fissural or peribronchial dissection.

ANATOMIC DISSECTION

Our preliminary work has found the minimum time required for successful migration of radioisotope is 10 minutes. During the time allowed for migration of the radioactivity, usual preparative dissection for resection is performed with a few considerations.

The fissure structures and peribronchial tissues known to be rich in lymphatics are to be left undisturbed until a minimum of 10 minutes after injection time. Dissection is generally commenced at the anteromedial hilum overlying the pulmonary vein and truncus branches of the pulmonary artery. The inferior pulmonary ligament and posterior mediastinal pleura are left intact until 10 minutes has elapsed.

SENTINEL NODE MAPPING

In Vivo Readings

The tumor specimen and nodal stations are initially surveyed in the thorax with the hand-held gamma probe (Navigator®), and background levels are recorded within the chest, distant from the primary tumor. The initial intrathoracic readings may be unreliable if there is high residual radioactivity in the primary tumor in close proximity to nodes within the chest (shine-through effect). To minimize this, the probe is angled away from the tumor if possible as it is generally exponentially more radioactive than the nodes (Figure 2).

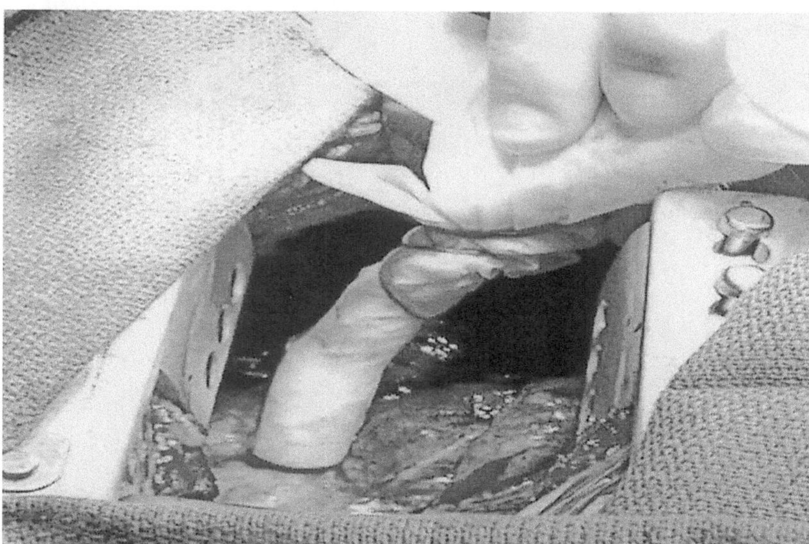

Figure 2. Intrathoracic SN reading for measurement of radioactivity background in chest. Hand-held gamma counter measures nodal stations.

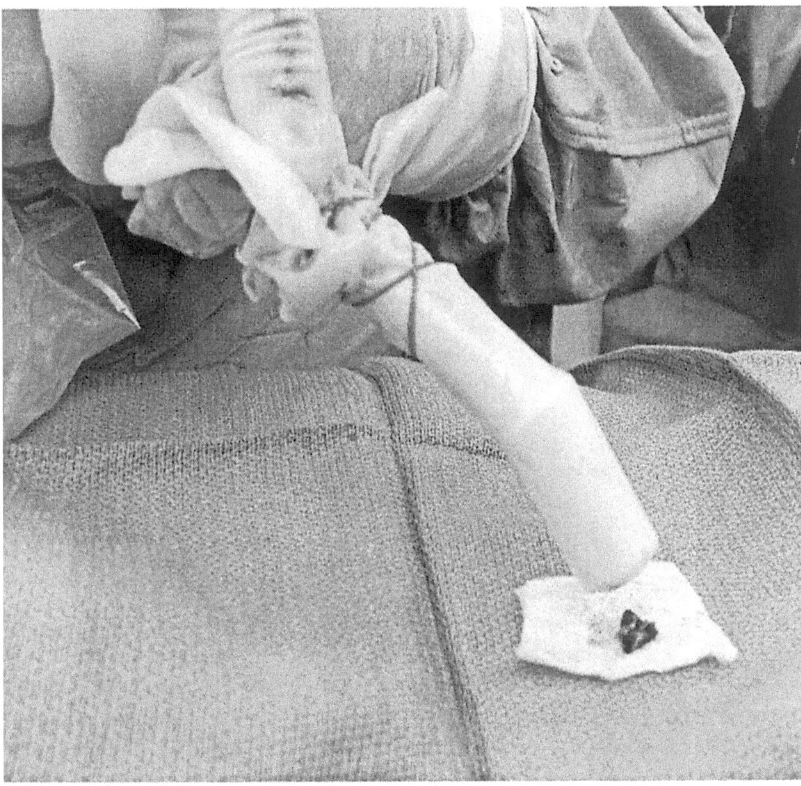

Figure 3. *Ex vivo* reading of dissected nodes. Nodes are separated from tumor on field. Highest CPS & 3x background = SN. The hemithorax is resurveyed postresection for residual CPS/nodes.

Ex Vivo Readings

Visible mediastinal, peribronchial, and hilar lymph nodes are dissected from the primary tumor and are also measured separately from the tumor specimen after removal from the chest (*ex vivo*). The time from injection of the tumor with the technetium-99m to the first *ex vivo* measurement of radioactivity is recorded.

The migration of the technetium sulfur colloid solution is considered successful if a specific nodal station registered counts per second (CPS) greater than 3 times background values. The most accurate reading of nodal radioactivity appears to be the *ex vivo* readings taken after separating the nodes from the tumor/lobar specimen. All lymph nodes with the requisite radioactivity 3-fold greater than intrathoracic background are classified as sentinel nodes. Our average number of sentinel nodes has been 1.5 (range 1–4) (Figure 3).

RESURVEY FOR RESIDUAL RADIOACTIVITY

After the initial scintigraphic readings and standard anatomic resection with ipsilateral mediastinal node dissection is completed, a repeat examination with the gamma probe is performed to assess for residual radioactivity and potentially overlooked lymph nodes. The remaining radioactivity levels are recorded and re-resections of nodal stations performed if indicated by the handheld gamma counter readings and visual inspection.

GAMMA PROBE

The Navigator GPS® gamma probe is used and set up according to the manufacturer's recommendations. The isotope selector switch is set to Tc99m. The Navigator Top Gun® external collimator is used to facilitate identification of hot nodes in close proximity to the injection site. The Count button initiates the required 10-second timed counts on the nodes and background. A sterile plastic sheath is used to cover the probe.

SPECIAL CONSIDERATIONS

Our experience to date suggests that sentinel node mapping in potentially resectable lung tumors may have its most important role in the staging and treatment of clinically early stage I tumors. [3,4] Large tumors with central necrosis or those patients with clinically positive lymph nodes had less accurately detected sentinel nodes and whatever information is gained in these advanced tumors, the detection of micrometastases appears less important to their treatment plans.

We have been successful less than 60% of the time in predicting a sentinel node station based solely on the intrathoracic *in vivo* readings in the thorax. This is due to the shine-through effect from the radioactivity of the tumor and in addition the aerosolization of technetium into the airways causing inaccurate readings.

This has led some to question the utility of this technique where limitation of node dissection is not possible with the methods described. [3,5]

While we await advances in the field to aid in limiting thoracic lymphadenectomy, the ability to select a few sentinel nodes for further study in search of micrometastatic disease from an average of 20–30 nodes allows pathologists to focus their efforts on the most promising tissues.

A multicentered trial is opening in the Cancer and Leukemia Group B to test the applicability of this promising technique in patients with potentially resectable clinical stage I lung cancers.

REFERENCES

1. Liptay MJ, Masters G, Winchester DJ, et al. Intraoperative radioisotope sentinel lymph node mapping in non-small cell lung cancer (NSCLC). *Ann Thorac Surg* (2000 Aug) 70:384-390.
2. Liptay MJ, Grondin SC, Fry WA, et al. Intraoperative sentinel lymph node mapping in non-small cell lung cancer improves detection of micrometastases. *J Clin Oncol* (April 15, 2002) 20:1984-1988.
3. Ueda K, Suga K, Kaneda Y, et al. Radioisotope lymph node mapping in non small cell lung cancer: can it be applicable for sentinel node biopsy? *Ann Thorac Surg* (2004 Feb) 77(2): 426-430.
4. Sugi K, Kaneda Y, Sudoh M, et al. Effect of radioisotope sentinel node mapping in patients with cT1N0M0 lung cancer. *J Thorac Cardiovasc Surg* (2003 Aug) 126(2): 568-573.
5. Liptay MJ. Sentinel node mapping in lung cancer. *Ann Surg Oncol*: (2004 Mar) 11(3 suppl): 271S-274S.

Chapter 8

LYMPHATIC MAPPING AND SENTINEL LYMPHADENECTOMY IN UROLOGY

Ramon M. Cabanas
Victory Memorial Hospital, Brooklyn, New York

INTRODUCTION

The sentinel lymph node (SLN) concept can be feasibly applied in the investigation, diagnostics, staging, and treatment of almost all solid tumors in human pathology, but its development as well as validation has required scientific fundament provided by many investigators.

Twenty-seven years ago, I proposed an approach for the treatment of penile carcinoma after I had studied in detail and over the course of 8 years lymphangiograms, anatomic dissection, and microscopic reports of 100 patients, including 80 cases of penile carcinomas, 10 inflammatory diseases of the penis, and 10 normal volunteers in whom lymphangiography was performed via the dorsal lymphatic of the penis. The basic concept derived was that the lymphatic system of the penis drains to one or a group of nodes, the SLN, that appeared to be the primary site of metastases from penile carcinoma.

This experience was part of 400 lymphangiograms performed in malignant melanoma, lymphomas, head and neck pathology, breast carcinoma, lymphedema of extremities, testicular carcinoma, scrotal carcinoma, anal-rectal carcinoma, vulvar carcinoma, as well as cervical carcinoma. Today, SLN localization and biopsy (sentinel node procedure) in the early stages of malignant tumors is a reliable technique with widespread applications as a practical means of identifying patients with microscopic regional nodal metastases and thereby eliminating routine lymph node dissection in patients with no clinical evidence of nodal involvement.

Concept, Scientific Basis, and Development

In the last decade, significant new data on the diagnosis and treatment of the lymphatic system have been accumulated in the field of malignant melanoma and breast and penile cancer.

Application of these findings to the urological field generates ongoing studies investigating the impact of the SLN procedure (SLNP) for the diagnosis of micrometastasis founded by cytochemical and immunohistochemical techniques.

SLN procedure can be applied in the field of urogenital cancer for penile, scrotal, prostatic, bladder, and testicular carcinomas.[4,8,10,18,27,28,31,40,62,64,67,70,71] The controversies about the definitive treatment of each disease are not within the boundaries of this publication.

The gold standard for the treatment of penile carcinoma remains local control (partial or total amputation of the penis) followed by bilateral ilio-inguinal lymphadenectomy, but only in the early stage can the SLNP apply.[3,8,11,12,15,16,24,26,30,38,43,51,52,54,55,60,62,63]

The ideal situation would be performing the procedure without morbidity and without incapacitating lymphedema, but this hypothetical situation does not exist and controversial issues regarding the treatment of regional lymph nodes persist.[11,28,30,31,35,39,42,57-59,66]

Across the United States, the incidence of penile carcinoma is low and the number of cases so few as to prevent prospective, randomized studies.[3,12,59]

The lack of training to identify the SLN, the learning curve phenomenon observed in breast and melanoma cancers, the nonexisting national and international protocols for lymphatic mapping that guides as in other locations are absent in the United States for the study of penile carcinoma. These create controversies in the application of the concept of the SLN.

Also, it should be pointed out that there is an absence of a standard pathology protocol for examination of SLN such as cytochemical reaction and immunohistochemical reaction. Several authors reported conclusions based on a limited number of cases and personal hypotheses.[11-13,20,41,54,59] The SLN for penile carcinoma exists. The questions remain: Where is it located? How do you find it? Pre- and intraoperative lymph node mapping or SLN detection by means of methylene blue injection as well as radioactive tracer apply in early cases and will "maximize" the staging and "minimize" the surgical therapeutics.

The aim of this chapter is as follows:

1. Describe the anatomical and pathological fundaments of the SLN concept.
2. Provide guidelines of the technique.
3. Review the experience of investigators working in the SLN procedure.

THE TECHNIQUE OF SLN BIOPSY

For SLN biopsy in penile and in scrotal cancers, this author recommends a technique that combines preoperative lymphoscintigraphy (LSG) and intraoperative SLN mapping using both blue dye and radioisotope. Both cancers require a widelocal excision of the primary lesion, with preoperative injection of tracer (blue dye and/or isotope) around the primary site. Although the basic treatment of squamous cell carcinoma of the scrotum is widelocal excision, SLN biopsy allows the surgeon to rule out nodal micrometastasis and therefore the need for a formal ilioinguinal lymphadenectomy. The male genital organ has the advantage of being a midline structure in which both anatomical parameters and lymphatic mapping (by isotope and blue dye) can be used to identify the SLN.

Initial work, based on the injection of contrast agents into the dorsal lymphatic of the penis, demonstrates that these lymphatics drain to the superficial inguinal nodes medially and to the superomedial inguinal nodes in particular (Figures 1, 2A–C).

Figure 1. Direct injection of one lymphatic duct, via dorsal lymphatic of the penis. The SLN is visualized.

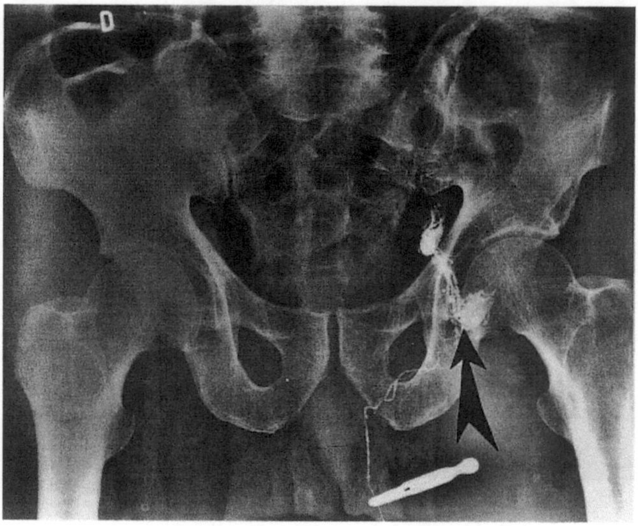

Figure 2. Completed lymphangiograms. (A) Right side: lymphatic system after injection of the dorsal lymphatic of the penis. Left side: visualization of lymphatics via dorsal lymphatics of the foot. Note that the lower nodes of the inguinal area do not collect lymph of the penis. The white line emphasizes this finding. (B) Completed or total visualization of the lymphatic system of the penis. Direct injection of two lymphatics via dorsal ducts of the penis. (C) Injection at the level of the lesion. Technetium -99m sulfur colloid. Similar result obtained.

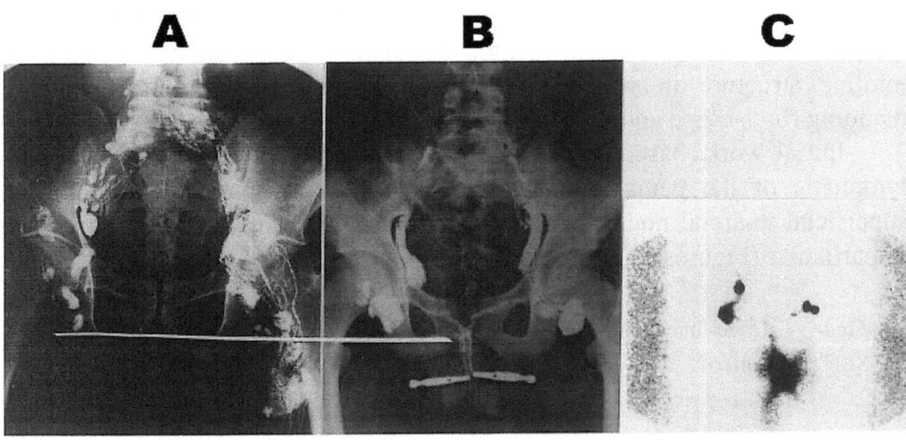

Because this particular technique of lymphangiography proved cumbersome, an alternative method is to identify the SLN by using anatomic parameters alone.[7,19,56,57] Here, a 5-cm incision is made parallel to the inguinal ligament, two fingers' breadth lateral and two fingers' breadth distal to the pubic tubercle, overlying the saphenofemoral junction. The SLN is identified by inserting the finger under the upper flap toward the pubic tubercle. The SLN lies among the lymph nodes associated with the superficial epigastric vein. The position of the SLN in relation to this vein may vary, but never by more than 1 cm. The superficial epigastric vein is absent in 1.4% of cases, and occasionally there is more than one lymph node in the superficial epigastric group. In this setting, all lymph nodes in this area (generally two or three) should be removed. The true SLN is always the larger and more medially situated (Figure 3A–C).[5-7,9,14,36,37,56]

Figure 3. (A) Total penectomy. Left radical ilioinguinal lymph node dissection. Surgical specimen, note SLN location. (B) The surgical specimen has been dissected. The inferior arrows are point to the lymph nodes without metastasis. They do not receive the lymphatic flow from the penis. (C) Anatomical details and landmarks of the location of the SLN.

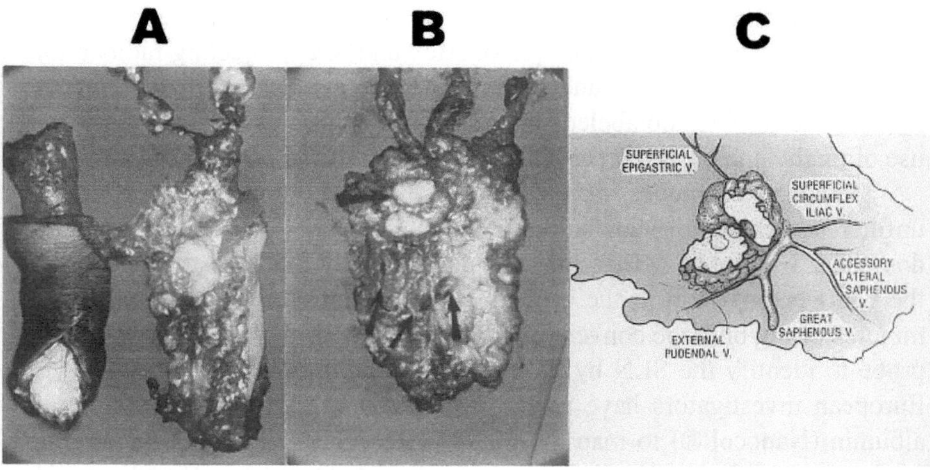

In lymphoscintigraphy (LSG), injected radioactive particles are imaged as they pass through lymphatic vessels to their respective lymph nodal drainage basins. Radionuclides such as ^{198}Au, ^{131}I, ^{197}HG, and ^{99m}TC attached to colloids, albumin, or other substances have been used in lymphoscintigraphy to study the anatomic pathways of lymphatic drainage for the planning of surgical or radiotherapeutic treatment.

Sherman and Ter Pogos in 1953 introduced the selective localization of regional lymph nodes with interstitially injected radioactive colloidal gold, marking the beginning of lymphoscintigraphy, although Walker published a work around 1950, on localization of radioactive colloid in lymph nodes.[2,17,25,32,53,61,69]

Pioneer investigation in LSG has been reported in the study of the lymph system of the breast, axillary and mammary intern lymph chain systems, malignant melanoma, prostate carcinoma, ilioinguinal nodes, and cervical nodes. Harper and colleagues first used ^{99m}TC.[25] Several other investigators continued the effort to find the draining system of the prostate gland.[21,22,29,33,44,73,74]

We welcome the procedure of Morton and associates using intradermal injection of "blue dye" at the primary tumor site in malignant melanomas.[46-48] We also welcome the technique of Alex and Krag, injecting radiocolloid at the level of the lesion, and using a manual gammaprobe as a guide to identify the SLN (radiolabeled) for excisional biopsy, as well as the pioneer use of methylene blue in breast cancer by Guiliano and co-workers.[1,20,23,34]

Modern techniques map the SLN by the preoperative injection of unfiltered technetium-99m sulfur colloid (Tc-99m-SC). We recommend a dose of 0.3 mCi (11 MBq), injected intradermally either in the foreskin of the penis or proximal to the cancer. The SLN is usually imaged within 30 minutes, using both the conventional gamma camera and a hand-held gamma probe to identify the SLN by its intense isotope uptake (Figures 4A–C).[5-10] European investigators have used 1.6 mCi (60 MBq) of Tc-99m colloidal albumin (Nanocoll®) to map the SLN.[68] Horenblas and co-workers report performing LSG the day before surgery.[28,31] A focal area of radionuclide accumulation, marking the location of the SLN, is easily discerned, and we recommend leaving a skin marker in this spot. Using the same technique, we search the opposite groin for SLNs as well. At the conclusion of the LSG procedure, anterior and lateral images are obtained (Figures 5–7).[5,10]

We have found that the time between the injection of the Tc-99m-SC and surgery could be at least 2 hours. At surgery, we first inject blue dye. While we have used Patent Blue V, Evans blue, and methylene blue in the past, we now use isosulfan blue dye. We inject 5 ml (cm^3) close to the tumor and gently massage the injection site in order to feel the lymphatic ducts after the blue dye has been injected. We then follow the standard steps of the SLN biopsy technique as for other anatomic sites. A skin incision is made at the point correlating with the "hot spot" identified on LSG and/or by the gamma probe. Dissection to the level of the radiolabeled SLN(s) is carried out, guided by the gamma probe and by blue staining of the lymphatic as they drain to the SLN. Once excised, the SLN can be confirmed by its high ex vivo counts, and by a low level of counts in the surgical bed (Figures 8 and 9).

Figure 4. Lymphangiograms taken at the end of the injection show the draining lymphatic system of the penis. Note the SLN. (A) Anatomical location of SLN. (B) Penile injection of technetium-99m sulfur colloid; SLN visualization bilaterally (tumoral-prepucium injection). (C) Lymphangiograms. End of the injection shows the draining lymphatic system of the penis.

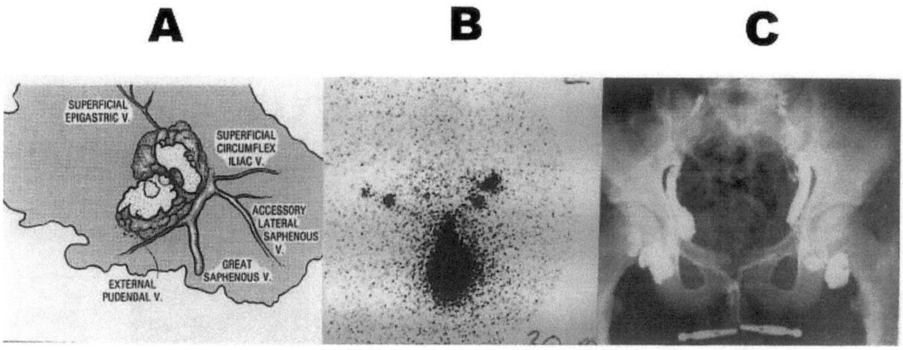

Figure 5. Lymphoscintigraphy reveals one SLN.

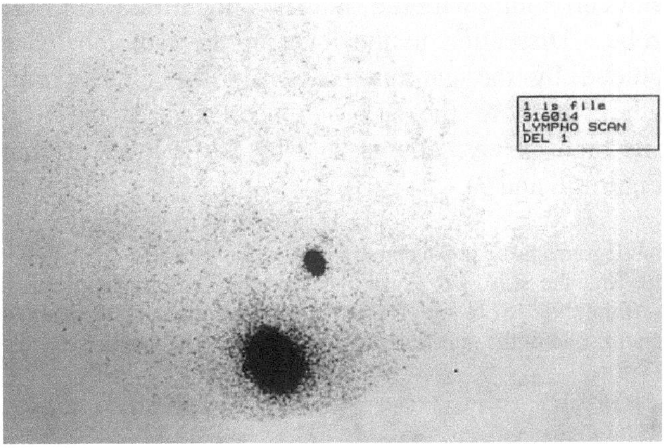

Figure 6. Lymphoscintigraphy reveals two SLN.

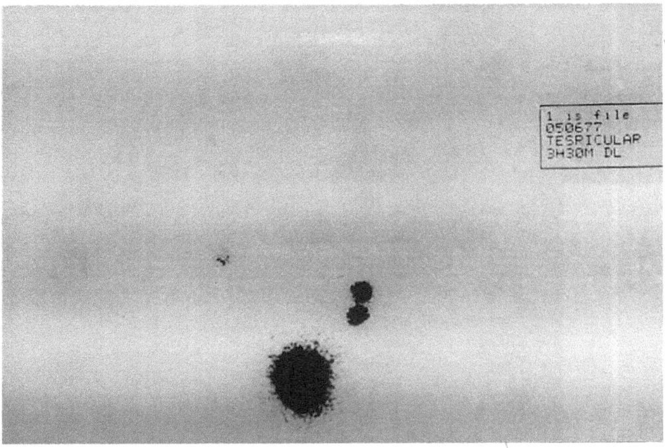

Figure 7. Injection of technetium-99m sulfur colloid visualizes the SLN.

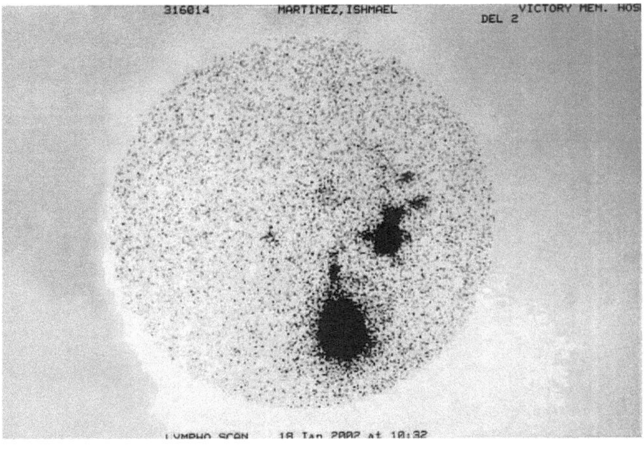

Figure 8. Penile carcinoma. Methylene blue injection. Injection of unfiltered technetium-99m sulfur colloid. The point of maximal emission was marked (SLN).

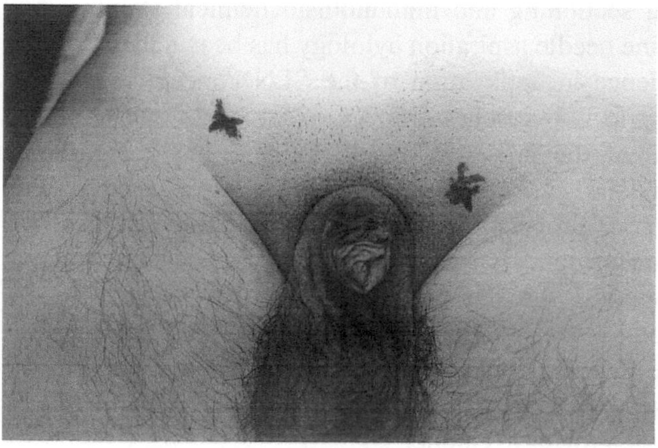

Figure 9. Transcutaneous localization of the SLN using the gamma probe.

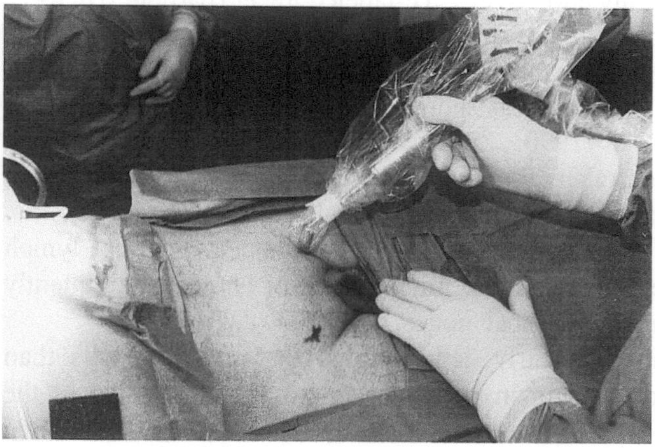

"Skip Metastasis" refers to nodes that are positive when the SLN is negative. Skip metastasis has been found to be related to the lack of experience with performing surgery for the SLN. The incidence decreases with the (greater) experience of the surgeon.[45]

Skip metastasis has been considered to be caused by collateral vessels and/or thick trunk providing a highway or bypass of one or some nodes of the lymphatic basin. Although some surgeons believe that skip metastasis limits the applications of the SLN procedure, we think that the SLN concept accommodates physiologic variations in individual patients, including the possibility of skip metastasis.[49,50]

Refinement of the sentinel node procedure was accomplished by Horenblas and colleagues to avoid false-negative SLN. Pathological analysis was extended by serial sectioning and immunohistochemical staining, and ultrasonography with fine needle aspiration cytology has been added.[35,41]

The larger experience in application of the SLN concept in prostate carcinoma cases belongs to Wawroschek.[70,71]

The identification of the prostatic lymph drainage has a significant clinical importance in the case of tumor spread: Pelvic lymph node metastases indicate a poor prognosis for patients with clinically localized prostate cancer. The prognosis depends on nodal cancer volume, extracapsular extension, and the number of affected lymph nodes. LSG remains the only method to visualize the physiologic lymphatic drainage.

For the first time, Menon and colleagues succeeded in verifying the controversially discussed existence of intraprostatic lymphatic pathways by intraprostatic injection of a tracer in canine.[44]

Gardiner and colleagues were the first to demonstrate lymphatic pathways by transrectal injection of a ^{99m}Tc-labeled tracer (particle size 4–12 nm) into the human prostate capsule.[21] Transperineal injections into the parenchyma and open and periprostatic injections were not successful. A uni- or bilateral lymph drainage was shown in all 40 patients with injections close to the capsule. In 1990, Zuckier and colleagues were able to demonstrate a partly contralateral, pelvic lymphatic drainage in eight out of nine patients with prostate cancer using a comparable technique (70,74).

As of spring 2003, 638 patients have been evaluated. Sentinel lymph nodes are located everywhere in the minor pelvis. The most frequently occurring location is the internal iliac nodes.[70,71]

Furthermore, it will be clearly demonstrated that more patients than previously believed are bearing in particular micrometastasis, also in the case of clinically localized prostate cancer. Those nodes are often exclusively located in the hypogastric region, a region that is normally not included in different forms of so-called modified pelvic (standard) lymphadenectomies.[70,71]

The day before pelvic lymphadenectomy, technetium-99m nanocolloid (Nanocoll, Sorin Co., Italy) was applied transrectally into the prostate under ultrasound guidance. The interval between injection and surgery varied between 18 and 22 hours. A 1-day protocol was an exception. A single central application was done per prostate lobe, rarely two. Depending on the interval between injection and surgery, the chosen activity attained 90–400 MBq (median 267.3 MBq) and the total injected volume was about 2–3 ml.

In the beginning, approximately 30 minutes later and a few hours after injection, scintigraphy (Sopha Camera, DSX, LEAP collimator) was performed in anteroposterior projections, and in single case lateral views.

The prostate was, in part, covered during this procedure. Later the taking of early images was abandoned, because they did not supply additional information about SLN identification. Initially, the SLN were seen to be covered by the inevitable overflow of radioactivity into urine of the bladder, especially in the early images. This problem was reduced by transurethral catheterization. After early imaging was abandoned, this measure was unnecessary.[70,71]

In relation to the intended therapy of prostate cancer (e.g., radiotherapy, perineal or retropubic prostatectomy), pelvic lymphadenectomy was carried out via different surgical accesses. In the majority of patients, a lymphadenectomy was directly followed by radical retropubic prostatectomy (n=282). In the beginning, all patients received sentinel lymphadenectomy (SLNE) plus the dissection of lymph nodes from the obturator fossa and the external iliac lymph nodes (so-called modified lymphadenectomy). Analysis of 121 patients showed that SLNE alone in comparison to modified lymphadenectomy has a sensitivity of about 96%. This result was statistically significant ($p<0.05$) compared to resection of the obturator lymph nodes only. Subsequently, we modified the protocol. In the following, the extent of pelvic lymphadenectomy varied depending on the preoperative risk factors between SLNE only (PSA <10 nm/ml, Gleason Score <7 in biopsy and clinical stage <T3) and SLNE with additional extended pelvic lymphadenectomy (PSA>10 nm/ml, Gleason Score >6 in biopsy or clinical stage >T2). Two cases received no operation after LSG.[70]

The radioactivity of the lymph nodes was measured intraoperatively by different gamma probes. The identification technique was similar to that used in other tumor entities.

Wawroschek in his extensive experience concluded[70,71] that homogeneous surgical standards of pelvic staging lymphadenectomy for prostate cancer cannot be gathered from the current literature. Because of the high morbidity due to extended pelvic lymphadenectomy and the average operating time of 2.5 hours, the area of dissection has been decreased at most centers. Published data on extended pelvic lymphadenectomy in prostate cancer point out that any limitation of the dissection area corresponds to a reduced detection rate of micrometastases. The widespread limitation of the dissection area to the so-called obturator fossa lymph nodes results in missing about 50% of the lymph node-positive patients. This and the at times rather surgically difficult to access locations (presacral, pararectal, paravesical, hypogastric lymph nodes) of the primary draining lymph nodes of the prostate explain the clinical need for radio guided lymph node surgery in prostate cancer.

Our investigation demonstrates that the number of lymph node-positive patients is considerably larger than mentioned in the current literature. Even with comparatively favorable preoperative prognostic factors (PSA<10 nm/ml, clinical stage <T3 and Gleason Score <7 in prostate biopsy) we found lymph node metastases in 11.8% of cases, although staging lymphadenectomy is no standard option in these patients.

As a consequence, lymph node surgery including the primary draining lymph nodes of the prostate is essential for most patients before or during therapy with curative intent (radiotherapy and prostatectomy). This may not only be of prognostic relevance for the patient, but also have a therapeutic background. Recent data from centers (Bern, Augsburg) that perform extended pelvic surgery in the case of radical prostatectomy demonstrate that patients with singular lymph node metastasis are possibly free of PSA recurrence in long-term follow-up.[70] The exploration of bladder and testicle carcinomas is still in the investigational stage.

CONCLUSION

The urological community needs a prospective multi-institutional and international protocol to enroll as many patients as possible so advances in the staging and treatment of solid urological tumors can be obtained.

REFERENCES

1. Alex J, Krag DN. Gamma probe guided localization of lymph nodes. Surg Oncol 2:137-144, 1993.
2. Boak JL, Agwunobi TC. A study of technetium-labeled sulfide colloid uptake by regional lymph nodes draining a tumor-bearing area. Br J Surg 1978. 65:374-378,
3. Bouchot et al. Morbidity of inguinal lymphadenectomy for invasive penile carcinoma. Euro Urol 45: 2004. 761-766.
4. Busch FM, Sayegh ES Roentgen graphic visualization of human testicular lymphatic, J Urol 89:106-110, 1963.
5. Cabanas RM Urologic cancers. The technique of SLN biopsy In: Sentinel Lymph Node Biopsy. Cody HS III (Ed.). Martin Dunitz, 2002, p. 333-338.
6. Cabanas RM, Whitmore WF Jr. The use of testicular lymphatics to bypass obstructed lymphatic in the dog. Invest Urol 18:262, 1981.
7. Cabanas RM. Thesis: Valoracion Quirurgica de la Linfoadenografia Facultad de Ciencias Medicas. Asuncion, Paraguay, 1969.
8. Cabanas RM. An approach for the treatment of penile carcinoma. Cancer 39:456-466, 1977.
9. Cabanas RM. Anatomy and biopsy of sentinel lymph nodes. Penile, urethral and scrotal cancer. Urol Clin of North Am 19:267-276, 1992.

10. Cabanas RM. Application of the sentinel node concept in urological cancer: The concept of the sentinel lymph nodes. Recent Results Cancer Res 157:109-120, 2000.
11. Catalona WJ. Modified inguinal lymphadectomy for carcinoma of the penis with preservation of saphenous veins; technique and preliminary results. J Urol 140:306, 1988.
12. Catalona WJ. Role of lymphadenectomy in carcinoma of the penis. Urol Clin North Am 7:785, 1980.
13. Cubilla A Atlas of Tumor Pathology. Tumor of Prostate Gland, Sentinel Vesicles, Male Urethra and Penis. Armed Forces Institute of Pathology, Washington, DC, 2002, p. 403-476
14. DiSaia PJ, Creasman WT, Rich WM. An alternative approach to early cancer of the vulva. Am J Obstet Gynecol 1979. 133:825-832.
15. Droller MJ: Carcinoma of the penis: An overview. Urol Clin North Am 7:783, 1980.
16. Ekstrom T, Edsmyr F. Cancer of the penis: A clinical study of 229 cases. Acta Chir Scand 115:25, 1958.
17. Fee HJ Robinson DS, Sanyle WF, Graham LS, Holmes EC, Morton DL. The determination of lymph shed by colloidal gold scanning in patients with malignant melanoma: A preliminary study. Surgery 84:626-632, 1978.
18. Fowler JE. Sentinel lymph node biopsy for staging penile cancer. Urology 23:352, 1984.
19. Funaoka S, Tachokawa R, Yamaguchi O, Fujita S. Kurze Mitteilung uber die Rontgenographie des Lymphgefabsystems sowie uber den Mechanismus der Lymphstromung. Arb Anat Inst Kais Univ Kyoto D 1:111, 1930.
20. Gallico E. Giacomelli V, Pricolo V. La colorazione vitale dei limfatici nella chirurgia lel Tumore. Chirurgia 9(3):1-8 1954.
21. Gardiner RA, Fitzpatrick JM, Constable AR et al, Human prostatic lymphoscintigraphy. A preliminary report. Br Urol 51:30-3, 1979.
22. Gervasi LA, Mata J, et al. Prognostic significance of lymph node metastases in prostate cancer. J Urol 142:332, 1989.
23. Giuliano AE, Kurgan DM, Guenther JM, Morton DL. Lymphatic mapping and sentinel lymphoadenectomy for breast cancer. Ann Surg 220:391-401, 1994.
24. Granstald H. Controversies concerning lymph node dissection for cancer of the penis. Urol Clin North Am 7:793, 1980.
25. Harper PV, Lathrop KA, Jimenez et al. Technetium 99m, as a scanning agent. Radiology 85:101-108 1965.
26. Hoppmann HJ, Fraley EE. Squamous cell carcinoma of the penis. J Urol 120:393, 1978.
27. Horenblas S, Jansen L, Meinhardt W, et al, Detection of occult metastasis in squamous cell carcinoma of the penis using a dynamic sentinel node procedure. J Urol 163:100-104, 2000
28. Horenblas S. Lymphanedectomy for squamous cell carcinoma of the penis. Part 1. Diagnosis of lymph node metastasis. BJU Int 88: 467-472, 2001.
29. Horenblas S, Nuyten MJ, Hoefnagel CA, et al. Detection of lymph node invasion in prostatic carcinoma with iliopelvic lymphoscintigraphy. Br Urol 69:180-182, 1992.
30. Horenblas S. Surgical management of carcinoma of the penis and scrotum. Medical Radiology. Diagnostic Imaging and Radiation Oncology. Petrovich Z, Baert L,

Brady LW (Eds.).Carcinoma of the Kidney and Testis, and Rare Urologic Malignancies. Innovations in Management. Springer-Verlag, Berlin, 1999.
31. Horenblas S, The role and technique of lymph node dissection. BJU Int 88: 473-483, 2001.
32. Kaplan WD. Iliopelvic lymphoscintigraphy. Semin Nucl Med 13:42-53, 1983.
33. Kaplan WD, Whitmore WF, Gittes RF. Visualization of canine and human prostatic lymph node following intraprostatic injection of technetium-99m-antimony sulfide colloid. Invest Radiol 15:4-8, 1980.
34. Krag D, Weaver DL, Alex JC, Fairbank JT. Surgical resection and radiolocalization of the sentinel node in breast cancer using gamma probe. Surg Oncol 2:335-340, 1993.
35. Kroon BK, Horenblas S et al. How to avoid false-negative dynamic sentinel node procedures in penile carcinoma. J Urol. 171: 2191-2194, 2004.
36. Levenback C. Intraoperative lymphatic mapping and sentinel node identification: Gynecologic applications. Recent Results Cancer Res 157:150-158, 2000.
37. Levenback C. Gynecologic cancers. In:. Sentinel Lymph Node Biopsy. Cody HS III (Ed.). Martin Dunitz, 2002, p. 339-350.
38. Levi, Dancona, et al. Long-term follow-up of penile carcinoma treated with penectomy and bilateral modified inguinal lymphadenectomy. J Urol. 172: 498-501, 2004.
39. Lima Pompeo AC, et al. Caracterizacao da lesao primaria e sua impotancia no risco de metastases linfonodais em cancer de penis. 29 Congresso Brasileiro de Urologia. TL-114.2003.
40. Lowe FC. Squamus cell carcinoma of the scrotum. Penile, urethral and scrotal cancer. Urol Clin of North Am 19:397-405, 1992.
41. Luciani L, Piscioli G, Scappini P, et al. Value and role of percutaneous regional node aspiration cytology in the management of penile carcinoma. Eur Urol 10:294, 1984.
42. Madeira Campos et al. Avaliacao do possivel valor da expressao imunohistoquimica da pan-caderina e metaloproteases da matriz exra-celular tipo 2 e tipo 9 como fatores preditivos do risco de metastases linfonodais em pacientes portadores de carcinoma epidermoide do penis. 29 Congresso Brasileiro de Urologia. TL-115.2003.
43. McDougal WS, Kirchner FK, Edwards RH, et al. Treatment of carcinoma of the penis: The case for primary lymphadenectomy. J Urol 136:38, 1986.
44. Menon M, Menon S, Strauss HW, Catalona WJ. Demonstration of the existence of canine prostatic lymphatics by radio isotope technique. J Urol 118:274-277, 1977.
45. Morita ET, Chang J, Leong SP. Sentinel lymph nodes in human solid cancer: Surg Clin North Am 80:1721-1739, 2000.
46. Morton DL, Wen D, Wong JH, et al. Technical details of intra-operative lymphatic mapping for early stage melanoma. Arch Surg 127:392-399, 1992.
47. Morton D L, Cagle LA, Wong JH, Economou JS, Foshag LJ, Wen DR, et al. Intraoperative lymphatic mapping and selective lymphadenectomy: technical details of a new procedure for clinical stage 1 melanoma. Presented at the Society of Surgical Oncology, March 1990, Washington, DC.
48. Morton D L, et al. Management of early stage melanoma by intraoperative lymphatic mapping and selective lymphadenectomy. An alternative to routine elective lymphadenectomy or watch and wait. Surg Oncol Clin North Am 1: 247, 1990.

49. Murakami G, Abe M, Abe T. Last intercalated node and direct lymphatic drainage into the thoracic duct from the thoraco-abdominal viscera. Jpn J Thorac Cardiovasc Surg 50:93-103, 2002.
50. Murakami G, Taniguchi I. Histologic heterogeneity and intronodal shunt flow in lymph nodes from elderly subjects: A cadaveric study. Ann Surg Oncol 11(3):278-284S.
51. Narayana AS, Olney LE, Loening SA, et al. Carcinoma of the penis: Analysis of 219 cases Cancer 49:2185, 1982.
52. Nelson AB, et al. Complications of inguinal and pelvic lymphadenectomy for squamos cell carcinoma of the penis: A contemporary series. J Urol 172:494-497, 2004.
53. Nieweg O, et al. (eds.). Lymphatic Mapping and Probe Applications in Oncology. Marcel Dekker, New York, 2000.
54. Perinetti E, Crane DB, Catalona WJ. Unreliability of sentinel lymph node biopsy for staging penile carcinoma. J Urol 124:734,1980.
55. Persky L, de Kernion JB. Carcinoma of the penis. CA 36:258, 1986.
56. Riveros M, Cabanas R, La lymphographie et le cancer due penis. SeM 23:1616, 1968.
57. Riveros M, Garcia R, Cabanas R. Lymphoadenography of the dorsal lymphatics of the penis: Technique and results. Cancer 20:2026, 1967.
58. Sampaio Ribeiro et al. Linfocintilografia na deteccao do linfonodo sentinela para carcinoma espino cellular do penis. 29 Congresso Brasileiro de Urologia. TL-116.2003.
59. Sánchez-Ortiz R, Pettaway CA. The role of lymphadenectomy in penile cancer. Urol Oncol 22(3): 236-244, 2004.
60. Schellhammer PF, Grabstald H. Tumors of the penis and urethra. In Walsh PC, Gittes RF, Perlmutter AD, et al. (eds.). Campbell's Urology, ed 5. Philadelphia, WB Saunders, 1986, p. 1171.
61. Sherman AI, Ter-Pogosian M, Tocus EC. Lymphnode concentration of radioactive colloidal gold following interstitial injection. Cancer 6: 1238-1240, 1953.
62. Sherif A, de la Torre M. et al. Lymphatic mapping and detection of sentinel node in patients with bladder cancer. J Urol 166: 812-815, 2001.
63. Spaulding JT, Grabstald H. Surgery of penile and urethral carcinoma. In Walsh PC, Gittes RF, Perlmutter AD, et al. (eds.). Campbell's Urology, ed 5. Philadelphia, WB Saunders, 1986, p. 2925.
64. Steinbecker KM, Muruve NA. Lymphoscintigraphy for penile cancer. J Urol 163: 1251-1252, 2000.
65. Stone AR, Merrick MV, Chisholm GD. Prostatic lymphoscintigraphy. Br J Urol 51: 556-560, 199 .
66. Tomas Filho et al. Uso intraoperatorio de sondas de deteccao de irradiacao gama para deteccao do linfonodo sentinela em cancer de penis. 29 Congresso Brasileiro de Urologia. TL-117.2003.
67. Tanis PJ Horenblas S, et al. feasibility of sentinel node lymphoscintigraphy in stage I testicular cancer. Eur JNucl Med 29:670-673, 2002.
68. Valdes-Olmos RA, et al. Penile lymphoscintigraphy for sentinel node identification. Eur J Nucl Med 28: 581-585, 2001.
69. Walker L. Localization of radioactive colloids in lymph nodes. J Lab Clin Med 36: 440-449, 1950.

70. Wawroschek F. Pelvic lymphadenectomy in clinically localized prostate cancer — Necessary or superfluous? The Fourth International Symposium — The Lymphatic System. Limburg, Germany, May 13-15, 2004.
71. Wawroschek F. Prostate lymphoscintigraphy and radio-guided surgery for sentinel node identification in prostate cancer. Urol Int 70:303-310, 2003.
72. Wespes E, Simon J, Shulman CC: Cabanas approach: Is sentinel lymph node biopsy reliable for staging penile carcinoma? Urology 28:278, 1986.
73. Whitmore WF, Blute RD, Kaplan WD, Gttes RF. Radiocolloid scintigraphic mapping of the lymphatic drainage for the prostate. J Urol 124:62-67, 1980.
74. Zuckier LS, Finkelstein M, Kreutzer ER, Stone PL, Freed SZ, Bard RH, Blaufox MD, Freeman LM. Technetium-99m antimony, sulphide colloid lymphoscintigraphy of prostate by direct transrectal injection. Nucl Med Com 11:589-596, 1990.

Chapter 9

SELECTIVE SENTINEL LYMPHADENECTOMY FOR GYNECOLOGIC CANCER

Charles Levenback
The University of Texas M. D. Anderson Cancer Center, Houston, Texas

INTRODUCTION

Lymphatic mapping and sentinel node biopsy are the greatest change in the clinical and surgical management of solid tumors since Halsted[1,2] popularized the concepts of radical resection of breast cancers with regional en bloc lymphadenectomy. In the last 10 years, gynecologic oncologists have begun to apply lymphatic mapping and sentinel node biopsy to patients with gynecologic cancers. In this chapter, I will review why vulvar and cervical cancers are good targets for the mapping strategy and review the published experience in patients with vulvar, cervical, and endometrial cancers.

VULVAR CANCER

Pathogenesis

Vulvar cancer is a relatively rare disease. In the United States, just over 3000 new cases of vulvar cancer occur each year, compared with over 175,000 new cases of breast cancer.[3] Over 90% of vulvar cancer patients have a squamous cancer; the rest have a melanoma, adenocarcinoma, or basal cell carcinoma. Two etiologic categories of squamous vulvar cancer have been proposed. In the first, which is related to infection with human papillomavirus (HPV), patients are typically young smokers who present with an invasive cancer within a larger carcinoma in situ. In the second, which is not related to HPV infection, patients are generally older and have no other lower-genital- tract lesions.[4]

Factors leading to chronic irritation of the vulva, including vulvar dystrophy and exposure to perfumes and chemicals, have been implicated in the development of non-HPV-related vulvar cancers. The incidence of vulvar cancer increases continually with age; the incidence does not plateau or decline, like the incidence of some other gynecologic cancers.

Treatment and Prognosis

At the start of the 20th century, Halstedian concepts of radical surgery for solid tumors were applied to vulvar cancer by pioneers including Stanley Way.[5] Radical vulvectomy and bilateral inguinal, femoral, and pelvic lymphadenectomy led to dramatically improved survival for women with vulvar cancers. This procedure was also, however, associated with very high incidence of infection, wound breakdown, and lymphedema. Numerous improvements in surgical techniques and the adoption of less radical surgery have maintained improved cure rates while reducing complications.[6,7] In spite of these improvements, though, lymphedema remains a common, underreported, and largely untreatable complication of treatment for vulvar cancer.

Fortunately, in addition to improvements in surgery, the last 100 years has also been marked by a relaxation of the social taboos associated with gynecologic cancers. Patients are much more likely to report vulvar symptoms, and primary care physicians have been educated regarding the importance of performing a biopsy on any suspicious vulvar lesion.

With earlier diagnosis of vulvar cancer, the prognosis is improved. The size of the primary lesion is directly related to the risk of lymph node metastases (Table 1), which is directly related to survival (Table 2). Metastases to inguinal lymph nodes are typically considered an indication for adjuvant therapy, although some authors believe that patients with only one positive lymph node require no additional treatment. Until recent years, inguinal and low pelvic radiotherapy was the most common adjuvant treatment; however, chemoradiation is now often prescribed.[8]

Table 1. Depth of invasion and risk of nodal metastases in patients with squamous cell cancer of the vulva

Depth of invasion, mm	Risk of metastases,%
≤ 1	0
1.1–2	7.6
2.1–3	8.4
3.1–5	26.7
>5	34.2

Adapted from Berek JS, Hacker NF, eds, *Practical Gynecologic Oncology,* 3rd ed. Philadelphia: Lippincott Williams & Wilkins, 2000.

Table 2. Five-year survival rates by stage for patients with vulvar cancer treated with curative intent

Clinical stage	5-year survival rate, %
I	90.4
II	77.1
III	51.3
IV	18.0
Overall	69.7

Adapted from Berek JS, Hacker NF, eds, *Practical Gynecologic Oncology*, 3rd ed. Philadelphia: Lippincott Williams & Wilkins, 2000.

Lymphatic Mapping

Classic anatomists studied lymphatic anatomy in cadaveric tissue using painstaking dissection and injection of a variety of compounds. The work of Sappey[9] is commonly identified as forming the basis for the radical vulvectomy performed by Way[10] and others. It was not until the mid-20th century that interest in *in vivo* lymphatic anatomy began to grow among gynecologists. In the early 1950s, Eichner[11] directly injected the dye sky blue into the ovaries, cervix, uterus, and vulva of some of his patients and then systematically described the results. The conclusions were not always correct. In the case of the vulva, Eichner preoperatively injected the dye into the deep subcutaneous tissues, although it is not clear how long prior to exploratory laparotomy. In addition, Eichner did not identify afferent lymphatic channels. Eichner reported finding blue staining along the major vessels of the pelvis but never in the inguinal area. Eichner thus concluded that the "labial and vulvar drainage does not go directly into the inguinal nodes..."[12]

In 1963, Parry-Jones published "Lymphatics of the Vulva,"[13] in which he described attempts to, first, determine if the vulvar lymphatics crossed the labial–crural fold, as classically described from cadaver studies, and, second, reveal the path of lymphatic drainage from the vulva directly to the pelvis. Thinking that Eichner had made his injections too deep and following the example of Kinmonth,[14] Parry-Jones approached his first goal by injecting patent blue into the vulvar dermis. In this way, he was able to show that no matter where in the vulva the dye was injected, the dye, and thus the lymphatic channels, never crossed the labial–crural fold. Consequently, Parry-Jones recommended modifying the vulvar incisions during radical vulvectomy so as to spare the skin of the inner thigh and allow primary wound closure.

Reaching his second objective—revealing the path of lymphatic drainage from the vulva to the pelvic—was not so easy. In none of his injected patients could Parry-Jones trace the drainage of patent blue into the pelvis. In fact, in a series of patients undergoing radical vulvectomy, he found that the dye was arrested in the groin and did not reach the pelvis. Unfortunately, Parry-Jones concluded that he had chosen the wrong dye, even though the lymphatic mapping concept as we currently know it was at his fingertips. So he began using Imferon, an iron-containing compound, and deeper injection sites. Histologic analysis of pelvic lymph nodes revealed microscopic evidence of iron particles in the pelvic nodes, leading him to conclude incorrectly that there was direct lymphatic drainage from the vulva to the pelvis. Although iron-containing compounds are now being studied as magnetic resonance lymphography agents, they are not suitable as mapping agents. Direct lymphatic drainage from the vulva to the pelvis has never been convincingly demonstrated.

Cabanas's work with penile lymphography in 1977 is often cited as the start of the modern interest in sentinel nodes.[15] His work was noticed by gynecologic oncologists who looked for application of this concept in the female genital tract. In 1979, DiSaia et al.[16] published "An Alternate Approach to Early Cancer of the Vulva," in which they emphasized the devastating and long-overlooked impact of radical vulvectomy on body image and sexual function. DiSaia et al. challenged the concept that radical vulvectomy was conservative and suggested that radical local excision with superficial inguinal lymphadenectomy was adequate treatment for patients with small vulvar cancers. They described how, in 79 cases, they never observed positive femoral nodes below the cribriform fascia if inguinal nodes above the cribriform fascia were negative. In describing this phenomenon, they cited the work of Cabanas and borrowed his term "sentinel nodes." In contrast to Cabanas's sentinel nodes—one or two nodes that directly drained the primary tumor as demonstrated by lymphography—DiSaia's sentinel nodes comprised the 8–10 inguinal nodes above the cribriform fascia and were identified without mapping procedures.

The Gynecologic Oncology Group protocol 74, reported in 1992, was a prospective study of wide radical vulvar resection and superficial inguinal lymphadenectomy in patients with stage I vulvar cancer.[17] Nine groin recurrences were seen in 121 patients with negative ipsilateral groin dissections (six on the ipsilateral side and three on the contralateral side). These results were supported by the series from The University of Texas M. D. Anderson Cancer Center[18] reported in 1995. These results led to the abandonment of superficial inguinal lymphadenectomy by the Gynecologic Oncology Group and most practicing gynecologic oncologists.

In spite of these results, DiSaia's group continued to report excellent outcomes with their techniques.[19] This led to suspicion that perhaps different groups and individuals were performing different procedures but calling them by the same name. This hypothesis was supported by

Levenback et al.[20] and Micheletti et al.,[21] who focused on the confusing nomenclature regarding groin anatomy.

In 1992, Morton et al. reported their now-well-known work with intraoperative lymphatic mapping and sentinel node identification with blue dye in patients with cutaneous melanoma.[22] Shortly thereafter, the first series of nine patients with vulvar cancer undergoing lymphatic mapping with blue dye confirmed the feasibility of sentinel node identification in this disease site.[23] Since that time, over 300 cases of lymphatic mapping in patients with vulvar cancer have been reported in the literature (Table 3). The general consensus emerging from the data so far is similar to those from lymphatic mapping at other disease sites, as shown in Table 4. Shortening the learning curve is a high priority for gynecologic oncologists since vulvar cancers are so rare. In addition, gynecologic oncologists will accept only a very low rate of false-negative sentinel nodes. Node status is the primary indication for adjuvant treatment. The cure rate for patients with positive regional nodes treated with radiotherapy or chemoradiation is high, with 5-year survival rates in the range of 50–70%.[8] The salvage rate for patients with recurrence in the groin is low, at best 30%.[24] For these reasons, most experts in the field still recommend full lymphadenectomy following sentinel node identification in patients with vulvar cancer.[25]

Two large prospective trials are under way that should provide additional data regarding lymphatic mapping in vulvar cancer and form the basis for phase III trials. Gynecologic Oncology Group protocol 173, "Intraoperative Lymphatic Mapping and Sentinel Node (SN) Identification in Patients with Squamous Cell Carcinoma of the Vulva," is a validation trial of sentinel node identification in the multi-institutional setting. There is also an observational trial of sentinel node dissection alone in selected patients in the Netherlands. Unfortunately, results from these trials will not be known for some time. Most likely, gynecologic oncologists will require a very low false-negative rate in order for sentinel node dissection to completely replace lymphadenectomy in patients with early vulvar cancer. On the other hand, sentinel node dissection helps assure that target nodes are removed and provides an opportunity for extended histologic analysis. I recommend sentinel node dissection to patients with vulvar cancer although I continue to perform regional lymphadenectomy. I perform sentinel lymph node dissection only in rare circumstances including patients with vulvar melanoma, and patients with comorbidities that increase the risk of complications from anesthesia or surgery. Patient preference may also dictate that sentinel node dissection alone be performed.

Table 3. Published studies of lymphatic mapping and sentinel node identification in patients with cervical cancer.

Reference	Stage	Mapping Technique	Surgical Technique	Technical Success (patients)	False (-) (patients)	NPV	Sensitivity	SN Only (+) node
Echt, 1999	IA-Ib	Blue dye	Laparotomy	2/13	0/2	0/0	2/2	1/2
Mendl, 2000	Ib-IIA	Blue dye	Laparotomy	3/3	0/3	0/0	3/3	2/3
Verheijen, 2000	Ib	Blue dye LS	Laparotomy	8/10	0/1	7/7	1/1	1/1
Oboyle, 2000	Ib-IIA	Blue dye	Laparotomy	12/20	0/3	9/9	3/3	2/3
Dargent, 2000	Ib	Blue dye	Laparoscopy	25/35	0/8	17/17	8/8	Unknown
Lantzsch, 2001	Ib	LS	Laparotomy	13/14	0/1	12/12	1/1	0/1
Malur, 2001	I-IV	Blue dye LS	Laparoscopy	39/50	1/6	33/34	5/6	Unknown
Levenback, 2002	Ib	Blue dye LS	Laparotomy	39/39	1/8	31/32	7/8	6/8
Rob, 2002	Ia-Ib2	Blue dye	Laparoscopy Laparotomy	50/65	0	Unknown	Unknown	Unknown
Rhim, 2002*	Ib	Blue dye LS	Laparotomy	25/26	1/5	20/21	4/5	Unknown
Barranger, 2002	Ib	Blue dye LS	Laparoscopy	9/10	0/0	9/9	0/0	0/0
Plante, 2003**	Ib	Blue dye LS	Laparoscopy Laparotomy	61/70	3/11	50/53	8/11	3/11
Marchiole, 2004***	Ia-Ib	Blue dye	Laparoscopy	29/29	3/8	21/24	5/11	2/3
Total				315/384 (82)	9/56 (16.1)	209/218 (95.9)	47/59 (80)	17/32 (53.1)

Technical success: number of patients in which SLNs were found at surgery/total number of patients.

Sensitivity: proportion of patients with pelvic metastases in whom the SLNs contained tumor (true positive/[true positive + false negative]).

Negative predictive value (NPV): proportion of patients without tumor in SLNs in whom the pelvis was free of tumor (true negative/[true negative + false negative]).

Accuracy: proportion of patients with successful SLN biopsy in whom the status of the SLN correlated with the status of the pelvis ([true positive] + true negative/[true positive + true negative + false positive + false negative]).

LS, lymphoscintigraphy; SN, sentinel node.
* Analysis of frozen section results.
** False-negative rate calculated by lymph node basin 0%.
*** Analysis based on serial sectioning and immunohistochemistry of sentinel and non-sentinel nodes.

Table 4. Incidence of pelvic and para-aortic lymph node metastasis by International Federation of Gynecology and Obstetrics stage in patients with cervical carcinoma

Stage	No. of patients	Positive pelvic nodes, %	Positive para-aortic nodes, %
IA1	179	0.5	0
IA2	178	6.2	<1
IB	1926	15.9	2.2
IIA	110	24.5	11
IIB	324	31.4	19
III	125	44.8	30
IVA	23	55.0	40

Adapted from Hatch KD, Cervical cancer. In Berek JD,ed, Practical Gynecologic Oncology, 2nd ed. Baltimore: Williams & Wilkins, 1994, p 243.

TECHNIQUE FOR LYMPHATIC MAPPING OF THE VULVA

Case Selection

Not all patients with vulvar cancer are suitable candidates for lymphatic mapping. Experience indicates that patients with suspicious palpable nodes are not good candidates since tumor or inflammatory reaction in the nodes may alter the lymphatic drainage of the vulva. Patients with tumors larger than 6 cm are not good candidates for similar reasons and because of some uncertainty regarding injection sites. Patients with tumors that extend into the vagina or anus may have lymphatic drainage to the pelvis and, therefore, are not good candidates for this technique. Patients with a small primary lesion and no suspicion of lymphatic metastases on physical examination or cross-sectional imaging are good candidates for lymphatic mapping.

Preoperative Lymphoscintigraphy

A major use of preoperative lymphoscintigraphy is in patients with tumors that may have lymphatic drainage to more than one lymphatic basin. This is a common clinical dilemma in patients with cutaneous melanoma.[26] For example, a patient with a melanoma of the trunk could have drainage to either groin or axilla. Similarly a breast cancer located in the medial third of the breast could have drainage to the axilla or internal mammary lymph nodes. Since all early vulvar tumors drain to the groin, is there any use for preoperative lymphoscintigraphy? The evidence to date suggests that preoperative lymphoscintigraphy may help gynecologic oncologists determine which patients with vulvar cancer require bilateral groin dissection and which patients can be treated with unilateral groin dissection.

The current definition of midline vs. lateral vulvar cancer is strictly arbitrary, yet this is the criterion used to decide whether to perform unilateral or bilateral groin dissections. The common clinical definition of a midline tumor is one within 2 cm of a midline structure, such as the clitoris, anus, urethral meatus, or perineum. The problem of defining midline tumors is further confounded by the fact that, in many patients, the area of invasive disease is surrounded by a zone of carcinoma in situ or inflammation. De Cicco et al.[27] performed preoperative lymphoscintigraphy and gamma probe-guided dissection in 37 patients with vulvar cancer. Eighteen had bilateral lymph node dissections because the tumor was located within 2 cm of the midline. Five of these 18 patients had unilateral drainage on preoperative lymphoscintigraphy. None of the five had a sentinel node or nodal metastasis on the nondraining side at surgery. de Hullu et al.[28] reported a similar experience. In their well-executed study, 12 patients had midline lesions by clinical criteria and unilateral drainage on preoperative lymphoscintigraphy. All 12 patients had bilateral groin dissections. No sentinel nodes or lymph node metastases were found in the 12 dissected groins that did not have lymphatic drainage from the primary tumor on the preoperative lymphoscintigram. Bowles et al.[29] described six patients with tumors located at sites where bilateral drainage would be expected. Five of the six had unilateral drainage on preoperative lymphoscintigraphy. All these studies suggest that preoperative lymphoscintigraphy in patients with vulvar cancer may help determine lymphatic basins at risk for metastases prior to surgery. Conversely, Stehman et al.[30] and Burke et al.[18] each described one patient in whom a vulvar lesion was believed to be unilateral, unilateral dissection was performed, all nodes were negative, and relapse occurred in the contralateral groin in the absence of a new vulvar lesion. Presumably these patients had contralateral lymph node metastases that were not recognized.

In summary, I recommend preoperative lymphoscintigraphy in all patients with vulvar cancer, especially patients with lesions close to the midline. This helps determine which patients require bilateral groin dissections and which patients may safely undergo unilateral groin dissection.

Intraoperative Management

Preoperative lymphoscintigraphy is performed the morning of surgery or perhaps the day before. If lymphoscintigraphy was performed more than 18 hours prior to surgery, the patient is reinjected with radionuclide in the operating room after anesthesia has been induced. The patient is prepped and draped in the usual manner, and then blue dye is injected around the lesion. If bilateral groin dissections are going to be performed by one team, one side is injected first and then the other side is injected when the team has completed the first side. Dye appears in the groin within about 5 minutes of injection and remains in the nodes for 30–45 minutes.

Figure 1. A blue sentinel lymph node in the left groin of a patient with invasive vulvar cancer.

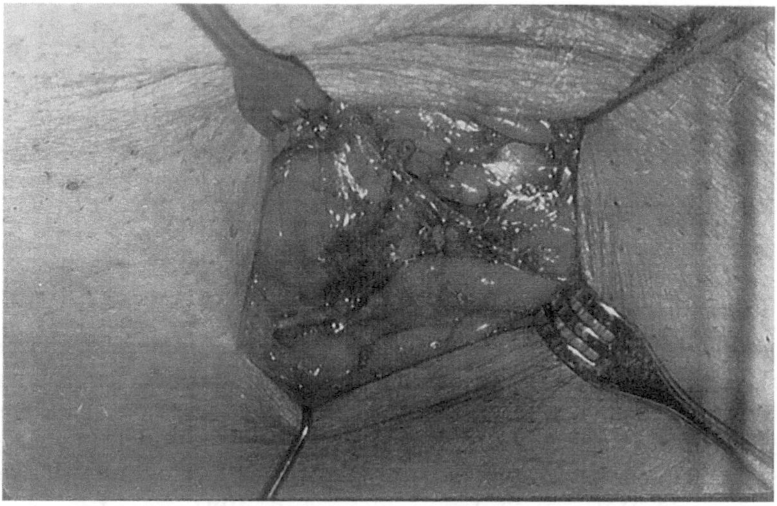

Gynecologic oncologists were commonly taught to mobilize the inguinal femoral fat pad from lateral to medial. Our experience at M. D. Anderson Cancer Center is that the sentinel node in patients with vulvar cancer is frequently found at the medial border of the femoral triangle. If the dissection proceeds lateral to medial, the blue dye will be faint or gone from the sentinel node by the time the medial border is reached. We now carry the incision through the superficial fascia (Camper's fascia) and then immediately start looking for lymphatic channels and the sentinel node in the medial portion of the fat pad. When the sentinel node is central or lateral, an afferent lymphatic channel is usually quickly apparent just below the superficial fascia. The hand-held gamma probe is used, in a fashion similar to how it is used in other disease sites, to help locate the sentinel node and confirm that all significant radioactivity in the lymphatic basin is gone.

CERVICAL CANCER

The incidence of cervical cancer varies throughout the world, but in many regions, it is the leading cause of cancer death in women. In the United States it is estimated that there will be 10,520 new cases of cervical cancer and 3900 deaths from this disease in 2002.[31] This compares with over 200,000 new cases of breast cancer in 2004. The incidence of cervical cancer for the general female population in the United States is 2.5 cases per 100,000 women per year, but it is as high as 43 cases per 100,000 women per year among Vietnamese women. The incidence for Hispanic women is 16.2 cases per 100,000 women per year and for African-American women is 13.2 cases per 100,000 women per year.[32]

The introduction of the Papanicolaou smear in the 1940s led to a dramatic reduction in mortality from cervical cancer in well-screened populations and an increase in the detection of carcinoma in situ. In the United States, deaths from cervical cancer have remained steady in the 1980s and 1990s. Today in the United States, 50% of the patients with cervical cancer have never been screened, and another 10% have not been screened in the last 5 years.

Pathogenesis and Risk Factors

One feature of cervical cancer that distinguishes it from other cancers is that it resembles a sexually transmitted disease. Many epidemiological studies have found an association between sexual behavior of both men and women and the risk of developing cervical cancer. With over 90% of cervical tumors demonstrating HPV DNA, researchers believe that infection with HPV is a likely causative agent. HPV genes E6 and E7 incorporate into the host's genetic material, which results in malignant transformation. HPV has many subtypes, some of which are associated with carcinoma in situ and invasive disease more commonly than others.

HPV infection, however, is probably only one factor involved in the development of cervical cancer. Diet, contraceptive methods, and smoking have also been linked to cervical cancer in women with and without HPV infection. In addition, the timing of HPV infection may be important. In the years following menarche, the cervical epithelium undergoes metaplasia, a process by which glandular epithelium is tranformed into squamous epithelium. This is apparently a vulnerable period, and coitus during this time increases the risk of cervical cancer .[32]

Treatment and Prognosis of Patients with Stage I Cervical Cancer

Cervical cancer is staged clinically. Stage I disease encompasses a wide range of clinical situations and risk categories. Virtually all of the experience with lymphatic mapping in cervical cancer involves patients undergoing radical hysterectomy and pelvic lymphadenectomy. Radical hysterectomy is reserved for patients with clinical stages 1a2, 1b1, 1b2, and occasionally IIa. Radical hysterectomy includes removal of the uterus, cervix, upper vagina, parametrium, and paravaginal tissue to obtain adequate margins around the cervix. Pelvic lymphadenectomy usually refers to all the lymph nodes below the bifurcation of the common iliac arteries. Lymphadenectomy should be extended to include the common iliac and low para-aortic lymph nodes if the pelvic nodes are involved or if the size of the tumor and its histologic feature indicated increased risk of metastatic disease. As is the case with most solid tumors, lymph node status is related to stage and is the most powerful prognostic factor.

Cervical cancer was the first cancer to be cured with radiotherapy. Treatment is initiated with external-beam radiation to parallel opposed fields encompassing the pelvic lymph nodes for a total of 45 Gy. With modern high-energy equipment, skin complications are nonexistent. Modern brachytherapy allows a high dose of radiation to be delivered to the cervix, which itself is relatively radioresistant. Two intracavitary treatments are given 2 weeks apart. The entire course should take about 7 weeks, and treatment should be delayed only if absolutely necessary.

In 1999, several randomized trials reached maturity that demonstrated improved survival with chemoradiation compared with radiation alone for patients with advanced cervical cancer {Morris, 1999 #1401;[33,34] and for patients treated with lymph node metastases found during radical hysterectomy and pelvic lymphadenectomy.[35] Chemoradiation has replaced radiation alone for most high-risk and some intermediate-risk situations.

Cure rates for stage I patients treated with radiotherapy or surgery are essentially the same. The choice of radiotherapy or surgery is based on multiple factors, including the size of the tumor, the likelihood of lymph node metastases, age, body habitus, comorbid conditions, the risk of radiation complications, and patient preference. There is a large range in practice patterns among gynecologic oncologists regarding indications for radical hysterectomy (Figure 2). The Gynecologic Oncology Group is currently conducting a randomized trial, GOG 201, "Treatment of Patients with Stage 1B2 Carcinoma of the Cervix: A Randomized Comparison of Radical Hysterectomy and Tailored Chemo-Radiation versus Primary Chemo-Radiation," to compare chemoradiation and radical surgery plus tailored chemoradiation for patients with stage 1B2 disease.

History of Lymphatic Mapping of the Cervix

The lymphatic drainage of the cervix is complicated and has been studied extensively. Early investigators used India ink[36] and blue dye.[11] The best comprehensive description of the lymphatics of the cervix was provided by Plentl and Friedman in 1971.[37] They described three major pathways of lymphatic drainage of the cervix. The largest and most significant pathway is the lateral trunks. Three branches of the lateral trunks drain to parametrial, obturator, and interiliac sites. The single most common site for sentinel nodes in cervical cancer is the interiliac nodes. These nodes are in contact with both the external iliac artery and vein. Posterior trunks drain to presacral or subaortic lymph nodes. Anterior trunks course along the superior vesical artery and round ligament to inguinal nodes.

The case for lymphatic mapping in cervical cancer is interesting. The cervix is accessible for injection; however, the sentinel node is more difficult to reach than in the groin. Three techniques are available: laparotomy, retroperitoneal dissection, and laparoscopy. In patients with stage 1b1 or 1b2 disease, knowledge of nodal status is the single most important factor in determining the need for adjuvant therapy. Sentinel lymph node dissection could assist with treatment selection in these patients. However, other facts argue against the use of sentinel node dissection in cervical cancer: lymphedema does not appear to be as common following pelvic lymphadenectomy as it is following groin dissection. In addition, the negative impact of radiotherapy on the incidence of lymphedema is not as great with pelvic irradiation as with groin irradiation. Another problem with lymphatic mapping in the cervix relates to the parametrial lymph nodes. One patient in the literature had negative sentinel nodes in the pelvis and multiple small microscopic lymph node metastases in medial parametrial nodes that were resected with the primary tumor.[38] The medial parametrial nodes are too close to the primary tumor to be imaged with lymphoscintigraphy or blue dye. More data will be required to determine if this circumstance occurs regularly or not.

Cervical cancer is an interesting target for lymphatic mapping since lymphatic mapping at this site can be combined with laparoscopy. Dargent et al.,[39] Roy et al.,[40] and Malur et al.[41] have reported excellent results with laparoscopic identification of sentinel nodes. This technique may allow identification of node-positive patients without laparotomy. Laparoscopy has also been combined with radical vaginal trachelectomy as a fertility-sparing procedure for women with early cervical cancers.[42] Patients eligible for this fertility-sparing procedure have a very low rate of node positivity, and lymphatic mapping and sentinel node identification appears to be a natural adjunct to this procedure. Institution of this procedure would permit less dissection in the pelvis and presumably reduce the number of fertility-compromising adhesions.

Early reports of lymphatic mapping of the cervix were limited to series with few patients.[43,44] More recently, larger series[41,45-47] have demonstrated high sensitivity and low false-negative rates. Most observers suggest that the use of radiocolloid and blue dye results in higher success rates.

Technique for Lymphatic Mapping of the Cervix

Case Selection

As is the case for lymphatic mapping of other disease sites, patients with lymph nodes congested with tumor metastases or inflammatory debris that alters lymphatic drainage are not good candidates for lymphatic mapping of the cervix. Patients with tumors that replace the cervix such that there is no visible normal cervical mucosa are also not good candidates, since the injection will be intratumoral. Intuitively, all patients with cervical cancer should have bilateral lymphatic drainage, yet 10–20% of patients in most series have sentinel nodes identified on only one side of the pelvis. It is unknown if previous cone biopsy, obstetrical trauma, or a history of pelvic inflammatory disease alters lymphatic drainage of the cervix.

Preoperative Lymphoscintigraphy

The utility of preoperative lymphoscintigraphy in patients with cervical cancer is limited. Both pelvic lymphatic basins can be inspected through the same incision, and therefore, preknowledge of the location of the sentinel node is not that valuable. In addition, sentinel nodes in the groin have not been described. Finally, the sentinel node is frequently close to the cervix and, therefore, difficult to see on a lymphoscintigram. The use of radiocolloid is extremely valuable; however, the additional time and expense of the scan is hard to justify except for patients in clinical trials.

Figure 2. Radical hysterectomy specimen in a patient with stage Ib1 cervical cancer. Injection of radiocolloid and blue dye was made into the submucosa at 3, 6, 9, and 12 o'clock.

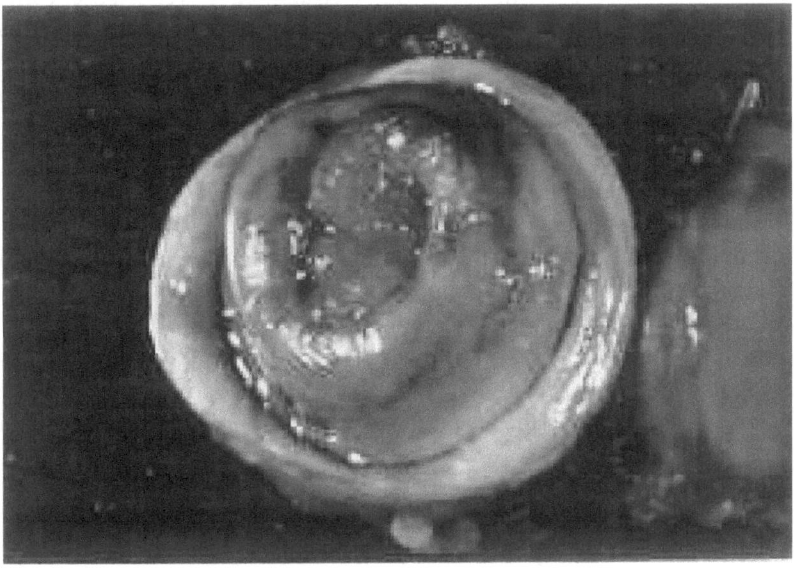

Intraoperative Management

After general anesthesia is induced, the patient is placed in a modified lithotomy position that permits intraoperative cervical injection. Before the patient is prepped and draped, a speculum is introduced into the vagina, and radiocolloid is injected peritumorally. The radiocolloid is injected submucosally. The routine prep and draping is performed, and the abdomen is opened. A vertical or low transverse incision can be used. The upper abdomen is manually explored, and then the bowel is packed out of the pelvis. Blue dye is then injected in a fashion similar to how the radiocolloid was injected. Within minutes, the dye can be seen filling afferent lymphatic channels and lymph nodes. Using a combination of the hand-held gamma probe and visualization of the blue dye, sentinel nodes are identified.

The most common site for sentinel nodes is along the external iliac vessels. Leveuf and Godard[48] were the first to describe this location as the primary lymphatic drainage site of the cervix based on their work with fetal cadavers. It is common to find blue or radioactive ("hot") nodes in the common iliac and low para-aortic regions in patients with sentinel nodes in the pelvis. Are these additional nodes sentinel or second-echelon lymph nodes? It is not possible to determine this with current technology, and both are possibilities. For this reason, I label all nodes that are blue or radioactive above well-accepted thresholds[49] sentinel nodes.

Histologic Evaluation of Sentinel Nodes

Extensive experience with sentinel nodes in patients with breast cancer and melanoma has demonstrated that extensive histologic evaluation with serial sectioning and immunohistochemical staining increases the rate of detection of metastatic disease by 40%.[50] Preliminary results in patients with vulvar cancer indicate that the increase in the rate of detection of nodal metastasis with extended histologic evaluation of the sentinel node(s) in patients with squamous cancers is much less, perhaps less than 10%.[51]

Intraoperative evaluation of sentinel nodes in patients with cervical cancer varies widely. Some gynecologic oncologists perform frozen sections on all pelvic lymph nodes and abandon radical hysterectomy in favor of chemoradiation if any positive node is encountered. Other gynecologic oncologists do not abort radical hysterectomy even when grossly positive nodes are encountered. In patients with vulvar cancer, some gynecologic oncologists curtail groin dissection when a grossly positive node is encountered, removing only the grossly involved nodes with the knowledge that the patient will undergo radiotherapy postoperatively. The rationale for this approach is that the overall morbidity of the combined treatment is reduced by limiting the extent of the dissection in the pelvis or groin.

Molecular studies of sentinel nodes in patients with gynecologic cancer are very limited. Van Trappen et al.[52] studied the presence of cytokeratin in pelvic nodes in patients with cervix cancer, and Malur et al.[41] searched for HPV DNA fragments in sentinel lymph nodes.[41] There is a need for further study of sentinel nodes in patients with squamous carcinomas of the vulva and cervix to improve the intraoperative and postoperative histologic and molecular analysis of sentinel nodes.

ENDOMETRIAL CANCER

Pathogenesis of Endometrial Cancer

The majority of endometrial cancers are the result of a hyperestrogenic state associated with obesity, early menarche, late menopause, nulliparity, or exogenous estrogen use. A small proportion of cases of the less common histologic subtypes, such as papillary serous carcinoma and carcinosarcoma, are probably random. There is increasing awareness of the role of heredity in endometrial cancer, especially in association with cancers of the colon in young patients.[53] All patients with endometrial cancer share a common presenting symptom, abnormal vaginal bleeding. Endometrial biopsy is an easy office procedure that is highly effective at diagnosing endometrial cancers and premalignant conditions.

Treatment and Prognosis

The primary treatment of endometrial cancer is removal of the uterus, fallopian tubes, ovaries, and pelvic and para-aortic lymph nodes. The risk of lymph node metastases is related to the grade of the primary tumor and depth of invasion. Patients with a grade 1 endometrioid endometrial adenocarcinoma limited to the endometrium have a 1–2% chance of pelvic node metastases, whereas patients with a high-grade lesion and deep invasion have a risk of 30–40%. Some gynecologic oncologists perform extended lymphadenectomy in all patients, while others tailor the dissection to the extent of uterine involvement based on intraoperative involvement.

History of Lymphatic Mapping of the Uterus

Plentl and Friedman[37] provided an in-depth analysis of the lymphatics of the uterus. The uterus has several lymphatic drainage routes, including along the uterine vessels to the pelvis, along the gonadal vessels to the high para-aortics, and along the round ligament to the groin. The latter route is rare since isolated metastases to the groin are extremely uncommon.

The uterus has proved to be a difficult target for lymphatic mapping. The tumor itself is not easily available for injection. Burke et al.[54] described serosal injections of blue dye in patients undergoing hysterectomy for endometrial cancer. These authors reported that sentinel nodes were found in the pelvis and between the renal vessels and origin of the inferior mesenteric artery but not between the inferior mesenteric artery and bifurcation of the aorta. Building upon this original work has proved difficult. Intraoperative injections of the uterus with radiocolloid with intraoperative lymphoscintigraphy have not been successful (Diane Bodurka, M.D., personal communication, 4/2004). The most innovative recent effort has been by Niikura et al.[55] This group performed preoperative hysteroscopy and intrauterine injection of radiocolloid and successfully identified pelvic and para-aortic radioactive sentinel nodes.

Lymphatic mapping in patients with endometrial cancer is confounded by the comorbid conditions frequently found in these patients, especially obesity. In addition, with the median patient age in the 60s, additional operative time must be carefully weighed and have a clear benefit to the patient. At present, there is no standardized technique for lymphatic mapping of the endometrium.

CONCLUSION

Sentinel node identification holds great promise for women with gynecologic cancers for reduction of surgical morbidity with improved identification of women with metastatic disease. Vulvar and cervical carcinomas are especially good targets for the sentinel node strategy, since chemoradiation improves survival for node-positive patients; however, when added to radical surgery, it also contributes significantly to morbidity. Progress in patients with cervical and vulvar cancer is hampered by the relative infrequency of patients with early disease most suitable for this approach. Much more work will be required in patients with endometrial cancer to overcome technical problems with sentinel node identification in this setting.

REFERENCES

1. Halsted, W., The results of operations for the cure of cancer of the breast performed at the Johns Hopkins Hospitals. Ann Surg, 1894. **20**: p. 497.
2. Halsted, W., The results of radical operations for the cure of carcinoma of the breast. Ann Surg, 1907. **46**: p. 1.
3. Landis, S.H., et al., Cancer statistics, 1999. CA Cancer J Clin, 1999. **49**(1): p. 8-31, 1.
4. Bloss, J.D., et al., Clinical and histologic features of vulvar carcinomas analyzed for human papillomavirus status: evidence that squamous cell carcinoma of the vulva has more than one etiology. Hum Pathol, 1991. **22**: p. 711-718.
5. Way, S., Carcinoma of the vulva. Malignant disease of the female genital tract. 1951, Philadelphia: The Blakiston Co. p. 27-28.
6. Hacker, N.F., et al., Radical vulvectomy and bilateral inguinal lymphadenectomy through separate groin incisions. Obstet Gynecol, 1981. **58**: p. 574-579.
7. Morris, J.M., A formula for selective lymphadenectomy: its application to cancer of the vulva. Obstet Gynecol, 1977. **50**: p. 152-158.
8. Katz, A., et al., The role of radiation therapy in preventing regional recurrences of invasive squamous cell carcinoma of the vulva. Int J Radiat Oncol Biol Phys, 2003. **57**(2): p. 409-418.
9. Sappey, P., Anatomie, physiologie et pathology, des vaisseaux lymphatiques consideres chez l'homme et les vertebres. 1885, Paris.
10. Way, S., Carcinoma of the vulva. Am J Obstet Gynecol, 1960. **79**: p. 692.
11. Eichner, E., I. Goldberg, and E.R. Bove, In vivo studies with direct sky blue of the lymphatic drainage of the internal genitals of women. Am J Obstet Gynecol, 1954. **67**(6): p. 1277-1286.
12. Eichner, E., L.P. Mallin, and M.L. Angell, Further experience with direct sky blue in the in vivo studies of gynecologic lymphatics. Am J Obstet Gynecol, 1955. **69**(5): p. 1019-1026.

13. Parry-Jones, E., Lymphatics of the vulva. J Obstet Gynaecol Br Commonw, 1963. **70**: p. 751-765.
14. Kinmonth, J., Lymphangiography in man. Clinical Science, 1952. **11**: p. 13-20.
15. Cabanas, R.M., An approach for the treatment of penile carcinoma. Cancer, 1977. **39**(2): p. 456-466.
16. DiSaia, P.J., W.T. Creasman, and W.M. Rich, An alternate approach to early cancer of the vulva. Am J Obstet Gynecol, 1979. **133**: p. 825-832.
17. Stehman, F.B., et al., Groin dissection versus groin radiation in carcinoma of the vulva: a Gynecologic Oncology Group study. Int J Radiat Oncol Biol Phys, 1992. **24**: p. 389-396.
18. Burke, T.W., et al., Surgical therapy of T1 and T2 vulvar carcinoma: further experience with radical wide excision and selective inguinal lymphadenectomy. Gynecol Oncol, 1995. **57**: p. 215-220.
19. Berman, M.L., et al., Conservative surgical management of superficially invasive stage I vulvar carcinoma. Gynecol Oncol, 1989. **35**: p. 352-357.
20. Levenback, C., et al., Potential applications of intraoperative lymphatic mapping in vulvar cancer. Gynecol Oncol, 1995. **59**(2): p. 216-220.
21. Micheletti, L., et al., A proposed glossary of terminology related to the surgical treatment of vulvar carcinoma. Cancer, 1998. **83**(7): p. 1369-1375.
22. Morton, D.L., et al., Technical details of intraoperative lymphatic mapping for early stage melanoma. Arch Surg, 1992. **127**(4): p. 392-399.
23. Levenback, C., et al., Intraoperative lymphatic mapping for vulvar cancer. Obstet Gynecol, 1994. **84**(2): p. 163-167.
24. Gordinier, M.E., et al., S-Phase fraction, p53, and HER-2/neu status as predictors of nodal metastasis in early vulvar cancer. Gynecol Oncol, 1997. **67**(2): p. 200-202.
25. Levenback, C., et al., Letter regarding Terada, E., et al., Sentinel node dissection and ultrastaging in squamous cell carcinoma of the vulva, T.e. al, Editor. 2000, Gynecol Oncol. p. 484-485.
26. Morton, D.L., Sentinel lymphadenectomy for patients with clinical stage I melanoma. J Surg Oncol, 1997. **66**(4): p. 267-269.
27. De Cicco, C., et al., Sentinel node biopsy in early vulvar cancer. Br J Cancer, 2000. **82**(2): p. 295-299.
28. de Hullu, J.A., et al., Sentinel lymph node procedure is highly accurate in squamous cell carcinoma of the vulva. J Clin Oncol, 2000. **18**(15): p. 2811-2816.
29. Bowles, J., et al., Preoperative lymphoscintigraphy in the evaluation of squamous cell cancer of the vulva. Clin Nucl Med, 1999. **24**(4): p. 235-238.
30. Stehman, F.B., et al., Sites of failure and times to failure in carcinoma of the vulva treated conservatively: a Gynecologic Oncology Group study. Am J Obstet Gynecol, 1996. **174**(4): p. 1128-1132; discussion 1132-1133.
31. Jemal, A., et al., Cancer statistics, 2002. CA Cancer J Clin, 2002. **52**(1): p. 23-47.
32. Levenback, C., Cancer of the uterine cervix, in Conn's Current Therapy, Rakel, Editor. 1999, W. B. Saunders: Philadelphia. p. 1066-1069.
33. Rose, P.G., et al., Concurrent cisplatin-based chemotherapy and radiotherapy for locally advanced cervical cancer. N Engl J Med, 1999. **340**: p. 1144-1153.
34. Keys, H.M., et al., Cisplatin, radiation, and adjuvant hysterectomy compared with radiation and adjuvant hysterectomy for bulky stage IB cervical carcinoma. N Engl J Med, 1999. **340**: p. 1154-1161.
35. Peters, W.A., III, et al., Concurrent chemotherapy and pelvic radiation therapy compared with pelvic radiation therapy alone as adjuvant therapy after radical surgery in high-risk early-stage cancer of the cervix. J Clin Oncol, 2000. **18**(8): p. 1606-1613.
36. Zeit, P.R. and G. Wilcoxon, In vivo coloring of pelvic lymph nodes with India ink. Am J Obstet Gynecol, 1950. **59**(5): p. 1164-1166.

37. Plentl, A.A. and E.A. Friedman, Lymphatics of the cervix uteri, in Lymphatic System of Female Genitalia. 1971, W. B. Saunders: Philadelphia. p. 75-115.
38. Levenback, C., et al., Intraoperative lymphatic mapping and sentinel node identification with blue dye in patients with vulvar cancer. Gynecol Oncol, 2001. **83**(2): p. 276-281.
39. Dargent, D., et al. Identification of a sentinel node with laparoscopy in cervical cancer, in Program and Abstracts of the 31st Annual Meeting of the Society of Gynecologic Oncologists, 2000, San Diego, California.
40. Roy, M., et al., Vaginal radical hysterectomy versus abdominal radical hysterectomy in the treatment of early-stage cervical cancer. Gynecol Oncol, 1996. **62**: p. 336-339.
41. Malur, S., et al., Sentinel lymph node detection in patients with cervical cancer. Gynecol Oncol, 2001. **80**(2): p. 254-257.
42. Dargent, D., et al., Laparoscopic vaginal radical trachelectomy. Cancer, 2000. **88**: p. 1877-1882.
43. Echt, M., et al., Detection of sentinel lymph nodes with lymphazurin in cervical, uterine, and vulvar malignancies. South Med J, 1999. **92**(2): p. 204-208.
44. Terada, K., D. Shimizu, and J. Wong, Sentinel node dissection and ultrastaging in squamous cell cancer of the vulva. Gynecol Oncol, 2000. **76**(1): p. 40-44.
45. Levenback, C., et al., Lymphatic mapping and sentinel node identification in patients with cervix cancer undergoing radical hysterectomy and pelvic lymphadenectomy. J Clin Oncol, 2002. **20**(3): p. 688-693.
46. Dargent, D., X. Martin, and P. Mathevet, Laparoscopic assessment of the sentinel lymph node in early stage cervical cancer. Gynecol Oncol, 2000. **79**(3): p. 411-415.
47. Plante, M., et al., Laparoscopic sentinel node mapping in early-stage cervical cancer. Gynecol Oncol, 2003. **91**(3): p. 494-503.
48. Leveuf, J. and H. Godard, Les lymphatiques de l'uterus. Revue de Chirurgie, 1923. **3**: p. 219-248.
49. Essner, R. and D.L. Morton, The blue-dye technique, in Sentinel Lymph Node Biopsy, H.S. Cody, Editor. 2002, Martin Dunitz Ltd: London. p. 91-104.
50. Cochran, A.J., The pathologist's role in sentinel lymph node evaluation. Semin Nucl Med, 2000. **30**(1): p. 11-17.
51. Moore, R.G., et al., Pathologic evaluation of inguinal sentinel nodes in vulvar cancer patients: a comparison of immunohistochemical staining versus ultra-staging with hematoxylin and eosin staining, in Programs and Abstracts of the 34th Annual Meeting of the Society of Gynecologic Oncologists, 2003, New Orleans, Louisiana.
52. Van Trappen, P., et al., Molecular quantification and mapping of lymph-node micrometastases in cervical cancer. Lancet, 2001. **357**(9249): p. 15-20.
53. Watson, P., et al., The risk of endometrial cancer in hereditary nonpolyposis colorectal cancer. Am J Med, 1994. **96**(6): p. 516-520.
54. Burke, T.W., et al:, Intraabdominal lymphatic mapping to direct selective pelvic and paraaortic lymphadenectomy in women with high-risk endometrial cancers: results of a pilot study. Gynecol Oncol, 1996. **62**(2): p. 169-173.
55. Niikura, H., et al., Sentinel lymph node detection in patients with endometrial cancer. Gynecol Oncol, 2004. **92**(2): p. 669-674.

Chapter 10

SELECTIVE SENTINEL LYMPHADENECTOMY FOR HEAD AND NECK SQUAMOUS CELL CARCINOMA

Jochen A. Werner
Department of Otolaryngology, Head and Neck Surgery, Philipps University of Marburg, Germany

INTRODUCTION

It is not new to describe the regional lymphatic drainage of malignant cancer in the head and neck by means of scintigraphic methods. First detailed examinations were performed by Fisch.[1,2] The objective initially associated with lymphoscintigraphy of the head and neck was to detect metastatic lymph nodes from malignant tumors. The investigation of this method was then neglected because it became obvious that especially metastatic lymph nodes could only be described insufficiently by scintigraphy or it was not possible at all.[3-5]

The renaissance of scintigraphic description that can be observed in the discussion of the value of the sentinel node concept is based on its application under another aspect and thus also objective. In earlier studies on lymphoscintigraphy, this examination method was generally performed in the case of suspected lymphogenic metastatic spread in order to determine the location of the metastases. In the context of the sentinel node concept, scintigraphy is performed on patients without clinical indication of lymphogenic metastatic spread in order to identify the lymph node draining the lymph fluid of the tumor region. This purpose is justified in patients who might develop occult metastatic spread into the first lymph node station due to the tumor size and location. Thus, the scintigraphic description of the lymphatic pathways draining a primary tumor of the upper aerodigestive tract serves to identify the so-called sentinel lymph node for which physiologic integrity is still intact. Only the following histological examination reveals a possible metastatic spread in the sense of micro- or limited macrometastasis.[6]

The detailed descriptions of the differences in density and the specific regional distribution pattern of the initial lymph vessels in the area of the upper aerodigestive tract are the basis for investigating the first question.[7-10] So individual modalities of the specific lymphatic drainage region of a primary tumor determine the location of the first draining lymph node. Basic principles for understanding the metastatic process of carcinomas located in the area of the upper aerodigestive tract were elaborated by Lindberg.[11] Lindberg neglected the grouping of the cervical lymph nodes mainly correlated anatomically as it was applied before his time and divided the lymphonodular system of the head and neck based on pathophysiological mechanisms. For this purpose, Lindberg performed a retrospective investigation of 2044 medical records of patients with squamous cell carcinomas of the head and neck who had not received prior treatment. Lindberg divided nine lymph node regions on each side and additionally the parotideal lymph nodes. With his investigations he created the bases for the understanding of a metastatic direction, which is predictable with a certain probability. This fact is of significant importance for the clinical application of the sentinel node concept in the head and neck.

The lymph fluid of the upper aerodigestive tract is drained via about 300 regional cervical lymph nodes, which are divided according to the current classification established by Robbins et al.[12] into nine lymph node levels (levels I–VI) (Figure 1). Level I is limited by the body of the mandible, the anterior belly of the contralateral digastric muscle as well as the anterior and posterior belly of the ipsilateral digastric muscle. Level II reaches from the skull base to the carotid bifurcation (surgical landmark). In the dorsal direction, it is limited by the posterior edge and in the ventral direction by the lateral edge of the sternocleidomastoid muscle. Level III reaches from the carotid bifurcation to the crossing of the omohyoid muscle with the internal jugular vein (surgical landmark). Level IV reaches from the crossing of the omohyoid muscle internation jugular vein to the clavicle. The dorsal and ventral borders of levels III and IV correspond to those of level II. Level V contains all lymph nodes of the so-called posterior triangle. In the posterior direction the borders are the anterior edge of the trapezius muscle, in the anterior direction the borders are limited by the posterior edge of the sternocleidomastoid muscle, and in the caudal direction by the clavicle. Level VI reaches from the hyoid bone to the jugulum. The lateral border is located on both sides medially to the carotid artery.

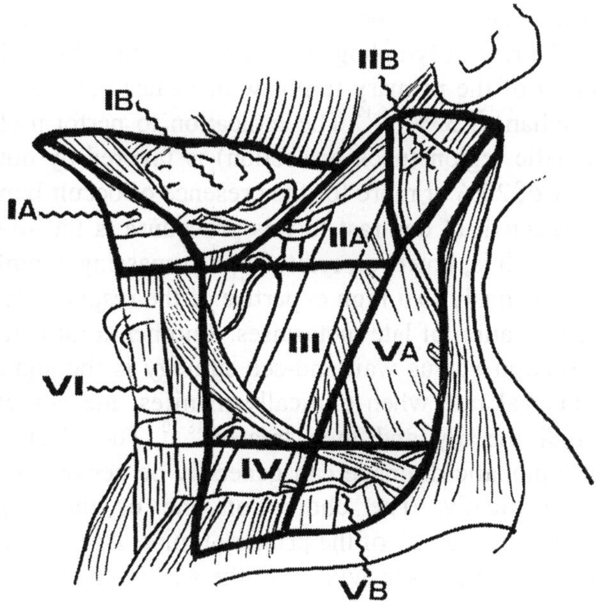

Figure 1. Actualized classification of the lymph node levels according to Robbins et al. (2002). From Ref. 78.

Depending on the density and direction of the initial lymph vessels in the region of the primary tumor, a preferred drainage exists in one or more of these lymph node groups for each tumor location of the upper aerodigestive tract.[13] At this point it must be mentioned critically that despite the lymphatic drainage along relatively constant and predictable lymph node groups, variations may arise in single cases even without prior therapeutical measures and even a skipping of the primarily draining lymph nodes can be observed in about 5% of the cervical metastases. Nonetheless the knowledge of the preferred drainage directions justifies a targeted investigation of those lymph nodes, which are located in the main drainage region of a primary tumor.[14]

Due to the fact that the prognosis of patients suffering from squamous cell carcinoma of the upper aerodigestive tract depends significantly on the presence or absence of lymphogenic metastatic spread the question of detecting clinically occult lymph node metastases is still the focus of discussion concerning the management of the clinical N0 neck. In the literature the rate of lymphogenic metastatic spread is indicated to depend on the location of the primary tumor with values between 12% and over 50% with a median of 33%.[15-17] The indication to perform elective treatment of the lymphatic region (neck dissection) is favored by numerous authors if a probability of 20% or more for the presence of occult lymph node metastases can be expected. In contrast to this procedure is the so-called wait-and-see strategy, which is, however, related to a surpassing compliance of the patient and simultaneously to a high expertise of the responsible physician allowing early identification of late metastases. Another argument in favor of elective neck dissection versus wait-and-see strategy is the significant deterioration of the survival rate when clinically manifest metastases are only detected after initial therapy and then treated.[18-20] The elective treatment of the regional lymphatic drainage can generally be performed either surgically or radiotherapeutically. The choice of one of these procedures depends generally on the therapy of the primary tumor. An advantage of elective neck dissection in comparison with radiotherapy is that histological examination of the neck dissection specimen can give important information for a decision as to therapy and prognosis, and in the sense of staging examination.[21]

The described problems make clear which difficulties arise in the context of the controversial discussion of the optimized therapy regime for clinical N0 neck. Regarding the efforts to find a consistent diagnostic and therapuetic procedure, reliable diagnostic methods for identification of possible occult metastatic spread become more and more important. The encouraging result concerning other tumor entities may explain the increasing interest in the so-called sentinel node concept for squamous cell carcinomas of the upper aerodigestive tract.

PREOPERATIVE DYNAMIC LYMPHOSCINTIGRAPHY AND TRANSCUTANEOUS IDENTIFICATION OF THE SENTINEL NODE

The classic concept of sentinel node biopsy as it is performed in cases of breast cancer and malignant melanoma consists of pretherapeutic dynamic lymphoscintigraphy in order to determine preoperatively the location of the sentinel node. Due to the mostly sufficient distance of the injection point (primary tumor) from the first draining lymph node station, this tumor entity generally allows a transcutaneous determination of the location of the sentinel node by means of a gamma probe. In comparison, the topographic relationships in the head and neck are significantly more complex. The main reasons for this are the high lymph node density of about 300 cervicofacial lymph nodes as well as the small distance between the injection point and the first draining lymph node station.

In contrast to breast cancer and malignant melanoma, the technical performance of the dynamic lymphoscintigraphy of the head and neck should not be limited to the isolated description of the injection point and the first draining lymph node station. An adequate evaluation and anatomic assignment of the draining lymph node station is favored by the additional description of the head and neck silhouette[22] which can be achieved by placing a radioactive phantom behind the patient's head. A simultaneous mapping of the bony structures by intravenous application of 8 mCi ^{99m}Tc-HDP allows an optimized anatomic orientation (Figure 2) and thus facilitates the topographic assignment of the described lymph node stations.[23]

Figure 2. Left-sided carcinoma of the tonsil (t) with neighboring sentinel node (s) close to the primary tumor.

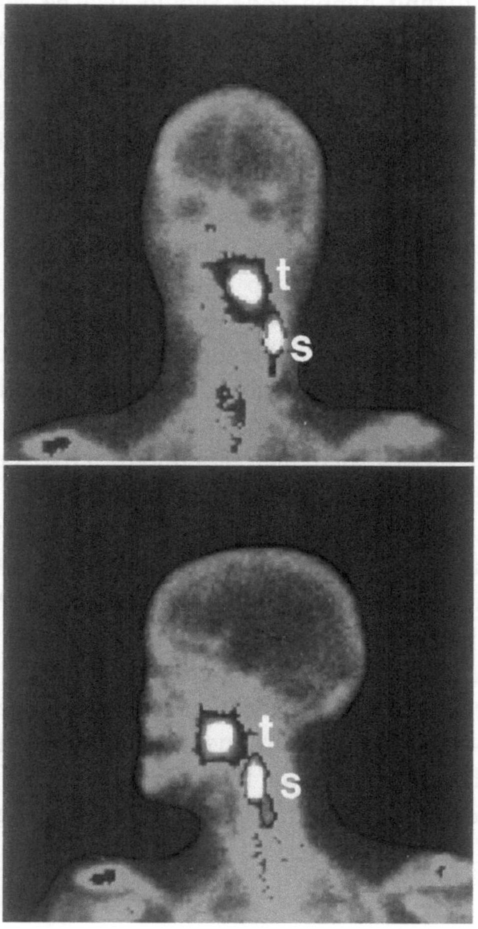

The dynamic lymphoscintigraphy with documentation under a double detector camera can visualize the lymphatic drainage into the regional lymph node stations by means of image processing techniques, which allow the demarcation of the first draining lymph node station from the injection point. The margin around the injection point and the sentinel nodes resulting from the summation effect illustrates the significant difficulties arising from the exact demarcation of the injection point and the sentinel lymph nodes performed transcutaneously by means of a gamma probe.

Because the value of this new diagnostic and therapeutic procedure is directly related to the reliable detection of the actual sentinel node, the last-mentioned statement represents an immense challenge for the detection technique of the sentinel node in the head and neck beside the disperse radiation of the directly neighboring primary tumor. In order to reliably detect the lymph node with the highest tracer uptake by means of transcutaneous measurement of the neck with a gamma probe, some of the requirements of the measurement system are obligatory.

A tracer-accumulating lymph node should also be selectable in tissue, which itself is radioactively concerned. The disperse radiation from the injection point must not falsify the location of the lymph node to be detected. If more lymph nodes are located in the direct surroundings of the sentinel node, a clear distinction must be made between nonsentinel and sentinel node. The local resolution must therefore allow an exact separation between two lymph nodes. The detection of the lymph node with the highest tracer uptake should be possible over several tissue layers.

With this background, the group at Marburg examined the detection spectrum of a gamma probe for identification of cervical lymph nodes in an in vitro model. It was found that a direct relationship between the number of radiation sources and their isolated detection could be shown. A measurement series with 0.4 cm muscle tissue and two radiation sources arranged in two rows revealed that if a more active radiation source is situated 1.5 cm behind the less active specimen, then the radiation sources can only be resolved with a maximal detector distance of Y=1 cm. Measurements with different tissue types and thicknesses show in this context that it is not the tissue type but the thickness that is decisive for differential detectability.[24]

These experimental data allowed the group to draw the conclusion that a measurement reflecting the exact location and tracer accumulation of the lymph nodes is not possible with sufficient reliability with increasing tissue thickness, especially in the area of the deep jugular lymph nodes, which represent the first draining lymph node station for pharyngeal and laryngeal lymph nodes.

Regarding the later transcutaneous identification of the first draining lymph node, a limited significance can be attributed to the preoperatively performed dynamic lymphoscintigraphy in cases of tumors of the upper aerodigestive tract. This method can demonstrate preoperatively an adequate functional capacity of the lymphatic drainage as well as the main lymphatic drainage direction of the primary tumor (ipsilateral or contralateral) due to a sufficient intranodal tracer uptake of the radiopharmacon. In order to clarify the lymphatic drainage in the case of suspected contralateral N0 neck and ipsilateral advanced lymphogenic metastatic spread, this procedure could also be indicated.[24] However, it must be mentioned critically that this method is not always appropriate to reliably identify transcutaneously the sentinel node in the region of the lymphatic drainage of deeper jugular lymph nodes of levels II–IV.

Value of Sentinel Lymphadenectomy

The first report on successfully identifying the sentinel node of supraglottic carcinoma crossing the midline was made by Alex and Krag in 1996.[25] On the basis of their examination of five partly pretreated patients with different cervical lymph node status, the authors drew the conclusion in another publication on this topic from 1998 that sentinel lymphadenectomy should only be performed in certain patients and could actually only be performed in cases of carcinomas in the area of the oral cavity and the oropharynx.[26] Also in 1998, Pitman and co-workers[27] were able to show in an examination of 16 patients with different cervical lymph node status that the dye injection method in the head and neck had only a subordinate significance for the description of the first draining lymph nodes. The first publication of Shoaib's group[28] concerning the detection of the sentinel node by means of tracer and dye application revealed that in 46.2% of the cases a histologically nonrepresentative sentinel node was found. However, it must be mentioned critically that the publication does not indicate the pretherapeutic N status. Thus, the representativeness of this examination seems to be doubtful with regard to the objective of verifying the validity of the sentinel node concept in the initial stage of lymphogenic metastatic spread by means of a patient population of whom suffer more than 65% histologically from an advanced lymphogenic metastatic spread.

The increasing popularity of this new diagnostic and therapeutic concept led to a significant increase of published investigations on this topic (Figure 3). Even though the reported results of different groups do not provide the opportunity to draw a final conclusion on the significance of sentinel lymphadenectomy in cases of squamous cell carcinomas of the upper aerodigestive tract, the early results of easily exposable carcinomas of the oral cavity[29,30,33,34] confirm the importance of this new diagnostic and therapeutic concept for the above-mentioned tumor entity. Groups with experience in the comparably easily accessible tumors of the oral cavity report a sensitivity of 94% in 57 examined patients suffering from oral or oropharyngeal carcinomas with clinical N0 neck[46] and 100% in 41 patients suffering from a T1-T2 carcinoma of the oral cavity.[47] The representativeness of the sentinel node concept is emphasized by the results of a recently published investigation by Hyde's group.[48] The study evaluated the utility of [^{18}F]fluorodeoxyglucose (FDG) positron emission tomography (PET) and sentinel lymph node imaging and biopsy in determining the true disease status of the loco-regional lymphatics in 19 patients. Hyde and co-workers could demonstrate that the sentinel node was representative in 18/19 patients with one false-negative result, while [^{18}F]FDG PET failed to identify nodal disease in all 4 patients with histologically proven lymph node metastases.

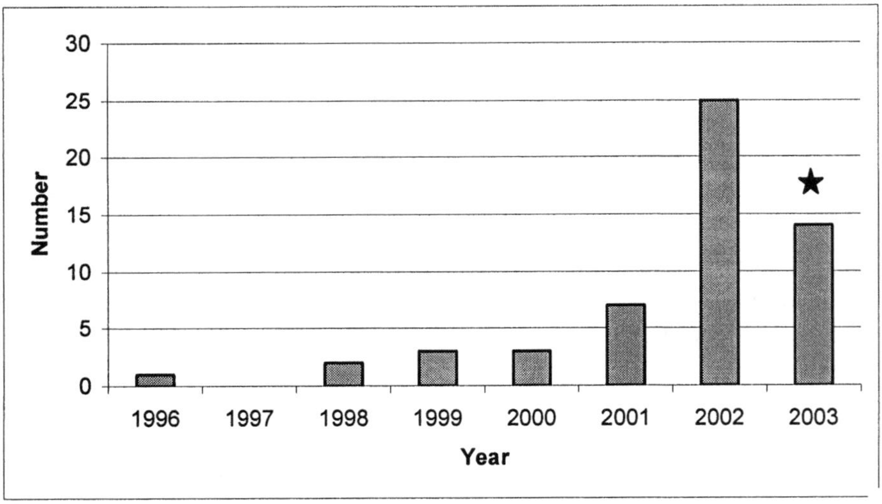

Figure 3. Publications on SN biopsy in HNSCC (MEDLINE listed).
★ (Status: August 2003)

In the majority of the cases the groups used exclusively radiotracers transported by lymph fluid[22,23,28,31-33,35,37,38,41,43] to mark the sentinel node of carcinomas located in the head and neck. Exceptions are Fang's group[49] which was able to identify the draining sentinel node(s) by isolated injection of Blue dye® in 29 patients with laryngeal and hypopharyngeal carcinomas, as well as the groups of Shoaib,[28,35,46,47] Mozzillo,[34] Hyde,[48] and Chiesa[29,37] who used Blue dye® besides radiotracers to mark the sentinel nodes. In this context Shoaib[51] mentioned self-critically in accordance with the first results of Pitman and co-workers[27] that the false-negative rate is not significantly reduced by additional color lymphography. He argued that in fact the radioactive marking of the sentinel nodes represented the base of sentinel lymphadenectomy in the head and neck.

The high sensitivity of the results achieved by means of radiotracer marking justifies no additional application of Blue dye® as do other complications associated with the application of colorings. An accidental injury of the lymph collector draining the dye would lead to an extravasation of the dye with resulting important reduction of the intraoperative sight.[61] Especially in the area of the cervical soft parts with their numerous neural and vascular structures this fact is of great importance. In 1985, Longnecker's group[61] reported on anaphylaxis after subcutaneous injection of Blue dye®. Data in the literature refer to 2% of the examined patients.[61] The clinical introduction and the proof of ^{99m}Tc radiotracers coupled with methylene blue for sentinel lymphadenectomy must be considered, as recently reported.[63]

The earlier mentioned explanations refer in particular to easily accessible carcinomas of the oral cavity. The modification developed in our own group concerning a merely intraoperative detection in the surgically opened neck (Figure 4) emphasized the appropriateness of sentinel lymphadenectomy also for limited (T1-T2) pharyngeal and laryngeal carcinomas for detection of clinically occult metastatic spread,[22,23,31,32,38] also including T3 glottic carcinomas.[41] The modification of an intraoperative detection technique can be justified as explained in the following paragraph.

Figure 4. Intraoperative view of radiolabeled identification of the sentinel nodes in a T2 carcinoma of the hard and soft palate (f, 57). SCM, sternocleidomastoid muscle.

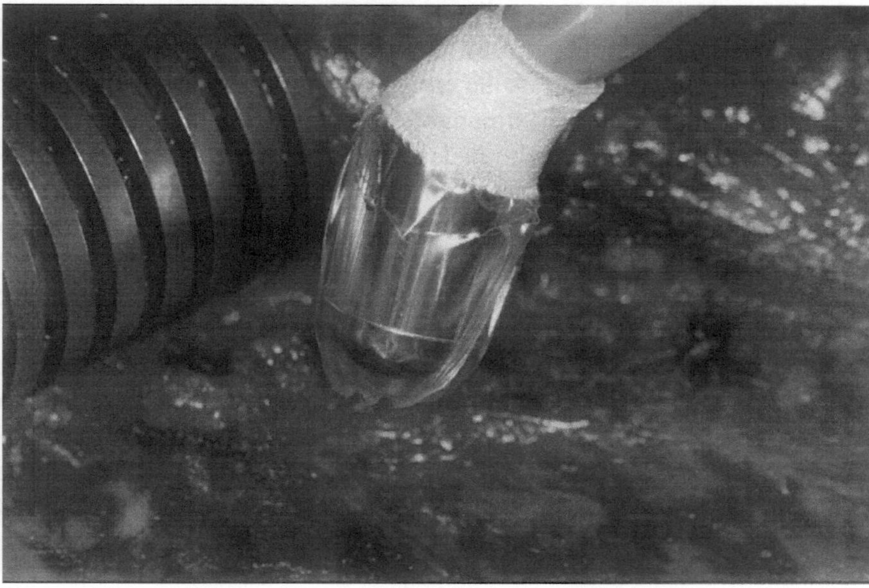

While easily accessible oral carcinomas allow an injection of the tracer in local anesthesia, pharyngeal and laryngeal carcinomas can only be completely exposed in the context of general anesthesia. It became obvious that also in cases of carcinomas of the oral cavity the injection reliability could be increased due to better exposure of the primary tumor and the missing, disturbing activity of the patient (e.g., nausea, motility of the tongue) when relaxed (Figure 4). This contributes to an increased representativeness of the marked drainage region and thus also to the reliability of this method.[22,23,31,38]

The last-mentioned statement is based on the knowledge of the well-examined differences in density of the regional distribution pattern of initial lymph vessels in the head and neck.[64-67] These directly influence the identification of the sentinel node(s). According to density and direction of the initial lymph vessels in the region of the primary tumor, a preferred drainage exists in one or more of those lymph node groups for every tumor site in the area of the upper aerodigestive tract.[66] Due to the narrowness of different lymphatic regions in the head and neck, the injection technique itself bears the risk of injecting in a drainage region adjacent to the main drainage area. A primary tumor can even drain in two or more neighboring lymphatic drainage regions because of its location and thus have more first draining lymph nodes.[31,32,66]

In conclusion, we think that one to three hot nodes should be resected and histologically examined in order to minimize the number of false-negative results.[23,38] Statements concerning the representativeness and significance of the discussed diagnostic concepts should be made on the basis of the histopathological examination of these one to three radiolabeled nodes (SN 1–3).[31,41] Because a further immunohistochemical coloring with cytokeratin antibodies performed additionally to H&E coloring can increase the detection of occult micrometastases,[68] an immunohistochemical examination of SN 1–3 would contribute to an increased reliability of the histological results. The limitation to a maximum of three sentinel nodes also would not strain too much the personally limited resources of pathologists.

In order to avoid deception in the application of a probably helpful technique in the case of correct indication, a critical and careful verification of the transferability of the method described for other tumor entities seems to be indispensable in dealing with the question of the significance of sentinel lymphadenectomy for carcinomas of the head and neck. A first step to achieve comparable examination results is standardization of the technical procedure. Table 1 gives an overview of the techniques performed by different groups that show a clear variation with partly far-reaching consequences for the oncological treatment concept of patients. In particular for an already performed isolated lymph node extirpation[46] no valid data exist until now. In view of the prognostic significance of ignored lymphogenic metastatic spread with partly significant reduction of the 5-year survival rate, such a procedure should be elaborated in the form of controlled prospective studies regarding the sentinel node concept, which is still at an experimental stage for this tumor entity.[58]

Table 1. Different techniques of sentinel node identification in head and neck cancer patients

References	First authors	Methods
14,15,23,24,30,33	Werner Dünne	Intraoperative tracer injection, radiolocalization and identification of the SN during elective ND[a]
17,45	Alex	Intraoperative tracer injection, radiolocalization and identification of the SN on the skin surface and in vivo during elective ND
18	Koch	Preoperative tracer injection, lymphoscintigraphy, open biopsy of the SN within 2 hours of injection after exstiration of the primary site, elective ND after SN biopsy
19,50	Pitman	Intraoperative blue dye injection, identification of the blue-stained SN during elective ND
20,25,27,35,38,43	Shoaib Ross von Buchwald	Preoperative tracer injection, lymphoscintigraphy and radiolocalization and identification of the SN on the skin surface, intraoperative blue dye injection, open biopsy of the SN: if the SN is found negative, there is no further treatment to the neck; if the SN tested positive, a therapeutic ND was performed
21,26,29,39	Chiesa Mozzillo Ionna	Tracer injection 4 weeks after primary resection, twice (tumor resection and ND) preoperative lymphoscintigraphy, radiolocalization and identification of the SN during elective ND

22	Zitsch	Intraoperative tracer injection, elective ND, ex vivo radiolocalization and identification of the SN
28	Stoeckli	Preoperative tracer injection, lymphoscintigraphy and radiolocalization and identification of the SN on the skin surface, elective ND after SN biopsy
40	Hyde	Preoperative [^{18}F]FDG PET, radiocolloid injection, preoperative lymphoscintigraphy and radiolocalization and identification of the SN on the skin surface, at operation blue dye injection, open biopsy of the SN, elective ND after SN biopsy
32,37,44,51,61	Nieuwenhuis van den Brekel Colnot Bilde	Resection of the primary, lymphoscintigraphy, radiolocalization and identification of the SN on the skin surface, USgFNAC of the SN
36	Barzan	Intraoperative tracer injection, selective ND, ex vivo radiolocalization and identification of the SN
41	Fang	Intraoperative blue dye injection, identification of the blue stained SN during elective ND
42,48	Civantos	Preoperative tracer injection, lymphoscintigraphy and radiolocalization and identification of the SN on the skin surface, open biopsy of the SN, elective ND after SN biopsy
47	Höft	Preoperative tracer injection, lymphoscintigraphy, radiolocalization and identification of the SN on the skin surface, USgFNAC of the SN, elective ND
49	Asthana	Intraoperative blue dye injection, identification of the blue stained SN during elective ND

[a]ND;neck dissection.

Limits and Pitfalls

Table 2 summarizes the limits and pitfalls resulting from the application of this method in cases of carcinomas of the upper aerodigestive tract. The limits refer to the technical difficulties of reliably identifying the hot nodes despite the disperse radiation of the primary injection point. The effort to shield the injection site by means of a lead plate[28,35] is often not possible due to the anatomical realities for deep oropharyngeal or laryngeal carcinomas and only incomplete for tumors located in the area of the oral cavity.[41]

Table 2. Limitations and pitfalls of sentinel lymphadenectomy in HNSCC

Dependent on investigator	Not related to investigator
Inadequate exposure of primary tumor	Poorly accessible primary tumor
Injection into neighboring basin	Lymphatic drainage into two parallel initial basins; drainage into two neighboring regions
Excessive volume of tracer substance with radioactive labeling of an excessive amount of non-representative lymph nodes	Missing accumulation of tracer substance in cases of tumor emboli in the afferent lymphatic vessel
Amount of sentinel node biopsies performed by the investigator (learning curve)	Close proximity of injection site and initial draining lymph node; risk of excision of a nonrepresentative lymph node
	Less or no tracer uptake due to extent of intranodal tumor disease with or without perinodal spread

With this background, our group as well as other groups[56] performed the resection of the primary tumor 15–20 minutes after injection. The associated reduction of the disperse radiation could directly contribute to an optimized procedure.[41] This technique is justified by findings of dynamic lymphoscintigraphy in the head and neck. Nieuwenhuis's group[69] was able to show in a detailed analysis of 82 patients that already 1 minute after injection a lymphatic drainage with description of the first draining lymph node could be detected by the double detector camera.

Another limit depends on the successful injection of the posterior or caudally situated tumor edge. This is especially true for pharyngeal and laryngeal carcinomas. In order to minimize this problem, the tracer injection can also be performed in retrograde direction via a so-called butterfly (e.g., Venofix®, 23G, 0.65x20 mm, Braun Melsungen) to increase the precision of the injection.[41]

Sentinel lymphadenectomy is contraindicated if ipsilateral advanced lymphogenic metastatic spread was detected. In accordance with Borgstein et al.,[70] our results illustrate that an advanced intranodal tumor growth, partly also with extracapsular metastatic spread, leads to a significant reduction of the radiopharmacon uptake and accumulation up to the complete loss of nodal storing capacity.[5,32] At this point it must not be forgotten that even small clinically unsuspected lymph nodes may reveal extracapsular tumor growth with resulting lack of radiopharmacon accumulation.[71,72]

Finally, the surgical or radiological pretreatment of the primary tumor region may lead to a lymphatic drainage of the radiopharmacon, which can be missing or which is not representative for the initial drainage direction.[73] Thus, pretreatments in the area of the first draining lymph node stations can result in a change of direction and a drainage of the radiopharmacon into a contralateral drainage region.[67] That is why sentinel lymphadenectomy should be indicated only in exceptional cases for patients who had received prior treatment.

Future Perspectives

The lymphatic drainage directions of the different primary tumor sites of the upper aerodigestive tract elaborated until now by our group using the earliermentioned method emphasize the validity of this procedure. The results correspond to the classic concept of regional lymphatic drainage. Thus, the dominating metastatic region of pharyngeal and laryngeal carcinomas is mainly level II and less commonly level III. Carcinomas of the anterior oral cavity drain mostly into level I and less commonly into level II. It may thus be expected that neck dissection of these lymph node levels will include the majority of clinically occult metastases.

With this background, it must still be clarified whether intraoperative identification of the radiolabeled sentinel node(s) is appropriate for reducing the extent of selective neck dissection in the suspected N0 neck or whether neck dissection can be completely avoided in the case of histologically proven tumor-free sentinel node. Opponents of such a procedure argue that selective neck dissection already has a morbidity that can nearly be neglected. Supporters of sentinel lymphadenectomy mention the most possible protection of the intact, i.e., nonmetastatic, cervical lymph node systems as well as the reduction of the extent of surgery. Scarring contractures, paresthesia, and partly also persisting lymphedemas could be reduced by a circumscribed extirpation of the sentinel node(s).

Other progress aims at optimized surgical access to the sentinel node(s). Alternative accesses such as video-assisted endoscopic surgery techniques are very interesting as they are already established especially in the fields of gynecology and visceral surgery.[74-76] The first results on endoscopically performed selective lymphadenectomy led to the assumption that this method of lymph node dissection could achieve some significance in the therapeutic regime of the clinical N0 neck, if based on the sentinel node concept.[77] However, the technical modalities would have to be optimized. Further, prospectively collected data should definitely be analyzed as a prerequisite. Within such an investigation it would make sense to send the excised lymph node to frozen section examination. Depending on the histopathological result, a surgical resection of the lymphatic drainage in the form of a selective neck dissection could then be indicated. At present, it can be stated that the technical diversity and importance of endoscopic lymphadenectomy in the neck shows scientific and clinical potential. The question about the significance of the procedure, however, can currently not be answered finally.

REFERENCES

1. Fisch UP (1964) Cervical lymphography in cases of laryngo-pharyngeal carcinoma. J Laryngol Otol 122: 712-726
2. Fisch UP (1966) Lymphographische Untersuchung über das zervikale Lymphsystem. Karger, Basel
3. Schwab W, Winkel K zum (1967) The current status of scintigraphy of the cervical lymphatic system. Nucl Med 6: 234-249
4. Zita G (1967) Contribution on cervical lymphoscintigraphy. Fortschr Geb Röntgenstr Nuklearmed 107: 644-654
5. Michailov V, Mlatschkov C (1969) Evaluation of cervical lymph node scintigraphy. Radiobiol Radiother 10: 769-777
6. Werner JA, Dünne AA, Moll T, Behr T (2003) Sentinel Lymphonodektomie bei Karzinomen der oberen Luft- und Speisewege. Onkologe 9: 635-642
7. Werner JA (1998) Aktueller Stand der Versorgung des Lymphabflusses maligner Kopf-Hals-Tumoren. Eur Arch Otorhinolaryng (Suppl) 1-85
8. Werner JA, Schünke M, Lippert BM, Koeleman-Schmidt H, Gottschlich S, Tillmann B (1995) Das laryngeale Lymphgefäßsystem des Menschen. Eine morphologische und lymphographische Untersuchung unter klinischen Gesichtspunkten. HNO 43: 525-531
9. Werner JA, Schunke M, Rudert H, Tillmann B (1990) Description and clinical importance of the lymphatics of the vocal fold. Otolaryngol Head Neck Surg 102: 13-19
10. Werner JA (1995) Untersuchungen zum Lymphgefäßsystem von Mundhöhle und Rachen. Laryngorhinootologie 74: 622-628

11. Lindberg RD (1972) Distribution of cervical lymph node metastasis from squamous cell carcinoma of the upper respiratory and digestive tracts. Cancer 29: 1446-1449
12. Robbins KT, Clayman G, Levine PA, Medina J, Sessions R, Shaha A, Som P, Wolf GT; American Head and Neck Society, American Academy of Otolaryngology - Head and Neck Surgery (2002) Neck dissection classification update: revisions proposed by the American Head and Neck Society and the American Academy of Otolaryngology-Head and Neck Surgery. Arch Otolaryngol Head Neck Surg 128: 751-758
13. Werner JA, Dünne AA, Lippert BM (2002) Indikationen zur Halsexploration bei nicht nachweisbaren Lymphknotenmetastasen. Teil II. HNO 50: 370-378
14. Werner JA (1995) Untersuchungen zum Lymphgefäßsystem der oberen Luft- und Speisewege. Shaker, Aachen
15. Hosal AS, Carrau RL, Johnson JT, Myers EN (2000) Selective neck dissection in the management of the clinically node-negative neck. Laryngoscope 110: 2037-2040
16. van den Brekel MW, van der Waal I, Meijer CJ, Freeman JL, Castelijns JA, Snow GB (1996) The incidence of micrometastases in neck dissection specimens obtained from elective neck dissections. Laryngoscope 106: 987-991
17. Teichgraeber JF, Clairmont AA (1984) The incidence of occult metastases for cancer of the oral tongue and floor of the mouth: Treatment rationale. Head Neck 7: 15-21
18. Gavilán J, Gavilán C, Herranz J (1994) The neck in supraglottic cancer. In: Smee R, Bridger GP (eds.) Laryngeal cancer. Elsevier, Amsterdam, pp. 576-581
19. DeSanto LW, Magrina C, O'Fallon WM (1990) The "second" side of the neck in supraglottic cancer. Otolaryngol Head Neck Surg 102: 351-361
20. Godden DR, Ribeiro NF, Hassanein K, Langton SG (2002) Recurrent neck disease in oral cancer. J Oral Maxillofac Surg 60: 748-753
21. Werner JA, Davis RK (in press) Metastasis in head and neck cancer. Springer, Heidelberg
22. Werner JA, Dünne AA, Brandt D, Ramaswamy A, Külkens C, Lippert BM, Folz BJ, Joseph K, Moll R (1999) Untersuchungen zum Stellenwert der Sentinel Lymphonodektomie bei Karzinomen des Pharynx und Larynx. Laryngorhinootologie 78: 663-670
23. Werner JA, Dünne AA, Ramaswamy A, Brandt D, Külkens C, Folz BJ, Moll R, Lippert BM (2002) Das Sentinel Node Konzept bei Plattenepithelkarzinomen der oberen Luft- und Speisewege – eine kritische Analyse an 100 Patienten. Laryngorhinootologie 81: 31-39
24. Wiesemann N (2002) Eignungstest eines Gamma-Messsondensystems bei der Simulation der ein Plattenepithelkarzinom der oberen Luft- und Speisewege drainierenden Lymphknoten. Thesis, Philipps University of Marburg, Germany
25. Alex JC, Krag DN (1996) The gamma-probe-guided resection of radiolabeled primary lymph nodes. Surg Oncol Clin North Am 5: 33-41
26. Koch WM, Choti MA, Civelek AC, Eisele DW, Saunders JR (1998) Gamma probe-directed biopsy of the sentinel node in oral squamous cell carcinoma. Arch Otolaryngol Head Neck Surg 124: 455-459
27. Pitman KT, Johnson JT, Edington H, Barnes EL, Day R, Wagner RL, Myers EN (1998) Lymphatic mapping with isosulfan blue dye in squamous cell carcinoma of the head and neck. Arch Otolaryngol Head Neck Surg 124: 790-793
28. Shoaib T, Soutar DS, Prosser JE, Dunaway DJ, Gray HW, McCurrach GM, Bessent RG, Robertson AG, Oliver R, MacDonald DG (1999) A suggested method for

sentinel node biopsy in squamous cell carcinoma of the head and neck. Head Neck 21: 728-733

29. Chiesa F, Mauri S, Grana C, Tradati N, Calabrese L, Ansarin M, Mazzarol G, Paganelli G (2000) Is there a role for sentinel node biopsy in early N0 tongue tumors? Surgery 128: 16-21
30. Zitsch RP 3rd, Todd DW, Renner GJ, Singh A (2000) Intraoperative radiolymphoscintigraphy for detection of occult nodal metastasis in patients with head and neck squamous cell carcinoma. Otolaryngol Head Neck Surg 122: 662-666
31. Dünne AA, Külkens C, Ramaswamy A, Folz BJ, Brandt D, Lippert BM, Behr T, Moll R, Werner JA (2001) Value of sentinel lymphonodectomy in head and neck cancer patients without evidence of lymphogenic metastatic disease. Auris Nasus Larynx 28: 339-344
32. Dünne AA, Jungclas H, Werner JA (2001) Intraoperative sentinel node biopsy in patients with squamous cell carcinomas of the head and neck—experiences using a well-type NaI detector for gamma ray spectroscopy. Otolaryngol Pol 55: 127-134
33. Ross GL, Soutar DS, Shoaib T, Camilleri IG, MacDonald DG, Robertson AG, Bessent RG, Gray HW (2002) The ability of lymphoscintigraphy to direct sentinel node biopsy in the clinically N0 neck for patients with head and neck squamous cell carcinoma. Br J Radiol 75: 950-958
34. Mozzillo N, Chiesa F, Botti G, Caraco C, La storia S, Giugliano G, Mazzarol G, Paganelli G, Ionna F (2001) Sentinel node biopsy in head and neck cancer. Ann Surg Oncol 8: 103S-105S
35. Shoaib T, Soutar DS, MacDonald DG, Camilleri IG, Dunaway DJ, Gray HW, McCurrach GM, Bessent RG, MacLeod TI, Robertson AG (2001) The accuracy of head and neck carcinoma sentinel lymph node biopsy in the clinically N0 neck. Cancer 91: 2077-2083
36. Stoeckli SJ, Steinert H, Pfaltz M, Schmid S (2001) Sentinel lymph node evaluation in squamous cell carcinoma of the head and neck. Otolaryngol Head Neck Surg 125: 221-226
37. Chiesa F, Tradati N, Calabrese L (2001) Sentinel node biopsy, lymphatic pattern and selective neck dissection in oral cancer. Oral Dis 7: 317-138
38. Werner JA, Dünne AA, Ramaswamy A, Folz BJ, Brandt D, Külkens C, Moll R, Lippert BM (2002) Number and location of radiolabeled, intraoperatively identified sentinel nodes in 48 head and neck cancer patients with clinically staged N0 and N1 neck. Eur Arch Otorhinolaryngol 259: 91-96
39. Hyde N, Prvulovich E (2002) Is there a role for lymphoscintigraphy and sentinel node biopsy in the management of the regional lymphatics in mucosal squamous cell carcinoma of the head and neck? Eur J Nucl Med 29: 579-584
40. Nieuwenhuis EJ, Castelijns JA, Pijpers R, van den Brekel MW, Brakenhoff RH, van der Waal I, Snow GB, Leemans CR (2002) Wait-and-see policy for the N0 neck in early-stage oral and oropharyngeal squamous cell carcinoma using ultrasonography-guided cytology: is there a role for identification of the sentinel node? Head Neck 24: 282-289
41. Werner JA, Dünne AA, Ramaswamy A, Folz BJ, Lippert BM, Moll R, Behr T (2002) Sentinel node detection in N0 cancer of the pharynx and larynx. Br J Cancer 87: 711-715
42. Maublant J, Cachin F, Mesta D, Geissler B (2002) Le repérage du ganglion sentinelle en médecine nucléaire. Bull Cancer 89: 671-680

43. Von Buchwald C, Bilde A, Shoaib T, Ross G (2002) Sentinel node biopsy: the technique and the feasibility in head and neck cancer. ORL J Otorhinolaryngol Relat Spec 64: 268-274
44. Barzan L, Sulfaro S, Albert F, Politi D, Marus W, Pin M, Savignano MG (2002) Gamma probe accuracy in detecting the sentinel lymph node in clinically N0 squamous cell carcinoma of the head and neck. Ann Otol Rhinol Laryngol 111: 794-798
45. Bilde A, von Buchwald C, Dreyer M, Eigtved AI (2002) Sentinel node biopsy in head and neck cancer. Is there an indication for use of this new surgical technique in the treatment of head and neck cancer? Ugeskr Laeger 164: 4276-4280
46. Ross G, Shoaib T, Soutar DS, Camilleri IG, Gray HW, Bessent RG, Robertson AG, MacDonald DG (2002) The use of sentinel node biopsy to upstage the clinically N0 neck in head and neck cancer. Arch Otolaryngol Head Neck Surg 128: 1287-1291
47. Ionna F, Chiesa F, Longo F, Manola M, Villano S, Calabrese L, Lastoria S, Mozzillo N (2002) Prognostic value of sentinel node in oral cancer. Tumori 88: S18-19
48. Hyde NC, Prvulovich E, Newman L, Waddington WA, Visvikis D, Ell P (2003) A new approach to pre-treatment assessment of the N0 neck in oral squamous cell carcinoma: the role of sentinel node biopsy and positron emission tomography. Oral Oncol 39: 350-360
49. Fang J, Wei X, Li S (2001) Clinical study of the sentinel lymph node of patients with laryngeal and hypopharyngeal carcinomas. Zhonghua Er Bi Yan Hou Ke Za Zhi 36: 244-246
50. Civantos FJ, Gomez C, Duque C, Pedroso F, Goodwin WJ, Weed DT, Arnold D, Moffat F (2003) Sentinel node biopsy in oral cavity cancer: Correlation with PET scan and immunohistochemistry. Head Neck 25: 1-9
51. Ross GL, Soutar DS, Shoaib T, Camilleri IG, MacDonald DG, Robertson AG, Bessent RG, Gray HW (2002) The ability of lymphoscintigraphy to direct sentinel node biopsy in the clinically N0 neck for patients with head and neck squamous cell carcinoma. Br J Radiol 75: 950-958
52. van den Brekel MW, Reitsma LC, Quak JJ, Smeele LE, van der Linden JC, Snow GB, Castelijns JA (1999) Sonographically guided aspiration cytology of neck nodes for selection of treatment and follow-up in patients with N0 head and neck cancer. Am J Neuroradiol 20: 1727-1731
53. Alex JC, Sasaki CT, Krag DN, Wenig B, Pyle PB (2000) Sentinel lymph node radiolocalization in head and neck squamous cell carcinoma. Laryngoscope 110: 198-203
54. Hyde NC, Prvulovich E, Keshtgar MR (2002) A needle free system for cervical lymphatic mapping and sentinel node biopsy in oral squamous cell carcinoma. Oral Oncol 38: 797-799
55. Hoft S, Muhle C, Brenner W, Sprenger E, Maune S (2002) Fine-needle aspiration cytology of the sentinel lymph node in head and neck cancer. J Nucl Med 43: 1585-1590
56. Civantos FJ, Gomez C, Duque C, Pedroso F, Goodwin WJ, Weed DT, Arnold D, Moffat F (2003) Sentinel node biopsy in oral cavity cancer: correlation with PET scan and immunohistochemistry. Head Neck 25: 1-9
57. Asthana S, Deo SV, Shukla NK, Jain P, Anand M, Kumar R (2003) Intraoperative neck staging using sentinel node biopsy and imprint cytology in oral cancer. Head Neck 25: 368-372

58. Pitman KT, Ferlito A, Devaney KO, Shaha AR, Rinaldo A (2003) Sentinel lymph node biopsy in head and neck cancer. Oral Oncol 39: 343-349
59. Colnot DR, Nieuwenhuis EJ, van den Brekel MW, Pijpers R, Brakenhoff RH, Snow GB, Castelijns JA (2001) Head and neck squamous cell carcinoma: US-guided fine-needle aspiration of sentinel lymph nodes for improved staging—initial experience. Radiology 218: 289-923
60. Peng HW, Zeng ZY, Chen FJ, Guo ZM, Zhang Q, Xu GP, Wei MW, Wu GH (2003) Optimized methods of sentinel node localization in cN0 tongue carcinoma. Ai Zheng 22: 286-290
61. Longnecker SM, Guzzardo MM, Van Voris LP (1985) Life-threatening anaphylaxis following subcutaneous administration of isosulfan blue 1%. Clin Pharm 4: 219-221
62. Cimmino VM, Brown AC, Szocik JF, Pass HA, Moline S, De SK, Domino EF (2001) Allergic reactions to isosulfan blue during sentinel node biopsy—a common event. Surgery 130: 439-442
63. Plut EM, Hinkle GH, Guo W, Lee RJ (2002) Kit formulation for the preparation of radioactive blue liposomes for sentinel node lymphoscintigraphy. J Pharm Sci 91: 1717-1732
64. Werner JA, Schunke M, Rudert H, Tillmann B (1990) Description and clinical importance of the lymphatics of the vocal fold. Otolaryngol Head Neck Surg 102: 13-19
65. Werner JA (1995) Untersuchungen zum Lymphgefäßsystem von Mundhöhle und Rachen. Laryngorhinootologie 74: 622-628
66. Werner JA, Dünne AA, Myers JN (2003) Functional anatomy of the lymphatic drainage system of the upper aerodigestive tract and its role in metastasis of squamous cell carcinoma. Head Neck 322-332
67. Werner JA (1998) Aktueller Stand der Versorgung des Lymphabflusses maligner Kopf-Hals-Tumoren. Eur Arch Otorhinolaryng (Suppl) 1-85
68. Barrera JE, Miller ME, Said S, Jafek BW, Campana JP, Shroyer KR (2003) Detection of occult cervical micrometastases in patients with head and neck squamous cell cancer. Laryngoscope 113: 892-896
69. Nieuwenhuis EJ, Pijpers R, Castelijns JA, Snow GB (2003) Lymphoscintigraphic details of sentinel lymph node detection in 82 patients with squamous cell carcinoma of the oral cavity and oropharynx. Nucl Med Commun 24: 651-656
70. Borgstein PJ, Pijpers EF, Comans PJ, van Diest PJ, Boom RP, Meijer S (1998) Sentinel lymph node biopsy in breast cancer: Guidelines and pitfalls of lymphoscintigraphy and gamma probe detection. J Am Coll Surg 186: 275-283
71. Croce A, Bianchedi M, Moretti A, Minni A (1992) The surgical treatment of laterocervical adenopathies due to malignant cervicofacial tumours. G Chir 13: 553-556
72. Coatesworth AP, MacLennan K (2002) Squamous cell carcinoma of the upper aerodigestive tract: The prevalence of microscopic extracapsular spread and soft tissue deposits in the clinically N0 neck. Head Neck 24: 258-261
73. Hildmann H, Kosberg RD, Tiedjen KU (1987) Lymphszintigraphische Untersuchungen der regionalen Lymphwege bei Patienten mit Kopf-Hals-Tumoren. HNO 35: 31-33
74. Beger HG, Schwarz A, Bergmann U (2003) Progress in gastrointestinal tract surgery: the impact of gastrointestinal endoscopy. Surg Endosc 17: 342-350
75. Liu Y, Zhang X (2002) Analysis of complications about gynecologic endoscopic procedures in 14 hospitals of Shanghai during 1992–2001. Zhonghua Fu Chan Ke Za Zhi 37: 646-649

76. Einarsson JI, Young A, Tsien L, Sangi-Haghpeykar H (2002) Perceived proficiency in endoscopic techniques among senior obstetrics and gynecology residents. J Am Assoc Gynecol Laparosc 9: 158–64
77. Werner JA, Sapundzhiev NR, Teymoortash A, Dünne AA, Folz BJ, Behr T (in press) Endoscopic sentinel lymphonodectomy as a new diagnostic approach in the N0 neck. Eur Arch Otolaryngol
78. Werner JA (2001) Historischer Abriss zur Nomenklatur der Halslymphknoten als Grundlage für die Klassifikation der Neck dissection. Laryngorhinootologie 80: 400-409

Chapter 11

ACCURATE EVALUATION OF NODAL TISSUES FOR THE PRESENCE OF TUMOR IS CENTRAL TO THE SENTINEL NODE APPROACH

Alistair J. Cochran, Alice Roberts, Duan-Ren Wen, Rong-Rong Huang, Eijun Itakura, Frank Luo, Scott W. Binder

Departments of Pathology and Laboratory Medicine and Surgery, David Geffen School of Medicine at UCLA and the Jonsson Comprehensive Cancer Center, Los Angeles, California

INTRODUCTION

Modern medicine is inescapably multidisciplinary and its effectiveness is greatly enhanced by interactions between specialists. The combined techniques of lymphatic mapping (LM) and sentinel node biopsy (SNB)[1] are highly influential and effective advances in the surgical management of malignant tumors. These approaches are particularly dependent on close collaboration between specifically trained and committed specialists in nuclear medicine, dermatology, surgery, and surgical pathology/dermatopathology. All such individuals should have received a specific period of training to develop the skills necessary for efficient performance of their roles within the management team. The best patient outcomes are achieved when the various specialists are in close communication and can readily discuss all aspects of the management of each individual patient.

There are two separate basic requirements for a successful sentinel node procedure: accurate identification of the true sentinel lymph node(s) (SLN) and precise and reliable determination of the presence of tumor within the sentinel node. The first step is the responsibility of nuclear medicine and surgical personnel. For many years lymphoscintigraphy, read several hours after introduction of isotope provided accurate information concerning the lymph node basin or basins that received lymph flow from a given area of the skin. If the lymphoscintigram is read "early," 30 minutes after radioisotope introduction, the actual afferent lymphatic(s) and individual SN are readily visualized. Skin markers can then be applied over the site of the SN to guide the surgeon in determining the optimum alignment for the initial skin incision. At surgery the surgeon injects blue dye (usually isosulfan blue) intradermally around the site of the primary tumor or (more usually) the scar from excision of that tumor. If the lymphoscintigram is performed immediately before the surgical operation, the surgeon need not add radioisotope to the blue dye injected at the beginning of the operation, as residual radioactivity from the lymphoscintigram will be sufficient to highlight the sentinel nodes. If the lymphoscintigram was performed more than 8 hours before surgery the intradermal injection should combine blue dye and radioisotope, as radioactivity from the lymphoscintigram will have faded. The surgeon places his incision according to the lymphoscintigraphy-based skin markings that localize the site of the sentinel node. Careful tissue dissection reveals the blue-colored afferent lymphatic(s) and these are followed until they terminate in one or more blue-colored sentinel node(s). Such nodes are more radioactive than adjacent nonsentinel nodes and adjacent fatty and connective tissues on assessment by a hand-held gammadetector. The sentinel node(s) is/are dissected and immediately sent to the pathology department for evaluation. The remaining tissues in the operative area are evaluated for residual additional foci of enhanced radioactivity that may represent further sentinel nodes. Any tissues showing enhanced radioactivity are dissected and sent to pathology for assessment as putative additional sentinel nodes.

The clinical protocol that identifies sentinel nodes is well described, logical, and permits high, though not perfect accuracy in sentinel node detection. The approach is by no means foolproof and there is at least a small possibility that a node claimed as sentinel on clinical grounds may not actually be the true sentinel node. There is thus a clear need for objective indices of sentinel node status that can be readily identified by the pathologist, permitting independent confirmation that a node is truly sentinel.

LABORATORY CONFIRMATION THAT A SUBMITTED NODE IS SENTINEL

Until recently the pathologist's ability independently to confirm the surgeon's claim that an excised node is sentinel was very limited. The blue marker dye, so readily visible in the operating room, has usually dissipated through the excised tissues by the time that the specimen arrives in pathology. Nonetheless the pathologist must examine the gross specimen for evidence of blue coloration. Blue coloration may be visible to the naked eye in fresh tissues (Figure 1a), in a frozen tissue block (Figure 1b), and even in a paraffin-embedded tissue block (Figure 1c). Since isosulfan blue does not survive the chemical exposures involved in preparation for staining and the staining process itself, it is not generally visible on microscopic inspection of stained tissue sections.

Figure 1. Residual blue dye in tissues examined in the laboratory. (a) A blue colored lymph node in an unfixed nodule of fat. (b) Blue color in tissue frozen for immediate sectioning (c) Blue color in paraffin-embedded tissue block.

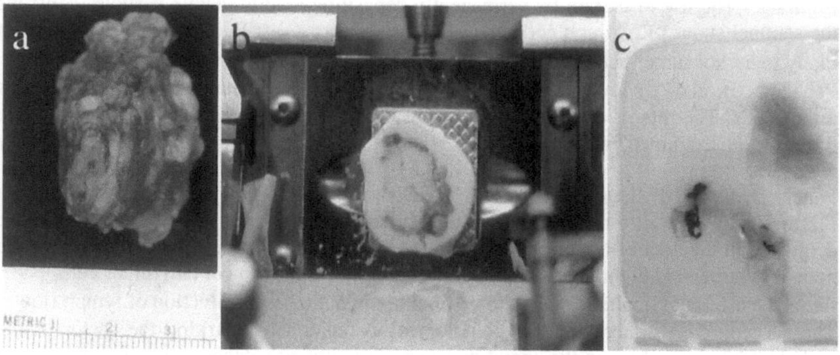

Laboratory confirmation of the sentinel status of a lymph node on the basis of its selective radioactivity is not really practicable. The isotope decays rapidly from the peak values measured in the operating room and pathology laboratories not usually equipped to measure tissue radioactivity.

The need is for an inert marker that could be included in the dye–isotope mixture that is injected prior to SN surgery. Such a marker should be retained selectively in the sentinel node and be readily visible to the inspecting pathologist. We have reported on the successful use of particulate carbon in this role.[2-4] The carbon particles accumulate preferentially and usually exclusively in the sentinel node. They settle in the subcapsular sinus and adjacent lymphoid tissues in the area where the afferent lymphatic that drains the area of dye injection (and thus the site of the primary melanoma) enters the node (Figure 2). Since this is likely to be the portal of entry of metastatic tumor cells that pass from the primary tumor to the sentinel node, the localization of the carbon particles neatly identifies the area of the sentinel node that is most likely to harbor tumor cells (Figure 2). This is a particularly valuable observation as the area of the SN that receives lymph and thus potentially metastatic cells from the primary tumor is often relatively limited in extent. Careful intraoperative inspection of blue stained sentinel nodes shows that, in some instances, the whole node may not be blue-colored. Blue coloration may be limited to half or less of the node, indicating that the node receives lymph from more than one lymphatic and tissue source (Figure 3). While one half of the node may receive lymph from the area of the tumor, the other may derive lymph from tissues remote from the tumor. Occult tumor cells are thus unlikely to be present in noncolored segments of a sentinel node.

Figure 2. The use of carbon by permanently depositing readily visible particles confirms the sentinel status of a lymph node and identifies the area(s) within the node that are most likely to harbor tumor cells and thus merit the closest scrutiny.
Panels A, B, and C show the passage of blue dye through a sentinel node that contains tumor cells. The rate of dye travel means that it has often traversed the SLN by the time the node is examined by a pathologist. Tumor is neither highlighted nor specifically identified.
Panels D, E, and F show the passage of blue dye containing carbon particles through a sentinel node. Despite the relatively rapid passage of the blue dye, carbon particles are deposited in the area of lymph inflow from the afferent lymphatic. This confirms that the node is sentinel and highlights the area of the node most likely to contain tumor cells.
AL is the afferent lymphatic. EL is the efferent lymphatic. → is direction of lymph flow.
The surgeon can further facilitate pathological evaluation by marking the sector of the node that is seen as blue in the operating room with clips or stitches of varying length and color and clearly indicating the significance of these markers in the requisition form.

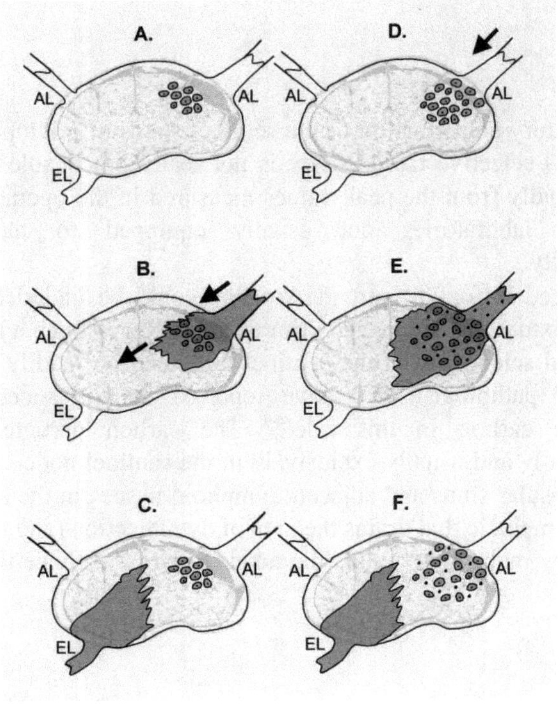

The carbon cannot be applied if the patient has a permanent tattoo in the relevant lymphatic drainage areas. Black pigmentation in tattoo is usually carbon-based and the regional nodes often display carbon-containing macrophages or free carbon in such patients.

Another approach to confirming that a submitted node is truly sentinel is to assess the presence of indices of immune down-regulation. We have shown that in sentinel nodes from patients with melanoma or breast cancer there is a significant reduction in the area of the node occupied by the paracortex and in the relative area of the paracortex occupied by dendritic leukocytes. We have also noted a significant reduction in the density of dendritic leukocytes, activated T lymphocytes, and high endothelial venules in the sentinel nodes. While these approaches are perhaps too complex for routine application, requiring a combination of immunohistochemistry and computer-linked morphometry, they provide unique insights into alterations in the microenvironment of the sentinel node.[5-8] These alterations are potentially of great importance, as they appear related to the susceptibility of sentinel nodes to early metastatic colonization.

Figure 3. **A.** A partially blue sentinel node that receives lymph from at least two separate afferent lymphatics. The right-side lymphatic drains dye-colored tissues, that on the left-side tissues remote from the site of blue dye injection and thus the primary melanoma. The probability of finding occult melanoma cells is greater in the right (colored) segment of the node.
B. This shows a completely blue-colored lymph node that has received lymph from two separate afferent lymphatics that both originate in the blue dye-injected tissues. In such a lymph node occult melanoma cells may be encountered throughout the entire structure of the node.

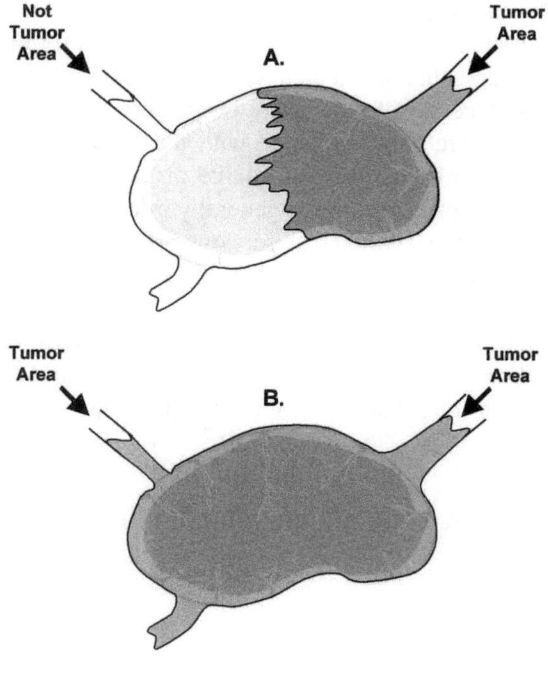

EVALUATION OF THE SENTINEL NODE FOR THE PRESENCE OR ABSENCE OF TUMOR

The role of intraoperative frozen sections

The main and cogent argument advanced for evaluation of sentinel nodes on the basis of intraoperative frozen sections is that it allows for the immediate performance of completion lymph node dissection if the sentinel node contains melanoma cells. This spares the patient a second anesthetic and a second operation. In the 1980s we developed the techniques of LM and SNB on the basis of intraoperative frozen sections and simultaneous rapid immunohistology.[1] As experience was gained with the technique, it became clear that the critical histologic evaluation of the sentinel node was more reliable when based on analysis of formalin-fixed and paraffin-embedded "permanent" preparations. Why is this the case? The number of melanoma cells in the sentinel node is often very small and they occur predominantly in the relatively narrow meridianal strip on either side of the bisecting section.[9,10] There is a real danger that limited diagnostic material may be lost during processing. The aim of the technologist preparing a frozen section is to provide the pathologist with a completely representative section that includes the whole cross section of the lymph node (full-face section). This is particularly desirable in the case of sentinel node tissues since single tumor cells or micrometastases are often confined to the peripherally located subcapsular sinus. In order to provide a full-face section it may be necessary to pare relatively substantial amounts of tissue from the cut surfaces of the node and in this process diagnostic tissue may be completely destroyed. The situation is compounded by the fact that once the frozen section process is completed the remaining tissue is thawed and placed in formalin at room temperature for fixation, a process that may lead to considerable tissue distortion. As a result it may be necessary to cut away even more tissue when full-face permanent sections are being prepared with the associated possibility of further loss of diagnostic tissue. The quality of preservation of tissue and cell morphology in frozen sections is generally inferior to that in formalin-fixed paraffin-embedded permanent sections. For all these reasons we strongly recommend that frozen section assessment of SN be avoided wherever possible. If an intraoperative opinion is desired it is possible to examine the cut faces of the node with a hand lens or dissecting microscope and/or evaluate the cytology of tumor imprints of cell smears derived by scraping the cut surfaces of the lymph node.

Examination of a sentinel node

To provide optimum specimens for analysis surgeons should minimize SLN crush and cautery artifacts and place the nodes in 10% formalin (at least ten times the SLN volume) immediately after excision (unless a frozen section is elected, when the node should remain unfixed) for transport to pathology. Surgeons should submit each putative SLN in a separate container and describe the node color and cpm as observed during the surgical procedure.

In pathology, the SLN specimen is immediately evaluated to minimize dissipation of any residual blue dye. The pathologist records the number of lymph nodes submitted and surgeon's description—color (blue) and counts (cpm)—for each node.

The dimensions of each SLN are recorded. If there is more than one node, and one is blue-colored and reported to be selectively radioactive, this is recorded and that node is accepted as the sentinel node and submitted separately for SLN workup. Additional nodes that are neither blue nor more radioactive than background are considered incidental non-sentinel nodes. These are also submitted individually for SLN workup. The pathologist may leave intact a thin rim of perinodal fat to preserve afferent lymphatics (that may contain tumor emboli) and to assess extra-nodal spread.

Melanomas metastasize first to the subcapsular space, particularly along the longest meridian of the node. Pathologists should accurately bisect the node through its longest meridian and evaluate both cut surfaces for tumor, blue coloration, and foci of carbon particles[4] (hand lens or dissecting microscope). Nodal halves are placed cut face down into cassettes, formalin-fixed for 24–48 hours, paraffin-embedded and serially sectioned at 4 μm intervals with minimal preparatory facing off of the block (Figure 4). Given the propensity of melanoma cells to affect the subcapsular sinus it is essential that "full-face" sections be prepared that fully represent the subcapsular tissues. A "melanoma-sentinel node" tag in the cassette reminds the technicians of the need for careful fully representative sectioning with minimal wastage of tissue. We prepare at least ten serial sections from each lymph node half: hematoxylin and eosin (H&E) staining alternates with immunohistochemistry with antibodies to S-100, HMB-45, and Melan-A/MART-1. If a sentinel node from a patient with a thick deep primary melanoma is negative (against expectation), we cut deeper into both halves of the node and repeat the sequence of cutting and staining noted above. It must be admitted that this additional sampling in our experience, seldom produces a positive result.

Figure 4. Technique for sampling the SLN. The node is cut into two equal halves through the longest meridian and ten full-faced sections are removed from each cut face of the node. Sections 1, 3, 5, and 10 are stained by hematoxylin and eosin (H&E). Section 2 is stained for S-100 protein, section 4 for HMB-45, and section 6 for Melan-A/MART-1. L, left; R, right.

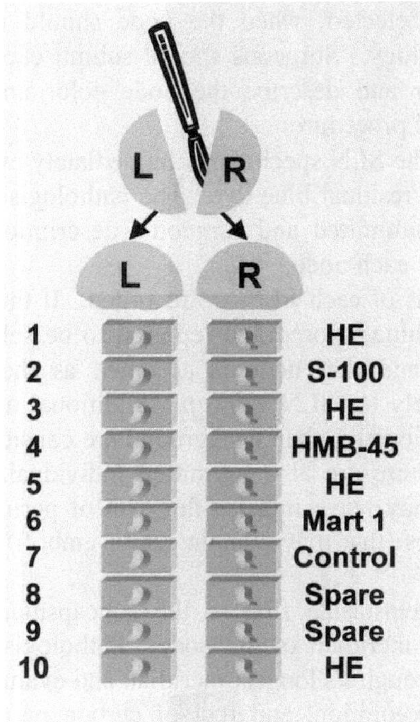

Melanoma metastases, other than substantial multicellular colonies, may be difficult to see on H&E staining. The entire slide is scanned at low power and the different nodal compartments assessed with particular attention to the subcapsular sinus. High-power (400X) fields are examined for single or clustered tumor cells (Figure 5). Melanoma metastases may later extend into the lymphoid parenchyma or central nodal sinus. Extracapsular invasion by tumor alters prognosis and is duly noted.[11] The pathologist records the number of metastatic foci and the greatest dimension of the largest focus, using a micrometer[12] or measures the percentage area of the node occupied by tumor.[13,23]

Colonies of melanoma cells often coexist with single tumor cells that are difficult to identify in H&E sections. Immunohistochemistry (S-100, HMB-45, and MART-1 or tyrosinase) is critical in the detection of micrometastases thereby improving the sensitivity of SLN analysis (Figure 5a,b). Without immunohistochemistry, even experienced observers fail to identify up to 12% of patients with SLN metastases.[14-16] With guidance from immunostained sections it is usually possible to identify even single tumor cells on reexamination of H&E sections.

Figure 5. Common patterns of melanoma metastases seen in sentinel nodes. (a) Single melanoma cells scattered along the subcapsular sinus (MART-1). (b) A micrometastasis in the subcapsular sinus and adjacent lymphoid tissue. These are often accompanied by single melanoma cells. Note the S-100-positive dendritic cells in the adjacent paracortical nodule (S-100 protein). (c) A larger colony of metastatic melanoma cells, based on the subcapsular sinus, but beginning to extend into the lymphoid tissue of the node (S-100 protein). (d) Larger metastases of melanoma involving the subcapsular region and the lymphoid tissues (S-100 protein).

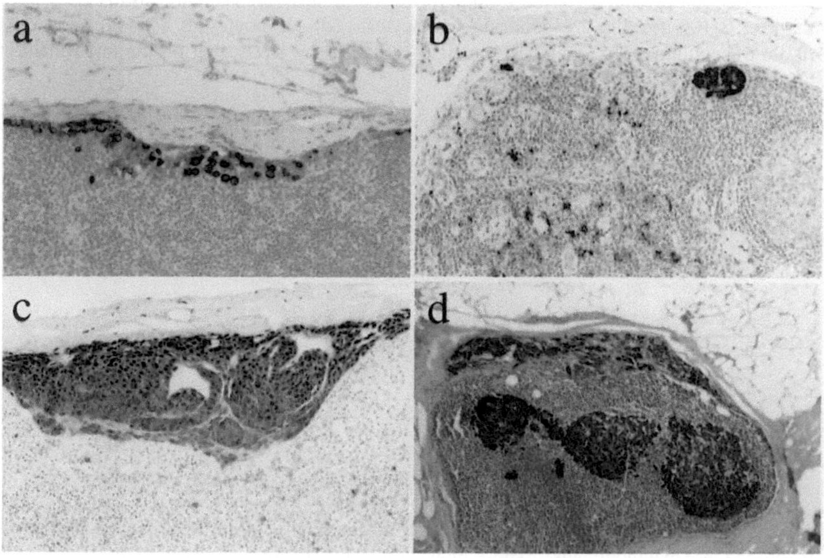

The proportion of SLN in which tumor is identified first in H&E sections increases with experience, but immunohistochemical analysis is still required. Tyrosinase and glycoprotein-100 are other markers of interest,[17,18] and there is some interest in the use of antibody cocktails. Antibodies to S-100 protein stain 100% of melanomas, whereas many other epitopes are not expressed by 10–20% of melanomas.[14] S-100 stains nodal cells that are not melanocytic, notably dendritic leukocytes of the paracortex, and separation of dendritic cells with reduced dendrites from small (and nevoid) melanoma cells can be difficult.[16] It is essential to use more than one immunomarker. We currently use S-100, HMB-45, and MART-1/Melan-A as single markers in parallel.

A potential pitfall in microscopic assessment of sentinel nodes for melanoma is misidentification of nonmelanoma cells in immunostained sections leading to a false-positive interpretation of the nodal tumor status. Confusion between (brown) melanin-containing macrophages and immunopositive melanoma cells may be reduced by the use of aminoethylcarbazole (red) rather than diaminobenzidine (brown) for antibody visualization. Other potential sources of false-positive interpretation are S-100 reactive dendritic cell (Figures 5b and 6c), capsular and trabecular nevi (Figure 6), histiocytes, intranodal and perinodal nerves and ganglion cells (Figure 7). HMB-45 reactivity in the absence of melanoma cells may be seen in the focally calcified trabeculae of inguinal or pelvic lymph nodes, most marked in older patients.

Figure 6. Node-associated nevocytes. (a) Nevocytes (possibly embolic) expanding an afferent lymphatic of a sentinel node (H&E). (b and c) Capsular nevocytes seen in an H&E stained section (b) and a section stained for S-100 protein (c). The subcapsular cells in (c) that are S-100-positive are dendritic leukocytes. (d) Nevocytes in a nodal connective tissue trabeculum. The image on the right is stained by H&E, that on the left for S-100 protein.

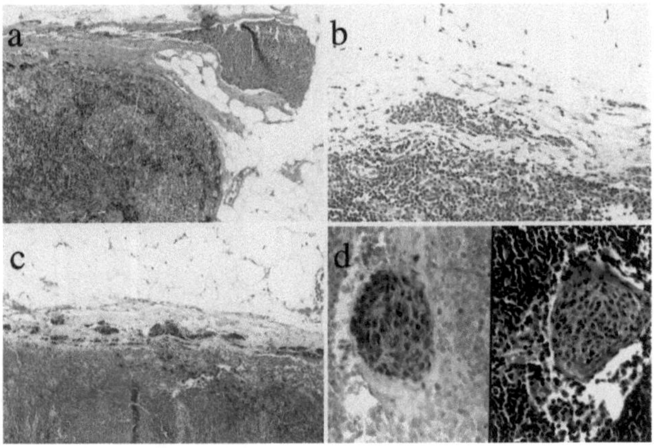

Figure 7. Some problems encountered in evaluating sentinel nodes. (a) Melanized macrophages (melanophages). These may show some reactivity with antibodies such as S-100 and MART-1. If may be necessary to bleach a section to assess the cytology. (b) Sinus macrophages may simulate melanoma cells but react with antibodies to macrophage markers and are usually nonreactive with antibodies to melanoma markers. (c) A large multinucleated macrophage reacting to the site of deposition of contrast medium. (d) Antibody to HMB-45 reacts nonspecifically to microcalcified structures in a groin lymph node. The structure at the extreme left is likely a single melanoma cell. This kind of reaction is relatively common in the calcified and sclerotic inguinal nodes of older patients.

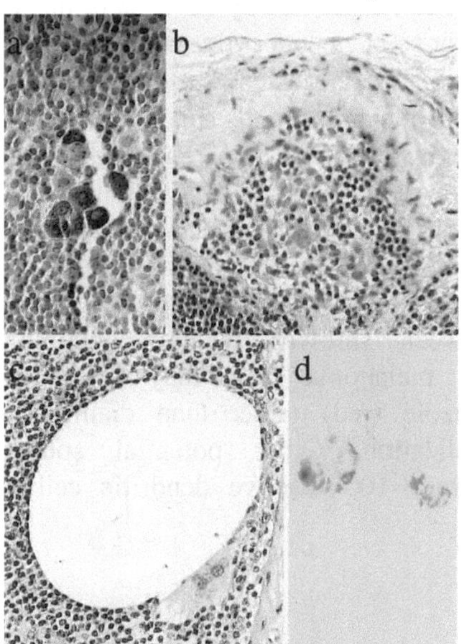

Discrimination of benign melanocytic and other cells from metastatic melanoma requires consideration of nodal architecture and cytologic features of the cells. Nevocytes typically occur in the nodal capsule around intracapsular vessels and in nodal trabeculae (Figure 6). When nevocytes appear to occur in the lymph node parenchyma, it is instructive to stain the section with Masson trichrome. This will usually demonstrate that such cells are actually present within subtle arborizations of the lymph node trabeculae. If this is not the case, consideration should be given to the possibility that the cells represent a metastasis of a nevocytically differentiated melanoma. Melanoma cells are usually larger than nevocytes and occur individually and in small aggregates within the subcapsular sinus and lymphoid tissues. Capsular/trabecular nevocytes have a low nucleus-to-cytoplasm ratio and lack prominent nucleoli. Histiocytes and macrophages have small, kidney bean-shaped nuclei with small nucleoli. Reactive histiocytes and endothelial cells may present cytologic appearances that raise the possibility of malignancy, requiring immunohistology for elucidation. Active antigen-presenting paracortical dendritic cells have readily visible elongated dendritic cell processes. The frequency, length, and complexity of dendrites may be sharply reduced in nodes that are immune down-regulated.[5-7]

Features that facilitate identification of melanoma cells include large size, a high nucleus-to-cytoplasm ratio, prominent nucleoli, mitotic figures (especially atypical forms) and the presence of the fine punctate melanin granules (single melanosomes that indicate melanogenesis by the cell) (as opposed to the coarse granules of melanin [aggregate melanosomes] that are seen in melanophages) (Figure 7).

Immunohistochemistry is of great assistance in distinguishing true metastases from other types of cells that may simulate melanoma. Nevocytic melanocytes are S-100$^+$, and MART-1$^+$, but have weak to absent reactivity for HMB-45 and are negative for Ki67. Paracortical dendritic cells, while S-100$^+$ are MART-1$^-$, HMB-45$^-$, and tyrosinase-negative. Intranodal nerves are S-100$^+$, but are negative for the other melanoma-associated markers.

The UCLA approach to SLN pathologic workup balances substantive assessment of each node with practical and economic constraints that impose limits on the extent of nodal sampling that is feasible. Tumor is detected in around 20% of SLN, a figure similar to the overall frequency of subsequent regional metastases in primary melanoma patients treated by wide excision alone.[19] Other approaches to SLN sectioning identify a similar frequency of positive SLN.[12,22]

The last word on pathological sampling has, however, yet to be written. We have recently shown that careful H&E section evaluation combined with immunohistochemistry detects occult metastatic melanoma in patients with primaries that are 2 mm thick or more at a frequency identical to the rate of regional nodal recurrence in thickness-matched patients treated by wide excision alone. In contrast the morphologic approach detects occult tumor in the sentinel nodes of patients with thinner primaries at a frequency that is lower than the regional nodal metastasis rate of patients who were treated by wide excision alone. Thus, conventional microscopy may fail to detect occult melanoma when that is present as a low amount of tumor. In the low-tumor-burden group it may be necessary to employ more extensive sampling[2] or supplement histology with studies by the real-time polymerase chain reaction.[4] This very important and practical concern further requires continuing study and will be examined in detail in the recently instituted NIH trial (Multicenter Selective Lymphadenectomy Trial-2). This trial is conducted by the John Wayne Cancer Institute, Santa Monica and proposals for participation are welcome. Information about the trial can be obtained by contacting Dr. Donald Morton at mortond@jwci.org. It will be essential to closely examine the reasons for the apparent underidentification of occult melanoma in patients with relatively thin primary melanomas. The explanation is likely to be complex. Factors involved will certainly include insufficient or inappropriate nodal sampling and misidentification of true sentinel nodes. Occult melanoma cell foci such as clinically inapparent satellites in tissues around the primary tumor excision site and in-transit lymphatic metastases may, in the presence of a tumor-free SLN, act as sources from which tumor cells may pass to nonsentinel nodes or other sites.

Molecular pathology

This topic is dealt with in detail elsewhere in this publication (Chapter 12). In this chapter it is appropriate to highlight the relationship of molecular approaches to conventional pathology as the two techniques will likely be used in the future to complement each other (see Morton et al.[4] for an up-to-date review). Molecular pathology detects the mRNA of melanoma-associated marker molecules. The markers that have been investigated to the present are not absolutely specific and may be expressed by cells other than melanoma cells. This fact is critical in attempting to interpret the meaning of an enhanced mRNA signal derived from lymph node or other tissues.

The majority of SLN from melanoma patients that have been investigated by both conventional pathology and RT-PCR neither contain visible melanoma cells nor have evidence of melanoma markers detected by RT-PCR. Such patients have a highly favorable outcome, very rarely recur, and can essentially be regarded as cured. Patients in whom tumor cells are identified by H&E/IPX and in whom melanoma markers are detected by RT-PCR have a distinctly poor prognosis and are likely to die from their melanoma. There is a third group with an intermediate prognosis who have detectable signal for one or more melanoma markers by RT-PCR, but no evidence of melanoma cells on microscopic evaluation. Thus, the two techniques are highly complementary and divide patients effectively on the basis of likelihood of melanoma metastasis and death. It is on this basis that we consider it likely that the two approaches will be used in parallel in the future. It has been suggested that increased sampling of the SLN may increase the detection of tumor to a frequency that is similar to that detected by conventional microscopy combined with RT-PCR.[20] Additional studies will be required to determine the truth of that assertion and the extent of sampling that will be practical and acceptable. Our data and those from Starz et al.[22] make a plausible case for the combined use of microscopy and RT-PCR.

Would it be feasible to abandon microscopy and simply analyze the nodes by RT-PCR? Probably not, because the preparative techniques required prior to performance of RT-PCR as presently performed require the destruction of the tissues. The cell of origin of any enhanced signal therefore cannot be identified. In various circumstances and with different markers it is possible that capsular and trabecular nevocytes, intranodal nerves, macrophages, and melanoma–macrophage hybrids could serve as the source of an enhanced signal. Overinterpretation of an enhanced mRNA signal as necessarily indicating the presence of metastatic melanoma would lead to a positive false interpretation that a patient is a tumor-positive and the likelihood of overtreatment.

REFERENCES

1. Morton DL, Wen D-R, Wong JH, Economou JS, Cagle LA, Storm FK, Foshag LJ, Cochran AJ. Technical details of intraoperative lymphatic mapping for early stage melanoma. Arch Surg 127(4):392-399, 1992.
2. Lucci A, Turner, RR, Morton DL. Carbon dye as an adjunct to isosulfan blue dye for sentinel lymph node dissection. Surgery 126:48-53, 1999.
3. Haigh PI, Lucci A, Turner RR, et al. Carbon dye histologically confirms the identity of sentinel nodes in cutaneous melanoma. Cancer 92:535-541, 2001.
4. Morton, DL, Hoon DSB, Cochran AJ, Turner RR, Essner R, Takeuchi H, Wanek LA, Glass E, Foshag LJ, Hsueh EC, Bilchik AJ, Elashoff D, Elashoff, R. Lymphatic mapping and sentinel lymphadenectomy for early-stage melanoma. Ann Surg 238:537-549, 2003.
5. Cochran AJ, Pihl E, Wen D-R, Hoon DSB, Korn EL. Zoned immune suppression of lymph nodes draining malignant melanoma: Histologic and immunohistologic studies. J Nat Cancer Inst 78:399-405, 1987.
6. Huang RR., Wen D-R, Guo J, Giuliano A, Turner R, Nguyen M, Cochran AJ Modulation of paracortical dendritic cells and T lymphocytes in breast cancer sentinel nodes. Breast J 6(4):225-232, 2000.
7. Cochran AJ, Morton DL, Stern S, Lana AM, Essner R, Wen D-R.. Sentinel lymph nodes show profound downregulation of antigen-presenting cells of the

paracortex: Implications for tumor biology and treatment. Mod Pathol 14:604-608, 2001.
8. Lana A-M, Wen D-R, Cochran A.J. The morphology, immunophenotype and distribution of paracortical dendritic leukocytes in lymph nodes regional to cutaneous melanoma. Melanoma Res 11:1-10, 2001.
9. Cochran A.J, Wen D-R, Herschman JR. Occult melanoma in lymph nodes detected by antiserum to S-100 protein. Int J Cancer 34:159-163, 1984.
10. Cochran A.J, Wen D-R, Morton DL. Occult melanoma cells in the lymph nodes of patients with pathological Stage I malignant melanoma: An immunohistological study. Am J Surg Pathol 12:612-618, 1988.
11. Singletary SE, Byers RM, Shallenberger R, McBride CM, Guinee VF. Prognostic factors in patients with regional cervical nodal metastases from cutaneous malignant melanoma. Am J Surg 152(4):371-375, 1986.
12. Starz H, Balda BR, Kramer KU, Buchels H, Wang H. A micromorphometry-based concept for routine classification of sentinel lymph node metastases and its clinical relevance for patients with melanoma. Cancer 91(11):2110-2121, 2001.
13. Cochran AJ, Morton DL, Johnson TD, et al. Prediction of outcome and tumor-status of the non-sentinel node in melanoma patients with a positive sentinel node (abstract). Mod Pathol 13:61, 2000.
14. Cochran AJ. Surgical pathology remains pivotal in the evaluation of 'sentinel' lymph nodes (review). Am J Surg Pathol 23(10):1169-1172, 1999.
15. Cochran AJ. The pathologist's role in sentinel lymph node evaluation (review). Semin Nucl Med 30(1):11–7, 2000.
16. Cochran AJ. Sentinel lymph node biopsy for melanoma: pathologic aspects. IN: Cody H (ed) Sentinel lymph node biopsy. Martin Dunitz, New York, pp 79-90, 2002.
17. Boyle JL, Haupt HM, Stern JB, Multhaupt HA. Tyrosinase expression in malignant melanoma, desmoplastic melanoma, and peripheral nerve tumors. Arch Pathol Lab Med 126(7):816-822, 2002.
18. Slominski A. Coming of age of melanogenesis-related proteins. Arch Pathol Lab Med 126:775-777, 2002.
19. Morton DL, Thompson JF, Essner R, Elashoff R, Stern SL, Nieweg OE, Roses DF, Karakousis CP, Mozzillo N, Reintgen D, Wang HJ, Glass EC, Cochran AJ. Validation of the accuracy of intraoperative lymphatic mapping and sentinel lymphadenectomy for early-stage melanoma: a multicenter trial. Multicenter Selective Lymphadenectomy Trial Group. Ann Surg 230(4):453-463; discussion 463-465, 1999.
20. Brady MaT, D. Sentinel lymph node biopsy for melanoma: review of published experience. IN: Cody H (ed) Sentinel lymph node biopsy. Martin Dunitz, New York, pp 161-173, 2002.
21. Cook MG, Green MA, Anderson B, Eggermont AMM, Ruiter DJ, Spatz AS, Kissin MW, Powell BW on behalf of the EORTC Melanoma Group. The development of optimal pathological assessment of sentinel lymph nodes for melanoma. J Pathol 200:314-319, 2003.
22. Starz H, Haas CJ, Schulz GM, Balda BR. Tyrosinase RT-PCR as a supplement to histology for detecting melanoma and nevus cells in paraffin sections of sentinel lymph nodes. Mod Patho 16(9):920-929, 2003.

Chapter 12

MOLECULAR DIAGNOSIS OF MICROMETASTASIS IN THE SENTINEL LYMPH NODE

Hiroya Takeuchi,[1] Robert A. Wascher,[1] Christine Kuo,[1] Roderick R. Turner,[2] Dave S.B. Hoon[1]
[1]Department of Molecular Oncology, [2]Department of Pathology, John Wayne Cancer Institute, Saint John's Health Center, Santa Monica, California

INTRODUCTION

The histopathological status of tumor-draining regional lymph nodes is one of the most significant predictors of recurrence and overall survival for most clinical stage I/II solid tumors, and is often used to justify stratification of patients for adjuvant therapy.[1-8]

The sentinel lymph node (SLN) is defined as one or more lymph nodes that first receive lymphatic drainage from the site of a tumor.[9] The SLN hypothesis was advanced to specifically address those patients at high risk of having lymph node (LN) metastasis based on the characteristics of their primary tumors, but who had no evidence of clinically detectable regional metastatic disease. SLN mapping and biopsy was first applied to melanoma, and was subsequently extended to breast cancer and, more recently, to many other solid tumors.10-28 The SLN concept for other solid tumors, including colorectal, esophageal, gastric, gynecologic, head and neck squamous cell, thyroid, urologic, and non-small-cell lung cancers, is still in the early stages of development. This concept has revolutionized the approach to the surgical staging of both melanoma and breast cancer, and has fundamentally resolved nagging questions as to the proper indications for extensive LN dissections in the former and, perhaps, in the latter disease as well.

For melanoma, breast cancer, and most other solid tumors, the morbidity of complete axillary, inguinal, and other regional LN basin dissections is significant, often disabling, and occasionally even life threatening.[29-34] The mapping and selective biopsy of the SLN(s) spares the patient significant potential morbidity, while simultaneously allowing the pathologist to perform a detailed and focused evaluation of a single or a few SLNs.[35-37] It has been estimated that, prior to the development of the SLN concept, as many as 80% of patients with primary melanomas < 4 mm thick who underwent elective lymph node dissection (ELND) did so without apparent benefit.[29,38]

Prior to the advent of the SLN concept, standard histopathologic assessment involved the cutting of several sections from multiple paraffin-embedded archival tissue (PEAT) lymph nodes, the staining of these sections with hematoxylin and eosin (H&E), and visualization under the light microscope by the pathologist. At this level of analysis, the detection of occult or small clumps of tumor cells within a background of mononuclear lymphoid cells in multiple LNs is a very tedious process and has been shown to have limitations in terms of sensitivity particularly for various carcinomas.[39,40] Before the advent of SLN mapping, the necessity of sampling multiple regional LNs for evidence of micrometastases was a labor-intensive and inefficient process, frequently resulting in "understaging" of the patient. The detailed analysis of multiple LNs, including serial sectioning, immunostaining, and assessing numerous serial LN sections, is costly, time-consuming, and also impractical for most community hospitals. In terms of today's health care logistics and costs, this is of major concern.

HISTOPATHOLOGICAL EVALUATION

Both H&E and IHC staining have been extensively used, in combination with thin serial sectioning of frozen and paraffin-embedded specimens, in the detection of micrometastatic disease in the SLN/LN.[40-47] The application of IHC has markedly improved the sensitivity of micrometastatic disease detection in the SLN/LN beyond the capability of routine H&E staining alone.[40-52]

The antibodies against tumor markers of interest must reproducibly be highly specific and sensitive for detection of tumor cells and virtually non-reactive to the adjacent nontumor cells in the SLN/LN. When searching for occult metastasis, the sensitivity of the antibody must be high. The most commonly used IHC target for epithelial carcinomas are the cytokeratins (CK), which are ubiquitously expressed as intermediate filaments in normal eukaryotic epithelial cells.[32,40-42,45,47,53] The risk of false-positive results with the use of individual anticytokeratin antibodies and some antibody cocktails has been well-described (54). An excellent review of the general topic of micrometastatic cancer detection has been written by Pantel and other colleagues, and should be considered complementary to our review.[42]

In comparison, the use of IHC to detect micrometastatic deposits of melanoma has been less problematic, due to the specificity of antibodies to HMB-45 and S-100 proteins.[38,55-57] Because these antibodies also have their limitations, new antibodies such as melanoma antigens recognized by T cells (MART-1) and microphthalmia-associated transcription factor (MITF) are being investigated.[58,59] IHC staining for detection of occult metastatic tumor cells in lymph nodes has been the "gold standard." More recently, molecular techniques have provided new approaches and demonstrated undetected metastatic tumor cells.

Figure 1. History of SLN micrometastasis diagnosis. ECL, electrochemiluminescence assay; CAE, capillary array electrophoresis.

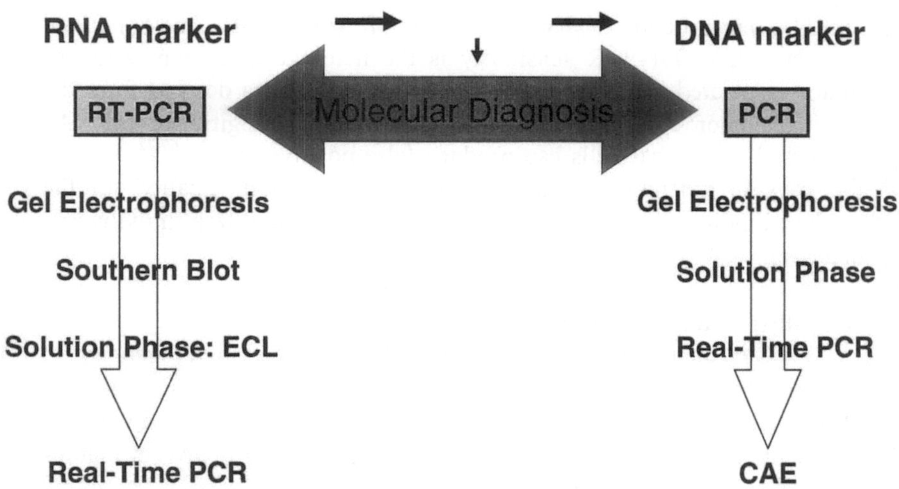

MOLECULAR DIAGNOSTIC APPROACHES FOR MICROMETASTIC DISEASE OF SLN/LN

Overview

The molecular detection of tumor cells using RNA or DNA markers with various PCR techniques has exponentially evolved in the last 10 years (Figure 1). The primary approach of molecular detection of tumor cells has been focused on mRNA of tumor markers using RT-PCR. Detection of metastatic tumor cells has been clearly demonstrated in lymph nodes, organs, and body fluids. Using RT-PCR, it is now possible to reliably detect 1–10 tumor cells within a background of 10^6–10^7 normal cells.[42,60-67] The high sensitivity of RT-PCR, as compared to H&E and IHC, allows for the detection of the histopathological equivalent of needles (i.e., occult tumor cells) in a haystack (SLN lymphoid cells). However, molecular-based techniques require the stringent optimization of sample processing, reagents, molecular targets, RT and PCR reactions, and PCR cDNA product detection assays. Meticulous attention to technique must be adhered to, throughout all stages of the assay, in order to ensure accurate results. As with IHC and its antigen targets, the specificity of molecular assays for tumor-associated targets depends on the selection of molecular target(s) expressed exclusively by tumor cells, and not expressed by the "normal cells" in the specimen being studied.[68] Contamination of reagents, particularly upstream of the PCR assay, can also produce flawed data and, therefore, inaccurate conclusions. False-negative results may arise when tissues are collected, processed, or stored under suboptimal conditions, or when reagents and reactions are not optimized. Small numbers of occult tumor cells that express only a few copies of the target mRNA may also prove difficult to detect within the "mRNA background" of many thousands of normal cells. Another factor that can affect RT-PCR sensitivity is the heterogeneous expression of tumor-associated genes by individual tumor cell clones derived from the original tumor. Additionally, the detection of "illegitimate mRNA" expressed by normal cells can produce false-positive results.[69-72] One of the keys to the most efficient RT-PCR assay is the "quality" of the marker. Finding a good marker(s) is the most important task in molecular detection.

Multiple marker RT-PCR

Our approach to the problem of tumor cell heterogeneity in marker expression is the use of a multiple marker RT-PCR assay, as developed by our laboratory for melanoma and breast cancer, and which is applicable to most solid tumors.[66] Tumors continue to evolve in marker expression and the strategy to detect this evolving target is complex. Targeting a panel of multiple mRNA markers increases the likelihood of detecting occult tumor cells that may not express a single tumor marker, or that express one or more markers at very low levels. This approach has been successfully applied to upstage patients with melanoma and breast cancer, and colorectal cancer more recently, with H&E/IHC-negative SLNs.[19,61,64,73-75] The use of a panel of multiple markers for RT-PCR has increased both the sensitivity and the reliability of results as compared to single marker RT-PCR assays.[19,61,66,76-81] We cannot overemphasize the importance of multiple marker assays for assessment of occult tumor cells. Another important consideration in performing either IHC or molecular studies on the SLN(s) is that of representative sampling, because failure to comprehensively sample the SLN can result in a high incidence of false-negative results.[82,83] Sampling of SLN/LN for analysis of IHC and RT-PCR remains a controversial field. This will continue to be so under the current guidelines of tissue usage and health care costs. We have developed a technique of cutting multiple thin sections, for the submission of alternating representative SLN sections to be analyzed by H&E/IHC or RT-PCR (Figure 2).[61,68,77]

Figure 2. Representation of SLN processing in our laboratory: the fresh SLN(s) are bisected and parallel thin serial sections are cut. Frozen section is performed on representative SLN sections, and submitted for Diff-Quick histopathology and RT-PCR analysis. The remaining sections are fixed in formalin and submitted for H&E and IHC staining and review.

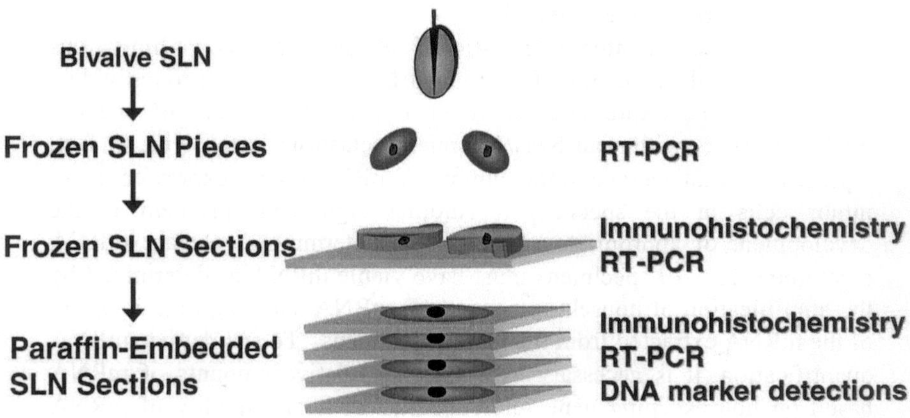

RT-PCR detection systems

A critical step in RT-PCR analysis is the detection of cDNA product(s). Currently, probe-based detection assays have now supplanted the older gel-based and hybridization assays (e.g., ethidium bromide gel and Southern blot assays). Recently, we have developed a highly sensitive high-throughput electrochemiluminescence (ECL) assay for PCR cDNA products (IGEN International, Inc., Gaithersburg, MD). This ECL solution phase system, when compared to ethidium bromide gel detection and Southern blot detection systems, is more sensitive, less labor intensive, and less subjective.[84] The ECL system is also semi-quantitative and more reproducible than traditional gel-based assays. TaqMan, also a probe-based detection system, allows for the real-time quantitative assessment of PCR cDNA products. Both ECL and TaqMan assays are representative of solution phase assays that allow for quantitative, repetitive, and high throughput analyses, and produce results that are much less subjective than previously used detection technologies.

Quantitative real-time PCR assay

Prior to the development of real-time PCR, it was difficult and arduous to perform quantitative molecular analysis. Quantitative real-time PCR assay is now being utilized more extensively to not only identify the presence of target mRNA but also to quantify the number of mRNA copies from tumor-associated genes of interest. Quantitative real-time PCR analysis permits the rapid molecular analysis of multiple mRNA targets expressed in tumor cells, and these results can then be correlated to clinical outcomes in order to study the relationship(s) between gene expression levels and prognosis.[64,76,85-87] Quantitative real-time PCR assay combined with multiple mRNA markers is an accurate, versatile, and sensitive technique. No other approach has reached this level of detection that can be reproduced easily to date.

However, quantitative real-time PCR assay has its own limitations with respect to the detection of micrometastatic disease. Due to individual tumor cell gene expression heterogeneity, copy numbers of specific mRNA markers within an SLN/LN micrometastasis lesion will, in fact, represent only an average of the number of mRNA copies expressed by all tumor cells in the specimen. Another significant problem is the development of appropriate standards for determining relevant mRNA copy numbers. All specimens must have viable mRNA as determined by the amplification of housekeeping gene(s) mRNA showing high integrity of the mRNA extracted from the tumor specimens. To standardize mRNA quantification, it is necessary to assess the relative amounts of mRNA based on housekeeping gene reference standards and quality of mRNA itself.[88] Specific mRNA expression is normalized with housekeeping gene mRNAs such as glyceraldehyde-3-phosphate dehydrogenase (GAPDH), porphobilinogen deaminase (PBGD), and β2-microglobulin.[88]

Because housekeeping gene mRNA expression can also vary significantly in tumor cells from their comparative normal cell counterparts, another method for mRNA quantification is to use an absolute value of the target mRNA copy number per specific amount of total RNA for analysis.[88] A standard curve with specific copy numbers of the target cDNA allows a more accurate estimate of mRNA copies in the amount of sample being tested (Figure 3). The method of reporting gene expression has yet to be standardized and can be a factor for variation in reporting assay results across different laboratories.

Figure 3. Representative qRT analysis for MART-1 mRNA copy levels. A: Serially diluted plasmids containing MART-1 cDNA (10^0 to 10^8 copies) were analyzed for controls. B: Standard curve (correlation coefficient, 0.998; PCR efficiency, 100%). ○ (blue): standards. □ (red): unknown samples. RFU, relative fluorescence unit.

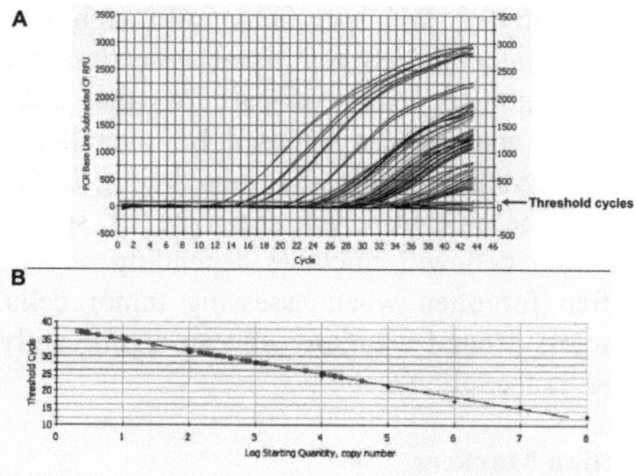

Real-time PCR assay which enables rapid analysis is currently being attempted for intraoperative molecular diagnosis.[89] Lymph nodes along the recurrent laryngeal nerves obtained from patients with esophageal cancer were assessed prospectively by intraoperative histopathologic examination and real-time RT-PCR assay using multiple markers (CEA, SCC, and MAGE-A3).[89] The whole procedure takes only 2.5 hours from the tissue sampling to completion of the real-time RT-PCR assay. Genetic diagnosis by intraoperative real-time PCR assay could predict cervical lymph node metastasis and may be used to indicate subsequent cervical lymphadenectomy. Further improvements of the assay may allow the PCR-based intraoperative diagnosis to be applicable to other cancer surgeries. Cepheid has instrumentation that allows rapid assessment of genes.[90] At the present time, this technique still requires further validation.

SLN specimen type and sampling

Traditional RT-PCR assays for assessing SLNs have been primarily based on analysis of frozen lymph node tissues using gel-based systems which are often subjective in interpretation and limited in sensitivity. Molecular analysis of frozen SLNs is limited by sampling error, logistic difficulties during multicenter studies, quality control, RT-PCR assay limitations, and most importantly specimen handling. False negatives occur when metastatic tumor cells are missed due to the bias of tissue sampling. On the other hand, contamination in the PCR reactions can occur during tissue preparation and produce false-positive results. Our laboratory therefore developed a more sensitive PCR-based assay using ECL or quantitative real-time PCR that utilizes PEAT SLN specimens.[91,92] A PEAT specimen is desirable because of its stability during storage and transport. Most importantly the approach of using PE SLN can be easily applied to multicenter trials.[92] In developing an RT-PCR assay for PE SLNs, primers and probes should be modified and redesigned to address RNA degradation, limited marker mRNA copy numbers, tumor heterogeneity, sensitivity, and specificity. Although RNA degradation occurs during the interval between tissue resection and fixation, the degree of degradation depends in part on the mRNA's half-life. Housekeeping gene analysis can be used for overall analysis of RNA degradation, but degradation time can vary among individual cells and gene transcripts. The mRNA level and type of specific gene being assessed in a tumor cell will fluctuate depending on its "physiological state." It is often forgotten when assessing tumor cells that the host environment factors around a tumor cell can significantly influence the "individual gene transcription state."

DNA Detection Markers

Molecular-based assays have historically been focused on mRNA targets as tumor-associated DNA markers are more problematic when assaying for micrometastases within the SLN/LN. The majority of potential DNA tumor markers include base substitutions, deletions, insertions, and chromosomal translocations (Table 1). However, they are difficult to assess on a small number of tumor cells detected among a large number of normal cells. In tumor types that are known to frequently express specific mutations, the mutation sites within the affected gene(s) are often multiple and variable in nature. However, there are exceptions.

K-*ras* is a useful DNA target in that the tumor-associated mutations in this gene are consistently and specifically limited to one or a few codons and occur frequently in CRC, pancreatic, and lung tumors.[93] Using a peptide nucleic acid (PNA)-clamping PCR assay for SLN analysis, K-*ras* mutation has been assessed in our laboratory as a DNA molecular marker in 72 primary CRC tumors and paired paraffin-embedded SLNs. Thirty (42%) of 72 tumors were found to be positive for K-*ras*. In 11 (92%) of 12 cases, SLNs histopathologically positive for metastatic disease were also positive for K-*ras* by PNA-clamping PCR (all primary tumors and SLNs were concordant for K-*ras* mutation). PNA-clamping PCR identified occult metastases in an additional six patients, upstaging 24% of K-*ras* positive primary CRCs. This study, therefore, demonstrated the potential utility of one potential DNA marker (i.e., K-*ras*) and suggests that genetic mutations arising from consistent single codon error and occurring frequently in specific cancers may be useful targets for molecular analysis.[94,95]

Table 1. Molecular markers for detection of micrometastasis of SLN/LN

Marker	Type	Target
RNA markers	Cancer specific	MAGE-A family, β-HCG, telomerase
		Tyrosinase, TRP-1, TRP-2, MART-1, MITF, PSA, PSMA, cytokeratin, CEA, SCC, muc-1, p97, AFP, mammaglobin
	Tissue specific	A/B, ER
DNA markers	Point mutation	p53, p16, ER, K-ras, B-raf
	Deletion	BRCA1, BRCA2, DCC
		c-erbB2, EGFR, myc, mdm2
	Amplification	cyclin D1
	Others	Translocations
		Hypermethylation in CpG island of tumor suppressor genes

AFP, alpha-fetoprotein; β-HCG, human chorionic gonadotropin β; BRCA, hereditary breast cancer gene; CEA, carcinoembryonic antigen; DCC, deleted-in-colorectal cancer gene; EGFR, epidermal growth factor receptor; ER, estrogen receptor; MAGE, melanoma antigen gene; MART-1, melanoma antigen recognized by T cell 1; MITF, microphthalmia-associated transcription factor; PSA, prostate-specific antigen; PSMA, prostate-specific membrane antigen; SCC, squamous cell carcinoma antigen; TRP, tyrosinase-related protein.

(These are some representative reported markers.)

Another potential DNA marker frequently confined to a single site is B-*raf* which has a mutation at V600E in exon 15.[96] B-*raf* mutation can be detected in > 60% of metastatic cutaneous melanoma. B-*raf* mutation is suggested to be a potential DNA marker to detect micrometastasis in the LN/SLN. We have detected B-raf mutations in metastatic tissues using capillary array electrophoresis (CAE) and also real-time PCR. The latter requires a clamping procedure with PNA.[97] CAE assays are useful for DNA sequencing, fragment sizing, and microsatellite marker analysis. DNA fragments are separated in gel-filled capillaries, and large numbers of samples can easily be loaded. CAE is a rapid and reproducible assay which can perform objective evaluations of the DNA fragments derived from metastatic tumor cells in LN/SLN.

Other Diagnostic Molecular Approaches

Other molecular-based techniques are also being adapted to the field of molecular oncology. The use of cDNA microarrays to screen large numbers of tumor cell gene changes in levels of expression has already provided important insights into the molecular profiles of tumor cells.[69,98-104] Currently, however, the sensitivity of cDNA microarrays is inefficient in consistently detecting and quantifying micrometastatic levels of tumor cells as the signal from the very small numbers of tumor cells is lost within the "background noise" of the very large number of normal cells.

One potential limitation of molecular analysis, when compared to H&E/IHC staining and light microscopy, is the lack of morphologic information. However, the use of *in situ* PCR and mRNA-probe *in situ* hybridization can provide detailed morphologic information while providing the exceptional sensitivity of a molecular detection assay.[105-107] The major problems with *in situ* PCR are reproducibility, lack of quantification, and labor technical requirements.

These significant technological improvements in the ability to detect micrometastatic LN/SLN disease have, perhaps, raised as many questions as they have answered. The most significant among these is the question of the clinical relevance of micrometastatic disease in the SLN.

MOLECULAR ANALYSIS OF THE SLN/LN

Overview

The current definition of SLN/LN micrometastasis is a deposit of tumor cells measuring ≤ 2 mm. However, this definition has become somewhat arbitrary due to the high degree of sensitivity of IHC and RT-PCR. With the advent of increasingly more sensitive detection assays for early metastasis, the actual definition of micrometastasis may need to be reconsidered. Does the detection of a single or a few occult tumor cells in the SLN/LN represent a biologically relevant micrometastasis? How many tumor cells must an LN/SLN micrometastasis contain for it to be of potential clinicopathological significance? Are tumor cells being detected active, dormant, dead or on a death pathway?

It has been demonstrated that the metastatic potential of individual tumor cells varies and that not all embolic tumor cells are capable of progressing to functional metastatic tumors.[70,108] There is also evidence to suggest that the number of tumor cells in the LN/SLN, as well as the location of nodal micrometastasis (i.e., single or few occult tumor cells versus clumps of cells, and cells located within the subcapsular sinus versus the nodal parenchyma), may be pathologically relevant factors.[43,56,109-113] A study by Nasser et al.[108] has suggested that the presence of rare occult breast cancer cells in LNs may have little or no prognostic significance. They reported that breast cancer patients with LN metastasis ≤ 0.2 mm in greatest dimension had the same clinical outcomes as patients without occult LN disease while those with ≥ 0.2 mm deposits of tumor in the LN experienced a worse recurrence rate (p=0.02), a worse disease-free survival (p=0.04), and a worse overall survival (p=0.07).

Page and colleagues [109] have described the phenomenon of benign transport of mammary epithelial cells into the sinus of axillary LNs following breast biopsy. Such translocated epithelial cells, whether benign or malignant, appear as occult metastases of the SLN by cytokeratin IHC. False-positive results arising from such translocated benign epithelial cells require the development of new PCR tumor markers that are more specific for tumor cells, but are not expressed by benign epithelial cells. This dilemma continues to challenge laboratories performing molecular studies of carcinomas, and its resolution awaits the discovery of more specific epithelial tumor markers. Another potential source of false-positive results is the expression of cytokeratins by reticulum cells and plasma cells in the SLN. Concerns regarding false-positive results by cytokeratin IHC apply to most epithelial tumors, including breast, CRC, gastric esophageal, squamous cell (head and neck and lung), urologic, and gynecologic carcinomas. There may be differences in interpretation and disease outcome of tumor cells in LN/SLN for individual cancer types.

At the present time, the presence of detectable tumor cells in the SLN/LN is considered a micrometastasis if the aggregate of such cells measures ≤ 2 mm. The issue of what constitutes a biologically significant SLN/LN micrometastasis, however, will remain subject to debate until our understanding of important occult tumor cell characteristics is further clarified, and more precise clinicopathological standards are established. At the present time, it appears that the current definition of SLN/LN micrometastasis may have already become too broad to be of clinical value, and may require further assessment and refinement, based on the sensitivity of current detection assays. New pathological standards will have to be adopted to take full advantage of the sensitivity offered by current detection approaches.

Historically, the clinicopathological relevance of micrometastatic SLN/LN disease (as it is presently defined) has been both unclear and controversial. There is, however, growing evidence that LN/SLN micrometastases may indeed portend a worse prognosis in melanoma, and in many other solid cancers, including breast, CRC, esophageal, gastric, lung, gallbladder, head and neck, gynecologic, and urologic cancers.[21,26,39-47,60-62,74,112-134]

Melanoma

The molecular detection of melanoma, using RT-PCR, is facilitated by the expression of melanogenesis-specific genes by melanoma tumors cells, including tyrosinase, gp-100/pmel-17, MART-1, MITF, and tyrosinase-related proteins 1 and 2 (TRP-1, TRP-2).[60,61,66,73,75,80,81,84,91,92,134-136] The expression of various mRNA transcripts of the human melanoma-associated antigen (MAGE-A) family of tumor-associated genes has also been demonstrated in a variety of tumors, including melanoma and cancers of the breast and gastrointestinal tract.[61,66,78]

Several studies have reported on the use of RT-PCR to detect micrometastatic melanoma in the LN/SLNs, and have shown that RT-PCR can significantly upstage patients with LN/SLNs that are negative by H&E and IHC (Table 2).[60,61,75,136,137] In addition to the accurate detection of micrometastatic melanoma cells in the SLN/LNs using molecular assays, there is persuasive evidence that the detection of such micrometastases by molecular means has prognostic significance as well. Regarding the SLN in particular, Reintgen et al.[138] followed 114 patients with melanoma for a mean duration of 28 months. Patients with SLNs that were histopathologically and RT-PCR negative had a recurrence rate of 2%, while patients with histopathologically negative but RT-PCR-positive SLNs had a 13% recurrence rate (p=0.02).

In 1999 Bostick et al.[61] reported on their study of the SLNs of 72 patients with early stage melanoma, using a multiple marker RT-PCR assay (tyrosinase, MART-1, and MAGE-3). Bisection and serial sectioning of SLNs, prior to H&E/IHC and molecular analysis, was performed to reduce the false-negative rate associated with random or limited sampling of the SLN. Twenty (36%) of 55 patients with SLNs negative by H&E and IHC stains were positive for at least two out of the three markers in the panel (44% of these 55 patients expressed MAGE-3, 36% expressed MART-1, and 29% expressed tyrosinase). By multivariate analysis, the presence of ≥ 2 RT-PCR markers in the SLN correlated with a significantly increased risk of recurrence (p=0.02).

Blaheta et al.[74] evaluated 214 SLNs from 116 patients with melanoma using IHC and single marker (tyrosinase) RT-PCR. Patients were followed up for a median of 19 months. Using H&E and IHC alone, 15 of 116 (13%) patients were confirmed to have SLN micrometastasis. Of the remaining 101 patients with histopathologically negative SLNs, 36 (36%) SLNs were positive by RT-PCR for tyrosinase. Of the 15 patients with histopathologically detected SLN micrometastases, 10 (67%) recurred, as compared to an overall recurrence rate of 20% among all 116 patients. During a 19-month median follow-up period, the recurrence rate for patients with RT-PCR-positive SLNs was 25%, and the recurrence rate in patients with negative SLNs by H&E, IHC, and RT-PCR was only 6%

(p=0.01). By multivariate analysis, histopathological and RT-PCR SLN tumor status were the only significant predictors of disease-free survival.

Table 2. SLN/LN RT-PCR studies: Melanoma

Study	Number of patients	Lymph node	PCR marker(s)	H&E/IHC positive (%)	RT-PCR positive (%)
Wang (1994)[137]	29	RLN[a]	Tyrosinase	38	66
Goydos (1998)[75]	45	SLN[b]	Tyrosinase, MART-1	22	29
Blaheta (1998)[62]	79	RLN	Tyrosinase	39	66
Shivers (1998)[138]	114	SLN	Tyrosinase	20	61
Blaheta (1999)[87]	73	SLN	Tyrosinase	18	49
Bostick (1999)[61]	72	SLN	Tyrosinase, MART-1, MAGE-A3	24	50[c]
Blaheta (2000)[74]	101	SLN	Tyrosinase	0	36
Shivers (2001)[60]	233	SLN	Tyrosinase	22	70
Ribuffo (2003)[134]	134	SLN	Tyrosinase, MART-1	11	63
Goydos (2003)[139]	175	SLN	Tyrosinase	19	58
Kuo (2003)[91]	77	SLN (PEAT)	Tyrosinase, MART-1, TRP-1, TRP-2	48	55[c]
Morton (2003)[92]	215	SLN (PEAT)	Tyrosinase, MART-1, TRP-2, MITF	25	47

[a]RLN, regional lymph nodes. [b]SLN, sentinel lymph nodes. [c]Percent of two or more markers positive.

(The authors regret not being able to cite all published studies. Studies were cited in this review based on sample size and/or the application of RT-PCR to previously unstudied tumors.)

Goydos et al.[139] reported on their study of 175 patients of stage I and II melanoma using single marker (tyrosinase) RT-PCR. At a median follow-up of 34 months, 17 of 34 (50%) patients with histologically positive SLNs had a recurrence. Of the 141 patients with histologically negative SLNs, 73 patients were negative for tyrosinase by RT-PCR, and none of these patients had a recurrence. Of the 68 patients with histologically negative but RT-PCR-positive SLNs, 14 patients (21%) had a recurrence.

Palmieri and colleagues[140] studied the PE SLNs from 16 melanoma patients with multiple marker (MART-1 and tyrosinase) RT-PCR. They found that both the stage of disease and the clinical progression of disease were significantly associated with both the presence and the number (p=0.001 and p=0.006, respectively) of positive RT-PCR markers found in the SLN of each patient.

Kuo et al.[91] reported on the PEAT SLNs of 77 patients with early-stage melanoma using a multiple marker RT-PCR by an ECL detection system. Four markers were used: tyrosinase, MART-1, TRP-1, and TRP-2. They initially demonstrated the capability of the assay in assessing PEAT SLN. At least one of the four melanoma markers could be detected in all PEAT metastatic melanoma specimens (n=45), and none of them was detected in any of the non cancerous PEAT lymph nodes (n=10) or tonsils (n=15). At a median follow-up of 55 months among 40 patients, patients with histopathologically negative SLNs had a significantly improved disease-free (p<0.002) and overall (p<0.03) survival if the SLNs expressed no more than one mRNA marker. Morton et al.[92] assessed the PEAT SLNs of 215 patients with AJCC stage I/II melanoma using a multiple marker quantitative real-time PCR assay. Tyrosinase, MART-1, TRP-2, and MITF were used as specific mRNA markers. Among 162 patients with histopathologically negative SLNs, 49 (30%) patients were PCR-positive and were upstaged. These patients had a significantly increased risk of disease recurrence and death compared to both histopathology and PCR marker negative patients by multivariate analysis (p<0.0001). These studies demonstrated the clinicopathological utility of detecting micrometastatic melanoma in PEAT SLNs.

The 5-year survival approaches 90% for patients with American Joint Committee on Cancer stage I malignant melanoma, 70% for stage II melanoma, but decreases significantly to 25–50% for stage III melanoma. Therefore, accurate staging is highly important for optimal management of early stage disease. Clinicopathological relevance of micrometastatic melanoma in SLNs detected by RT-PCR assay is still controversial because melanoma mRNA markers for RT-PCR assay are often expressed in melanocytes or nevus cells. A series of previous studies which reported prognostic significance of micrometastatic melanoma in SLNs detected by RT-PCR, however, may portend a clinical utility of molecular detection of micrometastasis in SLNs. Future investigations will prospectively validate clinicopathological importance of micrometastatic melanoma in SLNs.

Breast Cancer

A number of mRNA targets have been studied in breast cancer, including MAGE-A, MUC-1, C-MET, β1→4-N-acetylgalactosaminyltransferase (β1→4-GalNAc-T), β-hCG, carcinoembryonic antigen (CEA), prostate specific antigen (PSA), mammaglobin 1 and 2, c-myc, prolactin inducible protein (PIP), and various cytokeratin family markers.[77,78,141-148] However, the specificity of several of these markers for breast cancer, including CEA, CK-19, and MUC-1, appears to be poor based on positive results for RT-PCR performed on LNs and blood in healthy patients without breast cancer.[68,149,150] MAGE-A3 may be a promising breast cancer molecular marker, as it appears to be expressed by approximately 50% of breast cancers, but is not expressed in normal mammary epithelium, or in the LNs or blood of healthy volunteer donors.[78,151]

Although not as extensive as the work that has been done with melanoma, there is compelling evidence to suggest a clinically relevant impact of SLN/LN micrometastasis detected by molecular assays in breast cancer (Table 3).

Table 3. SLN/LN RT-PCR Studies: Breast Cancer

Study	No. of patients	Lymph node	PCR marker(s)	H&E/IHC Positive (%)	RT-PCR Positive (%)
Noguchi (1994)[142]	15	RLN	MUC-1	18	30
Lockett (1998)[148]	35	RLN	Cytokeratin-19, c-myc, prolactin inducible protein	0	40
Bostick (1998)[77]	41	SLN	β1→4-GalNAc-T, C-MET, p97	30*	95*
Masuda (2000)[141]	129	RLN	CEA	0	31
Wascher (2001)[152]	77	SLN	MAGE-A3	45	53
Manzotti (2001)[172]	123	SLN	Maspin, cytokeratin-19, CEA, MUC-1, mammaglobin	33	53*
Sakaguchi (2003)[173]	108	SLN	Cytokeratin-19, epithelial glycoprotein 2	26	30

*Percent of total number of SLNs found to be positive.

(The authors regret not being able to cite all published studies. Studies were cited in this review based on sample size and/or the application of RT-PCR to previously unstudied tumors.)

In 1998, Bostick et al.[77] demonstrated significant correlation between the presence of positive RT-PCR markers (C-MET, β1→4-N-acetylgalactosaminyltransferase, P97) in the SLN and primary tumor estrogen receptor status (p=0.04) and Bloom-Richardson histopathological grade (p=0.04), both of which are known prognostic factors.

Wascher et al.[152] assessed MAGE-A3 mRNA as a molecular marker for the detection of tumor cells in the SLN of breast cancer patients. Serial frozen sections of SLNs (n=121) obtained from 77 AJCC stage I–IIIA breast cancer patients were assessed by RT-PCR and Southern blot analysis. Forty-one of 77 (53%) patients were positive for MAGE-A3. MAGE-A3 mRNA expression in the SLN occurred more frequently with infiltrating lobular carcinoma than with infiltrating ductal carcinoma (p<0.001).

Others have studied non-SLN axillary LNs in breast cancer patients and have reported similar findings. Lockett et al.[148] assessed 61 consecutive breast cancer patients with H&E/IHC and a multiple marker RT-PCR assay (CK-19, c-myc, prolactin inducible protein). A total of 15 (40%) of 37 patients with H&E/IHC-negative LNs were positive by RT-PCR. An increasing number of positive RT-PCR markers correlated with increased primary tumor size (p<0.01) and decreased predicted 5-year survival (p=0.02).

In 2000, Masuda and colleagues[141] evaluated 149 breast cancer patients with negative LNs by both H&E and IHC evaluation. RT-PCR was performed using CEA as a marker, and 40 of 129 (31%) patients were found to have RT-PCR-positive LNs. Patients with RT-PCR-negative LNs had a 10-year disease-free survival rate of 88% versus 66% for RT-PCR-negative patients (p=0.0008) and an overall 10-year survival rate of 94% versus 68%, respectively (p=0.0024). On multivariate analysis, patients with RT-PCR-positive LN micrometastasis were found to have a hazard ratio of 3.992 (p=0.016) for relapse and 4.293 (p=0.0436) for death due to cancer. In view of the definition of the SLN, these compelling findings in the study of axillary LNs would be expected to be highly applicable to the molecular status of the SLN as well.

In general, the prognosis for breast cancer patients with early intervention is relatively more favorable than other carcinomas. Therefore, prognostic utility of molecular detection of micrometastasis in SLNs for breast cancer patients remains unclear. One major problem in evaluating the prognostic value of micrometastasis detection in SLN is that patients who had undergone SLND are often treated with postoperative adjuvant therapy. A minimum of 8 years is required for the follow-up of a large number of patients through a significant number of events. Detection of occult tumor cells in the SLN has not shown significant clinical utility to date.

Colorectal Cancer

The application of molecular analysis to the SLN in CRC is currently at an early stage (Table 4). However, with the recent and successful applications of the SLN concept to this disease, preliminary data from molecular-based assays are now being generated.[19,78,153-157]

Table 4. SLN/LN RT-PCR studies: Gastrointestinal cancers

Study	No. of patients	Tumor	Lymph node	PCR marker(s)	H&E/IHC positive (%)	RT-PCR positive (%)
Noguchi (1996)[164]	12	Gastric	RLN	Cytokeratin-19	7	21
Ichikawa (1998)[154]	15	Colon	RLN	MMP-7	19	26
Kijima (2000)[166]	21	Esophagus	RLN	CEA	52	86
Bernini (2000)[156]	43	Colorectal	RLN	MUC-2	0	28
Bilchik (2001)[19]	40	Colorectal	SLN	β-hCG, C-MET, MAGE-A	35	60
Yoshioka (2002)[89]	50	Esophagus	RLN	CEA, SCC, MAGE-A3	20 (intra-operative diagnosis)	48 (intra-operative diagnosis)
Noura (2002)[158]	64	Colorectal	RLN	CEA	55	30

(The authors regret not being able to cite all published studies. Studies were cited in this review based on sample size and/or the application of RT-PCR to previously unstudied tumors.)

Molecular markers for SLN/LN analysis in CRC studied so far include cytokeratin(s), CEA, MAGE-A, C-MET, β-hCG, MUC-2, and matrix metalloproteinases.[19,78,153-157]

Increasingly, CRC is being studied to evaluate the prognostic impact of micrometastatic SLN/LN disease. In 1998, Liefers et al.[157] analyzed 192 LNs from 26 stage II (i.e., with histopathologically negative LNs) CRC patients using nested RT-PCR and CEA as a molecular marker. In this study, 14 (54%) of 26 patients had LNs that were RT-PCR positive. The cancer-related 5-year survival rate for these 14 patients was 50%, while survival rate among the remaining 12 patients was 91% (p=0.03).

Table 5. SLN/LN RT-PCR studies: Other cancers

Study	No. of patients	Tumor	Lymph node	PCR marker(s)	H&E/IHC positive (%)	RT-PCR positive (%)
Deguchi (1993)[162]	22	Prostate	RLN	PSA	11	20
Edelstein (1996)[161]	57	Prostate	RLN	PSA	0	44
Ferrari (1997)[163]	33	Prostate	RLN	PSA, PSMA	12	94
Salerno (1998)[160]	28	Lung	RLN	MUC-1	0	38
Cortesina (2000)[159]	20	Head & neck	RLN	C-MET	24*	40*
Okami (2000)[168]	15	Biliary	RLN	CEA, mamma-globin	10*	21*
Van Trappen (2001)[23]	32	Cervix	RLN	Cytokeratin-19	4*	44*

*Percent of total number of SLNs found to be positive

(The authors regret not being able to cite all published studies. Studies were cited in this review based on sample size and/or the application of RT-PCR to previously unstudied tumors.)

Bernini et al.[156] recently studied the LNs of 43 CRC patients, using MUC-2 as a molecular target for RT-PCR. They found a correlation between RT-PCR LN positivity and the size of the primary tumor. None (0%) of the 10 Tis/T1 tumors and 1 (17%) of 6 T2 tumors had LNs positive by RT-PCR, while 10 (40%) of 25 T3 tumors and 1 (50%) of 2 T4 tumors were positive by RT-PCR. These results are of clinical significance, because primary tumor T-stage is a known prognostic factor for CRC.

Interim results from the first multicenter phase II trial evaluating the molecular staging of the SLN in early colon cancer (i.e., stage I/II) were recently reported by Bilchik and colleagues.[19] Forty patients with histopathologically negative (by H&E) SLNs were assessed by IHC for cytokeratin, and by a multiple marker RT-PCR panel (β-hCG, C-MET, and MAGE-A3) and ECL detection systems. A 100% SLN mapping success rate was demonstrated, with a 0% false-negative rate. Importantly, in 3 (8%) of 40 cases, the SLN was identified outside of the traditional oncologic resection margins, allowing for a modification of the operation (in one of these three cases, the SLN was positive by IHC). In 10 (25%) cases, the SN was positive by H&E. In 4 (10%) cases, the SLN(s) were positive by IHC and negative by H&E. Of the remaining 26 patients with negative SLNs by H&E and IHC, 12 (46%) were positive for at least two RT-PCR markers. This study, which is ongoing, also demonstrated a correlation between the number of markers detected and the tumor T-stage ($p<0.04$), which is, by itself, a significant prognostic factor for colon cancer. These intriguing results suggest that molecular staging can be successfully and meaningfully applied to the SLN in CRC, in addition to melanoma and breast cancer.

Noura et al.[158] recently reported a comparative study of detection of micrometastasis using IHC and RT-PCR assay in H&E-negative LNs of 64 AJCC stage II CRC patients. CEA was used for RT-PCR assay and compared to IHC study with anticytokeratin antibody. Micrometastases were detected in 19 (30%) of 64 patients by RT-PCR and in 35 (55%) of 64 patients by IHC. Patients who were PCR-positive in LNs showed significantly worse disease-free and overall survival (p=0.027 and 0.025) than PCR-negative patients. However, micrometastasis in LNs detected by IHC did not correlate with prognosis. Although larger prospective study may be required for the validation of the assay, the results suggested the prognostic utility of molecular detection of micrometastasis in LN/SLNs of CRC patients.

Other Carcinomas

Gastric, esophageal, prostate, biliary, head and neck, lung, and gynecologic cancers have also been upstaged following RT-PCR analysis medical therapy. Indeed, it is likely that the current definition of SLN micrometastasis has already become too broad in view of the highly sensitive detection assays now available. The routine application of molecular detection assays may further complicate the stratification of patients for additional—and potentially toxic—therapies, unless the true biology of SLN micrometastasis is further clarified for each tumor type. The balance between "inadequately sensitive" detection (i.e., understaging) and "excessively sensitive" (i.e., overstaging) assays can only be found through a better understanding of the clinicopathological significance of occult and micrometastatic SLN disease.

For all of the controversy, the ability to, ideally, detect a single cancer cell in a background of millions of normal cells offers a powerful tool with which to diagnose the presence of minimal metastatic disease, as well as to follow patient response to therapy. This clinical application of molecular biology-based technology is also poised to play a key role in defining the prognostic significance of SLN micrometastasis, within the context of prospective multicenter trials. When coupled with the SLN mapping concept, and all of its advantages to the patient, a powerful diagnostic combination results.

As the unraveling of the human genome completes, the number of known tumor-associated molecular targets will increase, providing a fertile field for the further evolution of molecular-based analysis of the SLN. It is possible that the combined application of molecular biology-based detection assays to the SLN, blood and bone marrow, and to the primary tumor as well, may someday allow clinicians to create a composite diagnostic and prognostic profile for individual cancer patients. Such a profile would, ideally, allow for highly individualized prognostic and adjuvant therapy algorithms to be developed and uniquely applied to a specific patient.

The development of PEAT sampling of SLN will allow better analysis for metastatic disease in SLN and provide a platform to design standard operating procedures applicable to any pathology laboratory around the world. It is strongly believed that molecular staging will be a significant part of pathology staging procedures in the near future. We have come a long way in a short time from our first molecular diagnosis using multiple markers for the detection of tumor cells in SLNs in 1991. Currently, we have started a National Cancer Institute (USA) funded International Randomized Trial (Multicenter Selective Lymphadenectomy Trial II; MSLT II) whereby molecular staging will be used to randomize a complete lymph node dissection. PEAT specimens will be used for multiple marker quantitative real-time RT-PCR analysis as described by Takeuchi et al.[171] The future for molecular staging of tumor draining lymph nodes looks promising and should benefit and improve patient managements.

medical therapy. Indeed, it is likely that the current definition of SLN micrometastasis has already become too broad in view of the highly sensitive detection assays now available. The routine application of molecular detection assays may further complicate the stratification of patients for additional—and potentially toxic—therapies, unless the true biology of SLN micrometastasis is further clarified for each tumor type. The balance between "inadequately sensitive" detection (i.e., understaging) and "excessively sensitive" (i.e., overstaging) assays can only be found through a better understanding of the clinicopathological significance of occult and micrometastatic SLN disease.

For all of the controversy, the ability to, ideally, detect a single cancer cell in a background of millions of normal cells offers a powerful tool with which to diagnose the presence of minimal metastatic disease, as well as to follow patient response to therapy. This clinical application of molecular biology-based technology is also poised to play a key role in defining the prognostic significance of SLN micrometastasis, within the context of prospective multicenter trials. When coupled with the SLN mapping concept, and all of its advantages to the patient, a powerful diagnostic combination results.

As the unraveling of the human genome completes, the number of known tumor-associated molecular targets will increase, providing a fertile field for the further evolution of molecular-based analysis of the SLN. It is possible that the combined application of molecular biology-based detection assays to the SLN, blood and bone marrow, and to the primary tumor as well, may someday allow clinicians to create a composite diagnostic and prognostic profile for individual cancer patients. Such a profile would, ideally, allow for highly individualized prognostic and adjuvant therapy algorithms to be developed and uniquely applied to a specific patient.

The development of PEAT sampling of SLN will allow better analysis for metastatic disease in SLN and provide a platform to design standard operating procedures applicable to any pathology laboratory around the world. It is strongly believed that molecular staging will be a significant part of pathology staging procedures in the near future. We have come a long way in a short time from our first molecular diagnosis using multiple markers for the detection of tumor cells in SLNs in 1991. Currently, we have started a National Cancer Institute (USA) funded International Randomized Trial (Multicenter Selective Lymphadenectomy Trial II; MSLT II) whereby molecular staging will be used to randomize a complete lymph node dissection. PEAT specimens will be used for multiple marker quantitative real-time RT-PCR analysis as described by Takeuchi et al.[171] The future for molecular staging of tumor draining lymph nodes looks promising and should benefit and improve patient managements.

REFERENCES

1. Yoshino I, Nakanishi R, Osaki T, Takenoyama M, Taga S, Hanagiri T, et al. Unfavorable prognosis of patients with stage II non-small cell lung cancer associated with macroscopic nodal metastases. Chest 1999;116:144-9.
2. Jatoi I, Hilsenbeck SG, Clark GM, Osborne CK. Significance of axillary lymph node metastasis in primary breast cancer. J Clin Oncol 1999;17:2334-40.
3. Gervasi LA, Mata J, Easley JD, Wilbanks JH, Seale-Hawkins C, Carlton CE Jr, et al. Prognostic significance of lymph nodal metastases in prostate cancer. J Urol 1989;142:332-6.
4. Morton DL, Wanek L, Nizze JA, Elashoff RM, Wong JH. Improved long-term survival after lymphadenectomy of melanoma metastatic to regional nodes. Analysis of prognostic factors in 1134 patients from the John Wayne Cancer Clinic. Ann Surg 1991;214:491-9.
5. Cohen AM, Tremiterra S, Candela F, Thaler HT, Sigurdson ER. Prognosis of node-positive colon cancer. Cancer 1991;67:1859-61.
6. Paik S, Bryant J, Park C, Fisher B, Tan-Chiu E, Hyams D, et al. erbB-2 and response to doxorubicin in patients with axillary lymph node-positive, hormone receptor-negative breast cancer. J Natl Cancer Inst 1998;90:1361-70.
7. Fisher B, Redmond C, Wickerham DL, Bowman D, Schipper H, Wolmark N, et al. Doxorubicin-containing regimens for the treatment of stage II breast cancer: The National Surgical Adjuvant Breast and Bowel Project experience. J Clin Oncol 1989;7:572-82.
8. Eifel P, Axelson JA, Costa J, Crowley J, Curran WJ Jr, Deshler A, et al. National Institutes of Health Consensus Development Conference Statement: adjuvant therapy for breast cancer, November 1-3, 2000. J Natl Cancer Inst 2001;93:979-89.
9. Morton DL, Wen DR, Wong JH, Economou JS, Cagle LA, Storm FK, et al. Technical details of intraoperative lymphatic mapping for early stage melanoma. Arch Surg 1992;127:392-9.
10. Morton DL, Wen DR, Foshag LJ, Essner R, Cochran A. Intraoperative lymphatic mapping and selective cervical lymphadenectomy for early-stage melanomas of the head and neck. J Clin Oncol 1993;11:1751-6.
11. Morton DL, Thompson JF, Essner R, Elashoff R, Stern SL, Nieweg OE. Validation of the accuracy of intraoperative lymphatic mapping and sentinel lymphadenectomy for early-stage melanoma: a multicenter trial. Multicenter Selective Lymphadenectomy Trial Group. Ann Surg 1999;230:453-63.
12. McMasters KM, Reintgen DS, Ross MI, Gershenwald JE, Edwards MJ, Sober A. Sentinel lymph node biopsy for melanoma: controversy despite widespread agreement. J Clin Oncol 2001;19:2851-5.
13. Krag DN, Meijer SJ, Weaver DL, Loggie BW, Harlow SP, Tanabe KK, et al. Minimal-access surgery for staging of malignant melanoma. Arch Surg 1995;130:654-8.
14. Giuliano AE, Kirgan DM, Guenther JM, Morton DL. Lymphatic mapping and sentinel lymphadenectomy for breast cancer. Ann Surg 1994;220:391-8.
15. Krag D, Weaver D, Ashikaga T, Moffat F, Klimberg VS, Shriver C, et al. The sentinel node in breast cancer—a multicenter validation study. N Engl J Med 1998;339:941-6.
16. Veronesi U, Paganelli G, Viale G, Galimberti V, Luini A, Zurrida S, et al. Sentinel lymph node biopsy and axillary dissection in breast cancer: results in a large series. J Natl Cancer Inst 1999;91:368-73.

17. Giuliano AE, Haigh PI, Brennan MB, Hansen NM, Kelley MC, Ye W, et al. Prospective observational study of sentinel lymphadenectomy without further axillary dissection in patients with sentinel node-negative breast cancer. J Clin Oncol 2000;18:2553-9.
18. Saha S, Wiese D, Badin J, Beutler T, Nora D, Ganatra BK, et al. Technical details of sentinel lymph node mapping in colorectal cancer and its impact on staging. Ann Surg Oncol 2000;7:120-4.
19. Bilchik AJ, Saha S, Wiese D, Stonecypher JA, Wood TF, Sostrin S, et al. Molecular staging of early colon cancer on the basis of sentinel node analysis: a multicenter phase II trial. J Clin Oncol 2001;19:1128-36.
20. Pelizzo MR, Boschin IM, Toniato A, Bernante P, Piotto A, Rinaldo A, et al. The sentinel node procedure with Patent Blue V dye in the surgical treatment of papillary thyroid carcinoma. Acta Otolaryngol 2001;121:421-4.
21. Hiratsuka M, Miyashiro I, Ishikawa O, Furukawa H, Motomura K, Ohigashi H, et al. Application of sentinel node biopsy to gastric cancer surgery. Surgery 2001;129:335-40.
22. Akduman B, Fleshner NE, Ehrlich L, Klotz L. Early experience in intermediate-risk penile cancer with sentinel node identification using the gamma probe. Urology 2001;58:65-8.
23. Van Trappen PO, Gyselman VG, Lowe DG, Ryan A, Oram DH, Bosze P, et al. Molecular quantification and mapping of lymph-node micrometastases in cervical cancer. Lancet 2001;357:15-20.
24. De Cicco C, Sideri M, Bartolomei M, Grana C, Cremonesi M, Fiorenza M, et al. Sentinel node biopsy in early vulvar cancer. Br J Cancer 2000;82:295-9.
25. Liptay MJ, Masters GA, Winchester DJ, Edelman BL, Garrido BJ, Hirschtritt TR, et al. Intraoperative radioisotope sentinel lymph node mapping in non-small cell lung cancer. Ann Thorac Surg 2000;70:384-9.
26. Tsioulias GJ, Wood TF, Morton DL, Bilchik AJ. Lymphatic mapping and focused analysis of sentinel lymph nodes upstage gastrointestinal neoplasms. Arch Surg 2000;135:926-32.
27. Kelemen PR, Van Herle AJ, Giuliano AE. Sentinel lymphadenectomy in thyroid malignant neoplasms. Arch Surg 1998;133:288-92.
28. Kitagawa Y, Fujii H, Mukai M, Kubota T, Ando N, Watanabe M, et al. The role of the sentinel lymph node in gastrointestinal cancer. Surg Clin North Am 2000;80:1799-1809.
29. Miliotes G, Albertini J, Berman C, Heller R, Messina J, Glass F, et al. The tumor biology of melanoma nodal metastases. Am Surg 1996;62:81-8.
30. Duff M, Hill AD, McGreal G, Walsh S, McDermott EW, O'Higgins NJ. Prospective evaluation of the morbidity of axillary clearance for breast cancer. Br J Surg 2001;88:114-7.
31. Schrenk P, Rieger R, Shamiyeh A, Wayand W. Morbidity following sentinel lymph node biopsy versus axillary lymph node dissection for patients with breast carcinoma. Cancer 2000;88:608-14.
32. Giuliano AE, Jones RC, Brennan M, Statman R. Sentinel lymphadenectomy in breast cancer. J Clin Oncol 1997;15:2345-50.
33. d'Amore ES, Wick MR, Geisinger KR, Frizzera G. Primary malignant lymphoma arising in postmastectomy lymphedema. Another facet of the Stewart-Treves syndrome. Am J Surg Pathol 1990;14:456-63.
34. Beitsch P, Balch C. Operative morbidity and risk factor assessment in melanoma patients undergoing inguinal lymph node dissection. Am J Surg 1992;164:462-5.

35. Giuliano AE, Dale PS, Turner RR, Morton DL, Evans SW, Krasne DL. Improved axillary staging of breast cancer with sentinel lymphadenectomy. Ann Surg 1995;222:394-9.
36. Cochran AJ, Essner R, Rose DM, Glass EC. Principles of sentinel lymph node identification: background and clinical implications. Langenbecks Arch Surg 2000;385:252-60.
37. Albertini JJ, Lyman GH, Cox C, Yeatman T, Balducci L, Ku N, et al. Lymphatic mapping and sentinel node biopsy in the patient with breast cancer. JAMA 1996;276:1818-22.
38. Cochran AJ, Balda BR, Starz H, Bachter D, Krag DN, Cruse CW, et al. The Augsburg Consensus. Techniques of lymphatic mapping, sentinel lymphadenectomy, and completion lymphadenectomy in cutaneous malignancies. Cancer 2000;89:236-41.
39. Hitchcock CL, Sampsel J, Young DC, Martin EW Jr, Arnold MW. Limitations with light microscopy in the detection of colorectal cancer cells. Dis Colon Rectum 1999;42:1046-52.
40. Cote RJ, Peterson HF, Chaiwun B, Gelber RD, Goldhirsch A, Castiglione-Gertsch M, et al. Role of immunohistochemical detection of lymph-node metastases in management of breast cancer. International Breast Cancer Study Group. Lancet 1999;354:896-900.
41. Czerniecki BJ, Scheff AM, Callans LS, Spitz FR, Bedrosian I, Conant EF, et al. Immunohistochemistry with pancytokeratins improves the sensitivity of sentinel lymph node biopsy in patients with breast carcinoma. Cancer 1999;85:1098-103.
42. Pantel K, Cote RJ, Fodstad O. Detection and clinical importance of micrometastatic disease. J Natl Cancer Inst 1999;91:1113-24.
43. Kamath VJ, Giuliano R, Dauway EL, Cantor A, Berman C, Ku NN, et al. Characteristics of the sentinel lymph node in breast cancer predict further involvement of higher-echelon nodes in the axilla: a study to evaluate the need for complete axillary lymph node dissection. Arch Surg 2001;136:688-92.
44. Chu KU, Turner RR, Hansen NM, Brennan MB, Giuliano AE. Sentinel node metastasis in patients with breast carcinoma accurately predicts immunohistochemically detectable nonsentinel node metastasis. Ann Surg Oncol 1999;6:756-61.
45. Turner RR, Ollila DW, Krasne DL, Giuliano AE. Histopathologic validation of the sentinel lymph node hypothesis for breast carcinoma. Ann Surg 1997;226:271-6.
46. Chen ZL, Wen DR, Coulson WF, Giuliano AE, Cochran AJ. Occult metastases in the axillary lymph nodes of patients with breast cancer node negative by clinical and histologic examination and conventional histology. Dis Markers 1991;9:239-48.
47. Schreiber RH, Pendas S, Ku NN, Reintgen DS, Shons AR, Berman C, et al. Microstaging of breast cancer patients using cytokeratin staining of the sentinel lymph node. Ann Surg Oncol 1999;6:95-101.
48. Hammond ME, Fitzgibbons PL, Compton CC, Grignon DJ, Page DL, Fielding LP, et al. College of American Pathologists Conference XXXV: solid tumor prognostic factors—which, how and so what? Summary document and recommendations for implementation. Cancer Committee and Conference Participants. Arch Pathol Lab Med 2000;124:958-65.
49. Bosman FT, de Goeij AF, Rousch M. Quality control in immunocytochemistry: experiences with the oestrogen receptor assay. J Clin Pathol 1992;45:120-4.

50. Bertheau P, Cazals-Hatem D, Meignin V, de Roquancourt A, Verola O, Lesourd A, Sene C, Brocheriou C, Janin A. Variability of immunohistochemical reactivity on stored paraffin slides. J Clin Pathol 1998;51:370-4.
51. Rhodes A, Jasani B, Barnes DM, Bobrow LG, Miller KD. Reliability of immunohistochemical demonstration of oestrogen receptors in routine practice: interlaboratory variance in the sensitivity of detection and evaluation of scoring systems. J Clin Pathol 2000;53:125-30.
52. Layfield LJ, Gupta D, Mooney EE. Assessment of tissue estrogen and progesterone receptor levels: a survey of current practice, techniques, and quantitation methods. Breast J 2000;6:189-96.
53. Kohlberger P, Gantert M, Volk-Orlowska T, Kieback DG, Gitsch G. Immunohistochemical detection of lymph node metastases in node-negative breast cancer patients. Anticancer Res 2001;21:697-9.
54. Xu X, Roberts SA, Pasha TL, Zhang PJ. Undesirable cytokeratin immunoreactivity of native nonepithelial cells in sentinel lymph nodes from patients with breast carcinoma. Arch Pathol Lab Med 2000;124:1310-3.
55. Cochran AJ, Wen DR, Herschman HR. Occult melanoma in lymph nodes detected by antiserum to S-100 protein. Int J Cancer 1984;34:159-63.
56. Cochran AJ, Wen DR, Morton DL. Occult tumor cells in the lymph nodes of patients with pathological stage I malignant melanoma. An immunohistological study. Am J Surg Pathol 1988;12:612-8.
57. Carson KF, Wen DR, Li PX, Lana AM, Bailly C, Morton DL, et al. Nodal nevi and cutaneous melanomas. Am J Surg Pathol 1996;20:834-40.
58. Yu LL, Flotte TJ, Tanabe KK, Gadd MA, Cosimi AB, Sober AJ, et al. Detection of microscopic melanoma metastases in sentinel lymph nodes. Cancer 1999;86:617-27.
59. King R, Weibaecher KN, McGill G, Cooley E, Mihm M, Fisher DE. Microphthalmia transcription factor. A sensitive and specific melanocyte marker for melanoma diagnosis. Am J Pathol 1999;155:731-738.
60. Shivers SC, Li W, Lin J, Stall A, Stafford M, Messina J, et al. The clinical relevance of molecular staging for melanoma. Recent Results Cancer Res 2001;158:187-99.
61. Bostick PJ, Morton DL, Turner RR, Huynh KT, Wang HJ, Elashoff R, et al. Prognostic significance of occult metastases detected by sentinel lymphadenectomy and reverse transcriptase-polymerase chain reaction in early-stage melanoma patients. J Clin Oncol 1999;17:3238-44.
62. Blaheta HJ, Schittek B, Breuninger H, Maczey E, Kroeber S, Sotlar K, et al. Lymph node micrometastases of cutaneous melanoma: increased sensitivity of molecular diagnosis in comparison to immunohistochemistry. Int J Cancer 1998;79:318-23.
63. Berois N, Varangot M, Osinaga E, Babino A, Caignault L, Muse I, et al. Detection of rare human breast cancer cells. Comparison of an immunomagnetic separation method with immunocytochemistry and RT-PCR. Anticancer Res 1997;17:2639-46.
64. Van der Velde-Zimmermann D, Roijers JF, Bouwens-Rombouts A, De Weger RA, De Graaf PW, Tilanus MG, et al. Molecular test for the detection of tumor cells in blood and sentinel nodes of melanoma patients. Am J Pathol 1996;149:759-64.
65. Hoon DS, Sarantou T, Doi F, Chi DD, Kuo C, Conrad AJ, et al. Detection of metastatic breast cancer by beta-hCG polymerase chain reaction. Int J Cancer 1996;69:369-74.

66. Hoon DS, Wang Y, Dale PS, Conrad AJ, Schmid P, Garrison D, et al. Detection of occult melanoma cells in blood with a multiple-marker polymerase chain reaction assay. J Clin Oncol 1995;13:2109-16.
67. Kuo CT, Bostick PJ, Irie RF, Morton DL, Conrad AJ, Hoon DS. Assessment of messenger RNA of beta ➡ 4-N-acetylgalactosaminyl-transferase as a molecular marker for metastatic melanoma. Clin Cancer Res 1998;4:411-8.
68. Bostick PJ, Chatterjee S, Chi DD, Huynh KT, Giuliano AE, Cote R, et al. Limitations of specific reverse-transcriptase polymerase chain reaction markers in the detection of metastases in the lymph nodes and blood of breast cancer patients. J Clin Oncol 1998;16:2632-40.
69. Morita R, Fujimoto A, Hatta N, Takehara K, Takata M. Comparison of genetic profiles between primary melanomas and their metastases reveals genetic alterations and clonal evolution during progression. J Invest Dermatol 1998;111:919-24.
70. Frost P, Fidler IJ. Biology of metastasis. Cancer 1986;58:550-3.
71. Price JE, Aukerman SL, Fidler IJ. Evidence that the process of murine melanoma metastasis is sequential and selective and contains stochastic elements. Cancer Res 1986;46:5172-8.
72. Kitadai Y, Ellis LM, Takahashi Y, Bucana CD, Anzai H, Tahara E, et al. Multiparametric in situ messenger RNA hybridization analysis to detect metastasis-related genes in surgical specimens of human colon carcinomas. Clin Cancer Res 1995;1:1095-1102.
73. Blaheta HJ, Schittek B, Breuninger H, Garbe C. Detection of micrometastasis in sentinel lymph nodes of patients with primary cutaneous melanoma. Recent Results Cancer Res 2001;158:137-46.
74. Blaheta HJ, Ellwanger U, Schittek B, Sotlar K, MacZey E, Breuninger H, et al. Examination of regional lymph nodes by sentinel node biopsy and molecular analysis provides new staging facilities in primary cutaneous melanoma. J Invest Dermatol 2000;114:637-42.
75. Goydos JS, Ravikumar TS, Germino FJ, Yudd A, Bancila E. Minimally invasive staging of patients with melanoma: sentinel lymphadenectomy and detection of the melanoma-specific proteins MART-1 and tyrosinase by reverse transcriptase polymerase chain reaction. J Am Coll Surg 1998;187:182-8.
76. Bilchik A, Miyashiro M, Kelley M, Kuo C, Fujiwara Y, Nakamori S, et al. Molecular detection of metastatic pancreatic carcinoma cells using a multimarker reverse transcriptase-polymerase chain reaction assay. Cancer 2000;88:1037-44.
77. Bostick PJ, Huynh KT, Sarantou T, Turner RR, Qi K, Giuliano AE, et al. Detection of metastases in sentinel lymph nodes of breast cancer patients by multiple-marker RT-PCR. Int J Cancer 1998;79:645-51.
78. Miyashiro I, Kuo C, Huynh K, Iida A, Morton D, Bilchik A, et al. Molecular strategy for detecting metastatic cancers with use of multiple tumor-specific MAGE-A genes. Clin Chem 2001;47:505-12.
79. Taback B, Morton DL, O'Day SJ, Nguyen DH, Nakayama T, Hoon DS. The clinical utility of multimarker RT-PCR in the detection of occult metastasis in patients with melanoma. Recent Results Cancer Res 2001;158:78-92.
80. Hoon DS, Bostick P, Kuo C, Okamoto T, Wang HJ, Elashoff R, et al. Molecular markers in blood as surrogate prognostic indicators of melanoma recurrence. Cancer Res 2000;60:2253-7.
81. Sarantou T, Chi DD, Garrison DA, Conrad AJ, Schmid P, Morton DL, et al. Melanoma-associated antigens as messenger RNA detection markers for melanoma. Cancer Res 1997;57:1371-6.

82. Hamakawa H, Takemura K, Sumida T, Kayahara H, Tanioka H, Sogawa K. Histological study on pN upgrading of oral cancer. Virchows Arch 2000;437:116-21.
83. Torrenga H, Rahusen FD, Meijer S, Borgstein PJ, van Diest PJ. Sentinel node investigation in breast cancer: detailed analysis of the yield from step sectioning and immunohistochemistry. J Clin Pathol 2001;54:550-2.
84. O'Connell CD, Juhasz A, Kuo C, Reeder DJ, Hoon DS. Detection of tyrosinase mRNA in melanoma by reverse transcription-PCR and electrochemiluminescence. Clin Chem 1998;44:1161-9.
85. Miyake Y, Fujiwara Y, Ohue M, Yamamoto H, Sugita Y, Tomita N, et al. Quantification of micrometastases in lymph nodes of colorectal cancer using real-time fluorescence polymerase chain reaction. Int J Oncol 2000;16:289-93.
86. Mitas M, Mikhitarian K, Walters C, Baron PL, Elliott BM, Brothers TE, et al. Quantitative real-time RT-PCR detection of breast cancer micrometastasis using a multigene marker panel. Int J Cancer 2001;93:162-71.
87. Blaheta HJ, Schittek B, Breuninger H, Sotlar K, Ellwanger U, Thelen MH, et al. Detection of melanoma micrometastasis in sentinel nodes by reverse transcription-polymerase chain reaction correlates with tumor thickness and is predictive of micrometastatic disease in the lymph node basin. Am J Surg Pathol 1999;23:822-8.
88. Takeuchi H, Kuo C, Morton DL, Wang HJ, Hoon DS. Expression of differentiation melanoma-associated antigen gene is associated with favorable disease outcome in advanced-stage melanomas. Cancer Res 2003;15:441-8.
89. Yoshioka S, Fujiwara Y, Sugita Y, Okada Y, Yano M, Tamura S, et al. Real-time rapid reverse transcriptase-polymerase chain reaction for intraoperative diagnosis of lymph node micrometastasis: clinical application for cervical lymph node dissection in esophageal cancers. Surgery 2002;132:34-40.
90. Raja S, El-Hefnawy T, Kelly LA, Chestney ML, Luketich JD, Godfrey TE. Temperature-controlled primer limit for multiplexing of rapid, quantitative reverse transcription-PCR assays: application to intraoperative cancer diagnostics. Clin Chem 2002;48:1329-37.
91. Kuo CT, Hoon DS, Takeuchi H, Turner R, Wang HJ, Morton DL, et al. Prediction of disease outcome in melanoma patients by molecular analysis of paraffin-embedded sentinel lymph nodes. J Clin Oncol 2003:21;3566-72.
92. Morton DL, Hoon DS, Cochran AJ, Turner RR, Essner R, Takeuchi H, et al. Lymphatic mapping and sentinel lymphadenectomy for early-stage melanoma: therapeutic utility and implications of nodal microanatomy and molecular staging for improving the accuracy of detection of nodal micrometastases. Ann Surg 2003;238:538-49.
93. Sanchez-Cespedes M, Esteller M, Hibi K, Cope FO, Westra WH, Piantadosi S, et al. Molecular detection of neoplastic cells in lymph nodes of metastatic colorectal cancer patients predicts recurrence. Clin Cancer Res 1999;5:2450-4.
94. Taback B, Nakayama T, Wiese D, Turner R, Bilchik A, Saha S, et al. Detection of colorectal micrometastasis in sentinel lymph nodes using the novel approach of PCR PNA clamping. Proc Am Assoc Cancer Res 2001;42:612.
95. Taback B. Bilchik AJ, Saha S, Nakayama T, Wiese DA, Turner RR, et al. Peptide nucleic acid clamp PCR: A novel K-*ras* mutation detection assay for colorectal cancer micrometastases in lymph nodes. Int J Cancer 2004, in press.
96. Shinozaki M, Fujimoto A, Morton DL, Hoon DS. Incidence of *BRAF* oncogene mutation and clinical relevance for primary cutaneous melanoma. Clin Cancer Res 2004;10:1753-7.

97. Shinozaki M, O'Day S, Kuo C, Hoon DS. Detection and clinical utility of BRAF mutation in serum of melanoma patients. Clin Chem, Abstract for CNAPS III, pp9 (on line).
98. Dong G, Loukinova E, Chen Z, Gangi L, Chanturita TI, Liu ET, et al. Molecular profiling of transformed and metastatic murine squamous carcinoma cells by differential display and cDNA microarray reveals altered expression of multiple genes related to growth, apoptosis, angiogenesis, and the NF-kappaB signal pathway. Cancer Res 2001;61:4797-808.
99. Chen JJ, Peck K, Hong TM, Yang SC, Sher YP, Shih JY, et al. Global analysis of gene expression in invasion by a lung cancer model. Cancer Res 2001;61:5223-30.
100. Zarrinkar PP, Mainquist JK, Zamora M, Stern D, Welsh JB, Sapinoso LM, et al. Arrays of arrays for high-throughput gene expression profiling. Genome Res 2001;11:1256-61.
101. Kannan K, Kaminski N, Rechavi G, Jakob-Hirsch J, Amariglio N, Givol D. DNA microarray analysis of genes involved in p53 mediated apoptosis: activation of Apaf-1. Oncogene 2001;20:3449-55.
102. Dales JP, Plumas J, Palmerini F, Devilard E, Defrance T, Lajmanovich A, et al. Correlation between apoptosis microarray gene expression profiling and histopathological lymph node lesions. Mol Pathol 2001;54:17-23.
103. Perou CM, Sorlie T, Eisen MB, van de Rijn M, Jeffrey SS, Rees CA, et al. Molecular portraits of human breast tumours. Nature 2000;406:747-52.
104. Li S, Ross DT, Kadin ME, Brown PO, Wasik MA. Comparative genome-scale analysis of gene expression profiles in T cell lymphoma cells during malignant progression using a complementary DNA microarray. Am J Pathol 2001;158:1231-7.
105. Macville MV, Van Der Laak JA, Speel EJ, Katzir N, Garini Y, Soenksen D, et al. Spectral imaging of multi-color chromogenic dyes in pathological specimens. Anal Cell Pathol 2001;22:133-42.
106. Tanner M, Gancberg D, Di Leo A, Larsimont D, Rouas G, Piccart MJ, et al. Chromogenic in situ hybridization: a practical alternative for fluorescence in situ hybridization to detect HER-2/neu oncogene amplification in archival breast cancer samples. Am J Pathol 2000;157:1467-72.
107. Ebina M, Martinez A, Birrer MJ, Ilona Linnoila R. In situ detection of unexpected patterns of mutant p53 gene expression in non-small cell lung cancers. Oncogene 2001;20:2579-86.
108. Nasser IA, Lee AK, Bosari S, Saganich R, Heatley G, Silverman ML. Occult axillary lymph node metastases in "node-negative" breast carcinoma. Hum Pathol 1993;24:950-7.
109. Carter BA, Jensen RA, Simpson JF, Page DL. Benign transport of breast epithelium into axillary lymph nodes after biopsy. Am J Clin Pathol 2000;113:259-65.
110. Siegel RJ. Surgical pathology of lymph nodes in cancer staging: routine and specialized techniques. Surg Oncol Clin North Am 1996;5:25-31.
111. Lilleng PK, Maehle BO, Hartveit F. The size of a micrometastasis in the axilla in breast cancer: a study of nodal tumour-load related to prognosis. Eur J Gynaecol Oncol 1998;19:220-4.
112. McGuckin MA, Cummings MC, Walsh MD, Hohn BG, Bennett IC, Wright RG. Occult axillary node metastases in breast cancer: their detection and prognostic significance. Br J Cancer 1996;73:88-95.

113. Sato F, Shimada Y, Li Z, Watanabe G, Maeda M, Imamura M. Lymph node micrometastasis and prognosis in patients with oesophageal squamous cell carcinoma. Br J Surg 2001;88:426-32.
114. Joosten JJ, Strobbe LJ, Wauters CA, Pruszczynski M, Wobbes T, Ruers TJ. Intraoperative lymphatic mapping and the sentinel node concept in colorectal carcinoma. Br J Surg 1999;86:482-6.
115. Miyake Y, Yamamoto H, Fujiwara Y, Ohue M, Sugita Y, Tomita N, et al. Extensive micrometastases to lymph nodes as a marker for rapid recurrence of colorectal cancer: a study of lymphatic mapping. Clin Cancer Res 2001;7:1350-7.
116. Braun S, Cevatli BS, Assemi C, Janni W, Kentenich CR, Schindlbeck C, et al. Comparative analysis of micrometastasis to the bone marrow and lymph nodes of node-negative breast cancer patients receiving no adjuvant therapy. J Clin Oncol 2001;19:1468-75.
117. Colpaert C, Vermeulen P, Jeuris W, Van Beest P, Goovaerts G, Weyler J, et al. Early distant relapse in "node-negative" breast cancer patients is not predicted by occult axillary lymph node metastases, but by the features of the primary tumour. J Pathol 2001;193:442-9.
118. Komukai S, Nishimaki T, Watanabe H, Ajioka Y, Suzuki T, Hatakeyama K. Significance of immunohistochemically demonstrated micrometastases to lymph nodes in esophageal cancer with histologically negative nodes. Surgery 2000;127:40-6.
119. Chen ZL, Perez S, Holmes EC, Wang HJ, Coulson WF, Wen DR, et al. Frequency and distribution of occult micrometastases in lymph nodes of patients with non-small-cell lung carcinoma. J Natl Cancer Inst 1993;85:493-8.
120. Izbicki JR, Passlick B, Hosch SB, Kubuschock B, Schneider C, Busch C, et al. Mode of spread in the early phase of lymphatic metastasis in non-small-cell lung cancer: significance of nodal micrometastasis. J Thorac Cardiovasc Surg 1996;112:623-30.
121. Harrison LE, Choe JK, Goldstein M, Meridian A, Kim SH, Clarke K. Prognostic significance of immunohistochemical micrometastases in node negative gastric cancer patients. J Surg Oncol 2000;73:153-7.
122. Mueller JD, Stein HJ, Oyang T, Natsugoe S, Feith M, Werner M, et al. Frequency and clinical impact of lymph node micrometastasis and tumor cell microinvolvement in patients with adenocarcinoma of the esophagogastric junction. Cancer 2000;89:1874-82.
123. Nagakura S, Shirai Y, Yokoyama N, Hatakeyama K. Clinical significance of lymph node micrometastasis in gallbladder carcinoma. Surgery 2001;129:704-13.
124. Hosch SB, Stoecklein NH, Pichlmeier U, Rehders A, Scheunemann P, Niendorf A, et al. Esophageal cancer: the mode of lymphatic tumor cell spread and its prognostic significance. J Clin Oncol 2001;19:1970-5.
125. Cochran AJ, Wen DR, Morton DL. Occult tumor cells in the lymph nodes of patients with pathological stage I malignant melanoma. An immunohistological study. Am J Surg Pathol 1988;12:612-18.
126. Gershenwald JE, Colome MI, Lee JE, Mansfield PF, Tseng C, Lee JJ, et al. Patterns of recurrence following a negative sentinel lymph node biopsy in 243 patients with stage I or II melanoma. J Clin Oncol 1998;16:2253-60.
127. Chu KU, Turner RR, Hansen NM, Brennan MB, Bilchik A, Giuliano AE. Do all patients with sentinel node metastasis from breast carcinoma need complete axillary node dissection? Ann Surg 1999;229:536-41.

128. International (Ludwig) Breast Cancer Study Group. Prognostic importance of occult axillary lymph node micrometastases from breast cancers. Lancet 1990;335:1565-68.
129. Dobashi K, Sugio K, Osaki T, Oka T, Yasumoto K. Micrometastatic P53-positive cells in the lymph nodes of non-small-cell lung cancer: prognostic significance. J Thorac Cardiovasc Surg 1997;114:339-46.
130. Clarke G, Ryan E, O'Keane JC, Crowe J, MacMathuna P. The detection of cytokeratins in lymph nodes of Duke's B colorectal cancer subjects predicts a poor outcome. Eur J Gastroenterol Hepatol 2000;12:549-52.
131. Tang R, Wang JY, Chen JS, Chang-Chien CR, Tang S, Lin SE, et al. Survival impact of lymph node metastasis in TNM stage III carcinoma of the colon and rectum. J Am Coll Surg 1995;180:705-12.
132. Kubuschok B, Passlick B, Izbicki JR, Thetter O, Pantel K. Disseminated tumor cells in lymph nodes as a determinant for survival in surgically resected non-small-cell lung cancer. J Clin Oncol 1999;17:19-24.
133. Nakajo A, Natsugoe S, Ishigami S, Matsumoto M, Nakashima S, Hokita S, et al. Detection and prediction of micrometastasis in the lymph nodes of patients with pN0 gastric cancer. Ann Surg Oncol 2001;8:158-62.
134. Ribuffo D, Gradilone A, Vonella M, Chiummariello S, Cigna E, Haliassos N, et al. Prognostic significance of reverse transcriptase-polymerase chain reaction-negative sentinel nodes in malignant melanoma. Ann Surg Oncol 2003;10:396-402.
135. Huang SK, Okamoto T, Morton DL, Hoon DS. Antibody responses to melanoma/melanocyte autoantigens in melanoma patients. J Invest Dermatol 1998;111:662-7.
136. Hatta N, Takata M, Takehara K, Ohara K. Polymerase chain reaction and immunohistochemistry frequently detect occult melanoma cells in regional lymph nodes of melanoma patients. J Clin Pathol 1998;51:597-601.
137. Wang X, Heller R, VanVoorhis N, Cruse CW, Glass F, Fenske N, et al. Detection of submicroscopic lymph node metastases with polymerase chain reaction in patients with malignant melanoma. Ann Surg 1994;220:768-74.
138. Shivers SC, Wang X, Li W, Joseph E, Messina J, Glass LF, et al. Molecular staging of malignant melanoma. JAMA 1998;280:1410-5.
139. Goydos JS, Patel KN, Shih WJ, Lu SE, Yudd AP, Kempf JS, et al. Patterns of recurrence in patients with melanoma and histologically negative but RT-PCR-positive sentinel lymph nodes. J Am Coll Surg 2003;196:196-204.
140. Palmieri G, Ascierto PA, Cossu A, Mozzillo N, Motti ML, Satriano SM, et al. Detection of occult melanoma cells in paraffin-embedded histologically negative sentinel lymph nodes using a reverse transcriptase polymerase chain reaction assay. J Clin Oncol 2001;19:1437-43.
141. Masuda N, Tamaki Y, Sakita I, Ooka M, Ohnishi T, Kadota M, et al. Clinical significance of micrometastases in axillary lymph nodes assessed by reverse transcription-polymerase chain reaction in breast cancer patients. Clin Cancer Res 2000;6:4176-85.
142. Noguchi S, Aihara T, Nakamori S, Motomura K, Inaji H, Imaoka S, et al. The detection of breast carcinoma micrometastases in axillary lymph nodes by means of reverse transcriptase-polymerase chain reaction. Cancer 1994;74:1595-1600.
143. Noguchi S, Aihara T, Motomura K, Inaji H, Imaoka S, Koyama H. Detection of breast cancer micrometastases in axillary lymph nodes by means of reverse transcriptase-polymerase chain reaction. Comparison between MUC1 mRNA and keratin 19 mRNA amplification. Am J Pathol 1996;148:649-56.

144. Mori M, Mimori K, Inoue H, Barnard GF, Tsuji K, Nanbara S, et al. Detection of cancer micrometastases in lymph nodes by reverse transcriptase-polymerase chain reaction. Cancer Res 1995;55:3417-20.
145. Ooka M, Sakita I, Fujiwara Y, Tamaki Y, Yamamoto H, Aihara T, et al. Selection of mRNA markers for detection of lymph node micrometastases in breast cancer patients. Oncol Rep 2000;7:561-6.
146. Kataoka A, Mori M, Sadanaga N, Ueo H, Tsuji K, Rai Y, et al. RT-PCR detection of breast cancer cells in sentinel lymph modes. Int J Oncol 2000;16:1147-52.
147. Hoon DS, Sarantou T, Doi F, Chi DD, Kuo C, Conrad AJ, et al. Detection of metastatic breast cancer by beta-hCG polymerase chain reaction. Int J Cancer 1996;69:369-74.
148. Lockett MA, Baron PL, O'Brien PH, Elliott BM, Robison JG, Maitre N, et al. Detection of occult breast cancer micrometastases in axillary lymph nodes using a multimarker reverse transcriptase-polymerase chain reaction panel. J Am Coll Surg 1998;187:9-16.
149. Yun K, Gunn J, Merrie AE, Phillips LV, McCall JL. Keratin 19 mRNA is detectable by RT-PCR in lymph nodes of patients without breast cancer. Br J Cancer 1997;76:1112-3.
150. Merrie AE, Yun K, Gunn J, Phillips LV, McCall JL. Analysis of potential markers for detection of submicroscopic lymph node metastases in breast cancer. Br J Cancer 1999;80:2019-24.
151. Fujie T, Mori M, Ueo H, Sugimachi K, Akiyoshi T. Expression of MAGE and BAGE genes in Japanese breast cancers. Ann Oncol 1997;8:369-72.
152. Wascher RA, Bostick PJ, Huynh KT, Turner R, Qi K, Giuliano AE, et al. Detection of MAHE-A3 in breast cancer patients' sentinel lymph nodes. Br J Cancer 2001;85:1340-6.
153. Aihara T, Fujiwara Y, Miyake Y, Okami J, Okada Y, Iwao K, et al. Mammaglobin B gene as a novel marker for lymph node micrometastasis in patients with abdominal cancers. Cancer Lett 2000;150:79-84.
154. Ichikawa Y, Ishikawa T, Momiyama N, Yamaguchi S, Masui H, Hasegawa S, et al. Detection of regional lymph node metastases in colon cancer by using RT-PCR for matrix metalloproteinase 7, matrilysin. Clin Exp Metastasis 1998;16:3-8.
155. Weitz J, Kienle P, Magener A, Koch M, Schrodel A, Willeke F, et al. Detection of disseminated colorectal cancer cells in lymph nodes, blood and bone marrow. Clin Cancer Res 1999;5:1830-6.
156. Bernini A, Spencer M, Frizelle S, Madoff RD, Willmott LD, McCormick SR, et al. Evidence for colorectal cancer micrometastases using reverse transcriptase-polymerase chain reaction analysis of MUC2 in lymph nodes. Cancer Detect Prev 2000;24:72-9.
157. Liefers GJ, Cleton-Jansen AM, van de Velde CJ, Hermans J, van Krieken JH, Cornelisse CJ, et al. Micrometastases and survival in stage II colorectal cancer. N Engl J Med 1998;339:223-8.
158. Noura S, Yamamoto H, Ohnishi T, Masuda N, Matsumoto T, Takayama O, et al. Comparative detection of lymph node micrometastases of stage II colorectal cancer by reverse transcriptase polymerase chain reaction and immunohistochemistry. J Clin Oncol 2002;20:4232-41.
159. Cortesina G, Martone T, Galeazzi E, Olivero M, De Stefani A, Bussi M, et al. Staging of head and neck squamous cell carcinoma using the MET oncogene product as marker of tumor cells in lymph node metastases. Int J Cancer 2000;89:286-92.

160. Salerno CT, Frizelle S, Niehans GA, Ho SB, Jakkula M, Kratzke RA, et al. Detection of occult micrometastases in non-small cell lung carcinoma by reverse transcriptase-polymerase chain reaction. Chest 1998;113:1526-32.
161. Edelstein RA, Zietman AL, de las Morenas A, Krane RJ, Babayan RK, Dallow KC, et al. Implications of prostate micrometastases in pelvic lymph nodes: an archival tissue study. Urology 1996;47:370-5.
162. Deguchi T, Doi T, Ehara H, Ito S, Takahashi Y, Nishino Y, et al. Detection of micrometastatic prostate cancer cells in lymph nodes by reverse transcriptase-polymerase chain reaction. Cancer Res 1993;53:5350-4.
163. Ferrari AC, Stone NN, Eyler JN, Gao M, Mandeli J, Unger P, et al. Prospective analysis of prostate-specific markers in pelvic lymph nodes of patients with high-risk prostate cancer. J Natl Cancer Inst 1997;89:1498-1504.
164. Noguchi S, Hiratsuka M, Furukawa H, Aihara T, Kasugai T, Tamura S, et al. Detection of gastric cancer micrometastases in lymph nodes by amplification of keratin 19 mRNA with reverse transcriptase-polymerase chain reaction. Jpn J Cancer Res 1996;87:650-4.
165. McDonald LA, Walker DM, Gibbins JR. Cervical lymph node involvement in head and neck cancer detectable as expression of a spliced transcript of type II keratin K5. Oral Oncol 1998;34:276-83.
166. Kijima F, Natsugoe S, Takao S, Aridome K, Baba M, Yoshifumi M, et al. Detection and clinical significance of lymph node micrometastasis determined by reverse transcription-polymerase chain reaction in patients with esophageal carcinoma. Oncology 2000;58:38-44.
167. Kano M, Shimada Y, Kaganoi J, Sakurai T, Li Z, Sato F, et al. Detection of lymph node metastasis of oesophageal cancer by RT-nested PCR for SCC antigen gene mRNA. Br J Cancer 2000;82:429-35.
168. Okami J, Dohno K, Sakon M, Iwao K, Yamada T, Yamamoto H, et al. Genetic detection for micrometastasis in lymph node of biliary tract carcinoma. Clin Cancer Res 2000;6:2326-32.
169. Taback B, Hashimoto K, Kuo CT, Chan A, Giuliano AE, Hoon DS. Molecular lymphatic mapping of the sentinel lymph node. Am J Pathol 2002;161:1153-61.
170. Morton DL. Lymphatic mapping and sentinel lymphadenectomy for melanoma: past, present and future (2nd International Sentinel Node Congress, 1-4 December 2000, Santa Monica, CA). Ann Surg Oncol (in press).
171. Takeuchi H, Morton DL, Kuo C, Turner RR, Elashoff D, Elashoff R, et al. Prognostic significance of molecular upstaging of paraffin-embedded sentinel lymph nodes in melanoma patients. J Clin Oncol (submitted).
172. Manzotti M, Dell'Orto P, Maisonneuve P, Zurrida S, Mazzarol G, Viale G. Reverse transcription-polymerase chain reaction assay for multiple mRNA markers in the detection of breast cancer metastases in sentinel lymph nodes. Int J Cancer 2001;95:307-12.
173. Sakaguchi M, Virmani A, Dudak MW, Peters GN, Leitch AM, Saboorian H, Gazdar AF, Euhus DM. Clinical relevance of reverse transcriptase-polymerase chain reaction for the detection of axillary lymph node metastases in breast cancer. Ann Surg Oncol 2003;10:117-25.

Chapter 13

CREDENTIALING OF NUCLEAR MEDICINE PHYSICIANS, SURGEONS, AND PATHOLOGISTS AS A MULTIDISCIPLINARY TEAM FOR SELECTIVE SENTINEL LYMPHADENECTOMY

Masaki Kitajima, Yuko Kitagawa, Hirofumi Fujii,
Makio Mukai, Atsushi Kubo
Keio University School of Medicine, Tokyo, Japan

Abstract There are several possible applications of the sentinel lymph node (SLN) concept with different technological aspects such as individualized surgical management of solid tumors, multidisciplinary treatments, and novel therapeutic approaches. To achieve these clinical applications, multidisciplinary teamwork with surgeons, nuclear medicine physicians, and pathologists would be critically required. Interdisciplinary issues should be resolved in order to develop optimal standard procedures of SLN dissection for various solid tumors.

INTRODUCTION

The sentinel lymph node (SLN) concept itself is very simple and attractive. Some pioneers had already attempted to utilize this concept in the middle of the 20th century for specific organs.[1,2] Although these brave challenges were extremely innovative, the procedures were not initially widely accepted as feasible and reproducible in clinical practice. Now we know that the hypothesis is basically and generally acceptable since Donald Morton and his colleagues demonstrated the clinical significance of the SLN concept in melanoma.[3] A number of advanced technologies and clinical circumstances played various roles in the realization of the clinical significance of this concept. For example, a gamma probe with high collimation enabled accurate detection of SLN, in addition to the traditional dye-guided method. An improvement of imaging technologies to visualize the distribution of SLN contributes to the individualized management of solid tumors. Now we have to try to detect the micrometastasis not only by histological procedure but also with molecular biological techniques. Intraoperative utilization of real-time RT-PCR technique is one of the challenging topics in this field. An emergence of endoscopic surgery has changed surgical thinking since the 1990s. Even in the field of surgical oncology, surgeons tend to pay attention not only to radical resection but also to minimal invasiveness and enhanced quality of life after surgery. Endoscopic surgery is a great tool to realize a minimally invasive approach for SLN-negative patients. As indicated in the official logo of the Japanese Society for Sentinel Node Navigation Surgery (SNNS), multidisciplinary cooperation of different fields is essential for the further development of SLN technologies (Figure 1). In this chapter, we would like to introduce current topics and issues for a multidisciplinary team of surgeons, nuclear medicine physicians, and pathologists.

Figure 1. Logo mark of the Japanese Society of Sentinel Node Navigation Surgery. A combination of three blue nodes symbolizes the credentialing of nuclear medicine physicians, surgeons, and pathologists as a multidisciplinary team for sentinel node navigation.

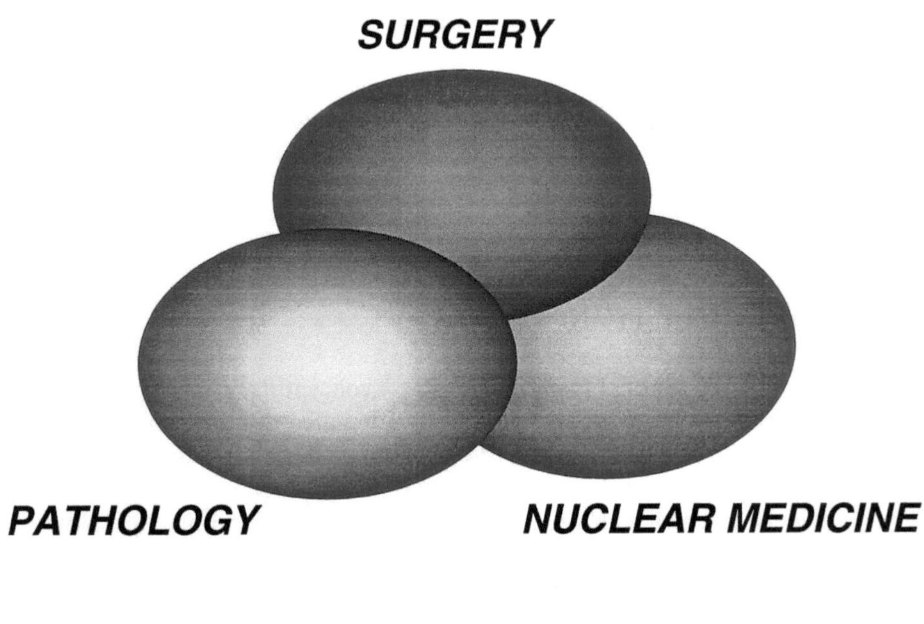

OPTIMAL COOPERATION OF MULTIDISCIPLINARY TEAM

Although several reports demonstrate the feasibility of dye-guided SLN mapping for certain organs,[4-6] a combination technique with dye and radioactive tracer is a more stable and reliable method to detect the SLN of various solid tumors. Therefore, the cooperation of nuclear medicine physicians is essential for performing this procedure. An accurate and adequate injection of tracer particles is one of the most important procedures in SLN mapping. In this phase of the procedure, nuclear medicine physicians and surgeons should cooperate to trace the lymphatic drainage routes from the primary lesion. Although preparation of radioactive tracer should be controlled by nuclear medicine physicians, surgeons have to provide detailed information of the characteristics of the primary lesion, and in some cases they should perform tracer injection themselves.

Interpretation of the preoperative lymphoscintigram is also critical for an accurate SLN sampling. Surgeons have to select the best surgical approach for each patient based on the SLN distribution demonstrated by the preoperative lymphoscintigram. For example, surgical approaches for SLN sampling for the patients with esophageal cancer, in which multiple SLNs are widely spread from cervical to abdominal areas, vary for each patient. In the case of the patient with the preoperative lymphoscintigram shown in Figure 2, the status of cervical SLN should be checked initially by cervical incision. On the other hand, in the case of the patient with the SLN distribution demonstrated in Figure 3, a transabdominal approach would be reasonable. Therefore, nuclear medicine physicians must strive to improve the quality of lymphoscintigrams and should discuss the interpretation of scintigrams with surgeons very carefully.

Figure 2. Lymphoscintigram: SLN in cervical area in patients with esophageal cancer.

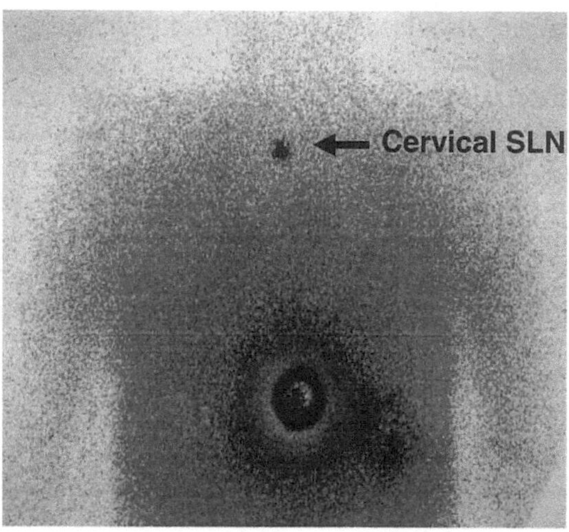

Figure 3. Lymphoscintigram: SLN in abdominal area in patients with esophageal cancer.

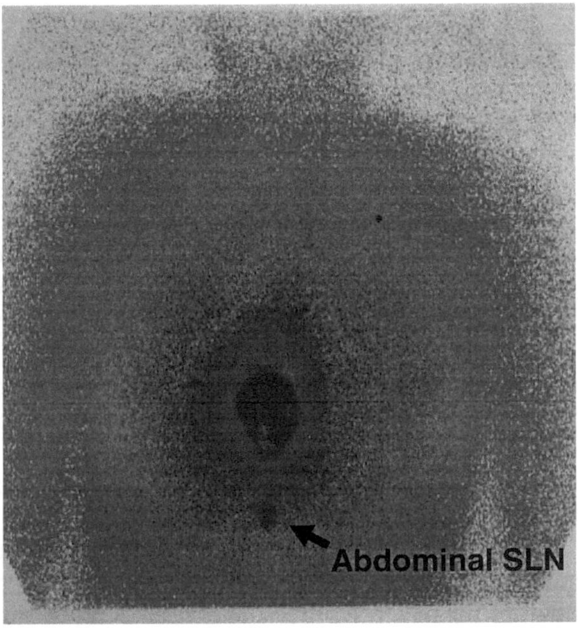

Surgeons are responsible for intraoperative detection of SLNs using hand-held gamma probes and dye-guided visualization of lymphatic flow. A shine-through effect from the injection site is one of the obstacles to performing intraoperative accurate SLN sampling by radio-guided method. The semiconductor-type portable camera is a useful device for detecting SLNs adjacent to the primary tumor, which could not be clearly visualized by a conventional gamma camera. Nuclear medicine physicians could contribute to the intraoperative accurate and complete sampling of SLNs using these devices.

Intraoperative pathological evaluation of harvested SLNs is another critical step in selective lymphadenectomy based on SLN status. Surgeons have to cooperate with pathologists in this stage. Surgeons must provide adequate samples of SLNs without any contamination of cancer tissues. Although optimal procedures of intraoperative pathological and/or molecular biological examinations are still controversial, the contribution of pathologists is essential to this team. Nuclear medicine physicians also have to know the final results of the location and status of SLNs to improve the technologies for imaging. The cooperative triangle as shown in Figure 1 clearly indicates the special multidisciplinary characteristics of this novel technology in clinical oncology.

REMAINING ISSUES AND CURRENT TOPICS

Improvement of the quality of preoperative lymphoscintigram

Lymphoscintigraphy is a very useful tool for confirming the locations of SLN preoperatively, making the SLN dissection less invasive and avoiding missing SLNs with unexpected locations.[7]

Simple acquisition of a lymphoscintigram, however, only depicts the hot areas due to the injected drugs and SLN, and the anatomic location of the SLNs remains unclear[8] (Figure 4). An outlining of the body contour is useful for understanding the anatomic location of the sentinel nodes. In our institute, the silhouette of the body is imaged using Compton's scattered photons originating in the body. We acquire lymphoscintigrams using dual-energy windows, namely, 130–150 keV for primary photons and 70–110 keV for scattered photons[8] (Figure 5). This method is easy and imposes no additional burden on patients or medical staff.

Figure 4. Original lymphoscintigram. Simple acquisition of lymphoscintigram shows only injected radionuclide and SLN with faint radioactivity. From Ref. 8.

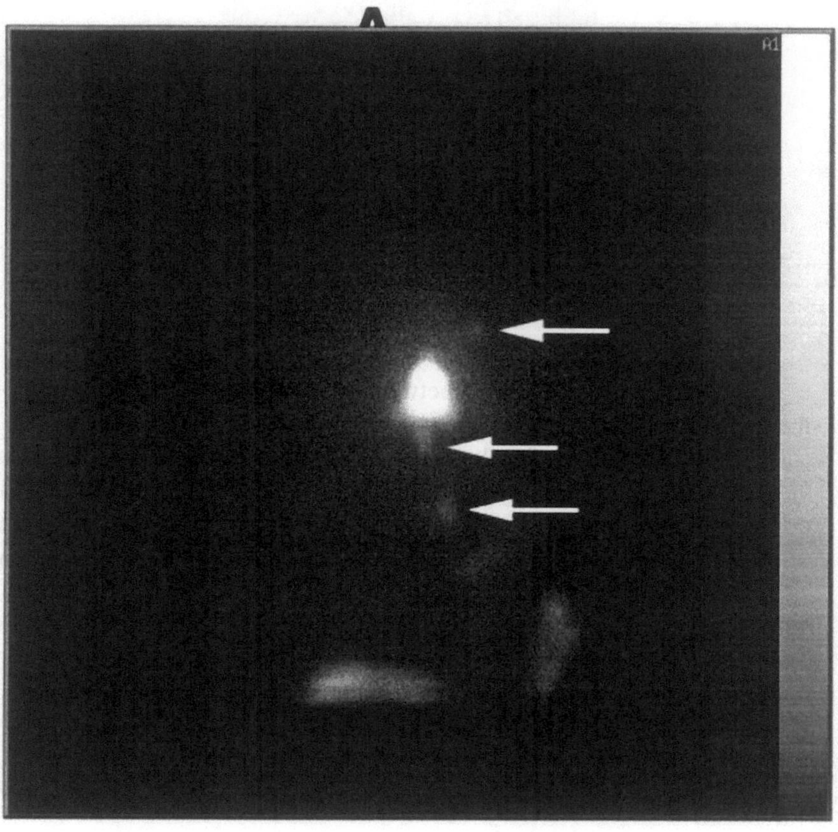

Figure 5. Outlining body contours using Compton scattered photons. Body contour can be imaged using second energy window for Compton scattered photons (70–110 keV). Superimposing the image with primary photons (a) and the image with scattered photons (b) clearly indicates the anatomical location of SLN (c). From Ref. 8.

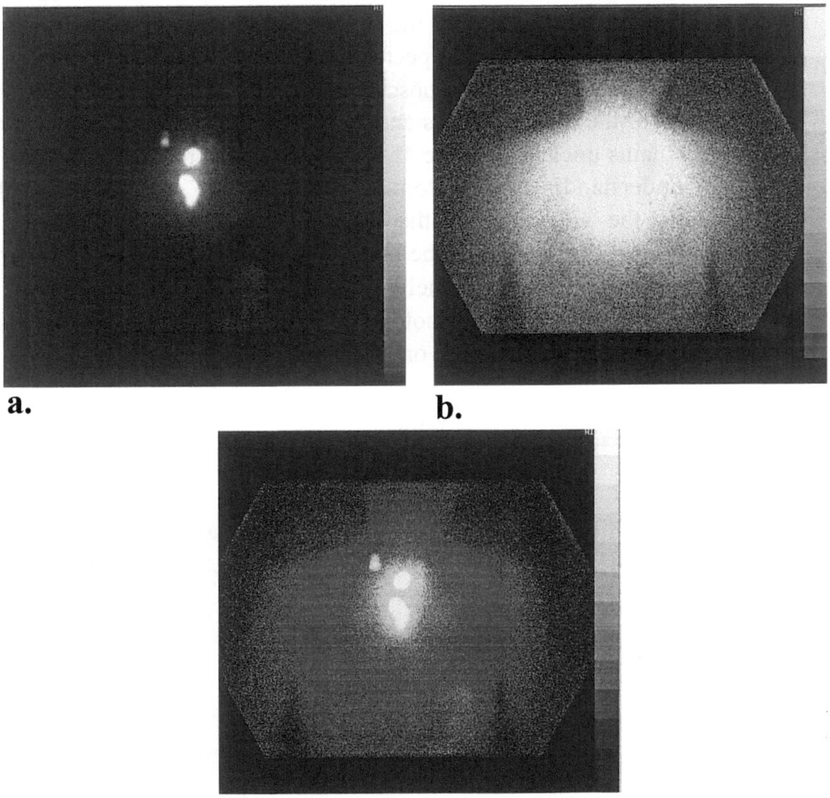

a. b. c.

Improvement of the contrast between the SLN and the injection site on the lymphoscintigram is another difficult problem.

Recently, we have developed a new simple method for the clear visualization of sentinel nodes.[9] With this method, the counts on the primary photon image are divided for each pixel by the count on the scattered photon image that is acquired to outline the contour of the body. The counts on the scattered photon image show a gentle distribution, whereas the SLN on the primary photon image shows a sharp peak. Therefore, the division of the counts of both images enhances the locally protruded count of the SLNs. This method is simple, and it takes only a few minutes to process scintigrams of one patient when a standard workstation is used[8] (Figure 6).

Figure 6. Simple method for clear visualization for both body contour and SLN. The division of the counts on the primary photon image (a) by those on the scattered photon image (b) makes image with good visualization of both body contour and SLN (c). From Ref. 8.

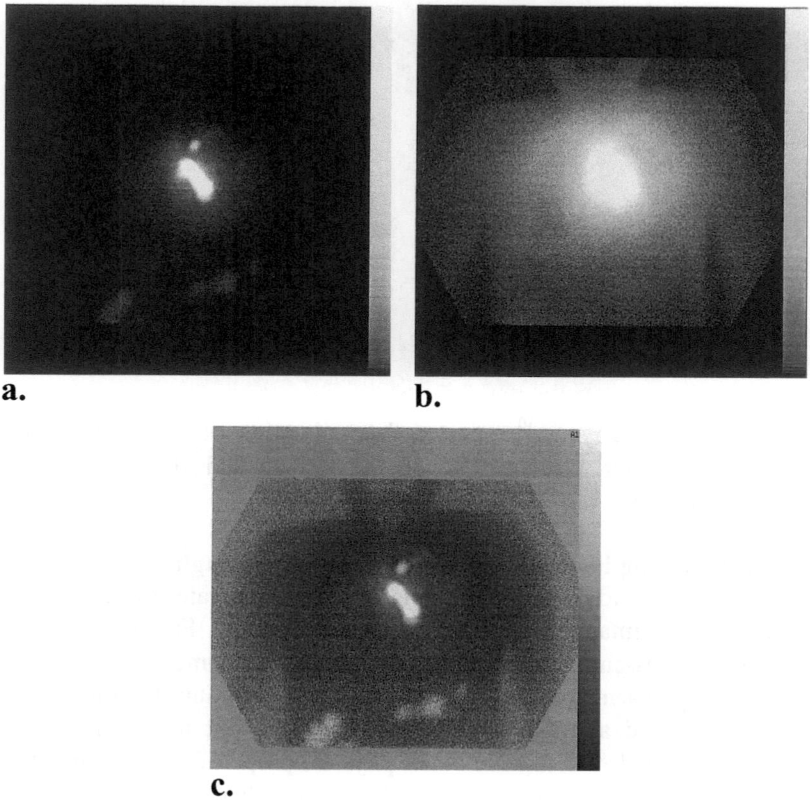

Currently, we usually acquire only planar images. In some cases, SLNs located at adjacent sites are imaged as a single fused nodule. SLNs of the alimentary tract are often located in the deep portion of the body. If the depth of the sentinel nodes can be measured, surgeons can access them more easily. SPECT images would provide useful information about the depth of the SLNs (Figure 7). However, good-quality SPECT images of lymphoscintigraphy for SLNs are difficult to obtain because of artifacts due to strong activity that is concentrated locally at the injection site. Our experiences revealed that the SPECT images have poor quality, even if the acquisition data were reconstructed by the ordered subsets-expectation maximization (OS-EM) algorithm. When good-quality SPECT images are available, fusion of the CT images and these SPECT images will provide highly valuable information.

Figure 7. Fusion image of SPECT and CT. When good-quality SPECT images are available, fusion of the CT images and these SPECT images will provide highly valuable information.

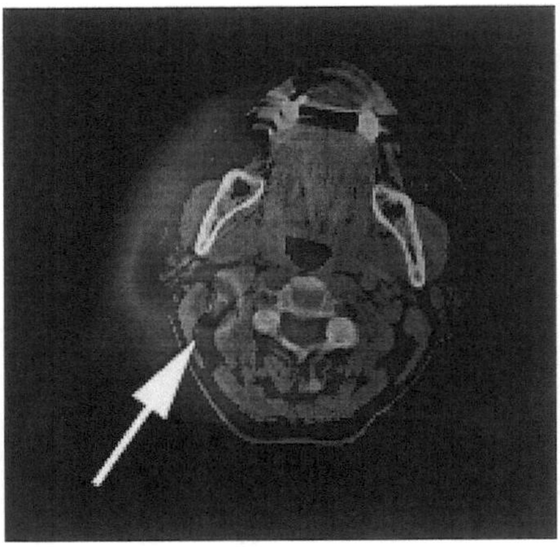

Recently, Yokoyama[10] reported that animation of projection images resulted in better visualization of SLNs than did the reconstructed sectional images.

New imaging instruments for intraoperative imaging

Surgeons and nuclear physicians may cooperate to develop an intraoperative imaging system for SLN sampling. For intraoperative imaging, it is essential to develop a portable gamma camera.

Recently, a semiconductor detector utilizing cadmium telluride, which can be operated at room temperature, has been put to practical use.[11] Semiconductor detectors have better physical properties than scintillation detectors, and they are compact enough to render them portable.

A hand-held imaging device called "eZ-SCOPE" has been developed in Japan recently.[12] This, small gamma camera includes detectors that consist of cadmium zinc telluride (CZT). We have tried this device using model sources sealed with Tc-99m pertechnetate. The SLN model with 1% of radioactivity of the injected dose located 1 cm from the injected site could be clearly depicted with only 10 seconds of acquisition time under conditions where no background activity exists.[13]

eZ-SCOPE includes a unique system to measure the depth of the radioactive focus. When this device is equipped with a specific collimator called a coded aperture, sectional images are available at 3- to 4-mm intervals.[14] Tsuchimochi and co-workers[15] also have developed a new semiconductor gamma camera using cadmium telluride, which shows better physical properties than CZT as shown in Figure 8.

Figure 8. Image of model sources obtained by a hand-held semiconductor gamma camera using cadmium telluride. Two microcuries of radioactive source mimicking SLN located 1 cm from 0.2 mCi of main source is clearly drawn by 10 seconds of acquisition.

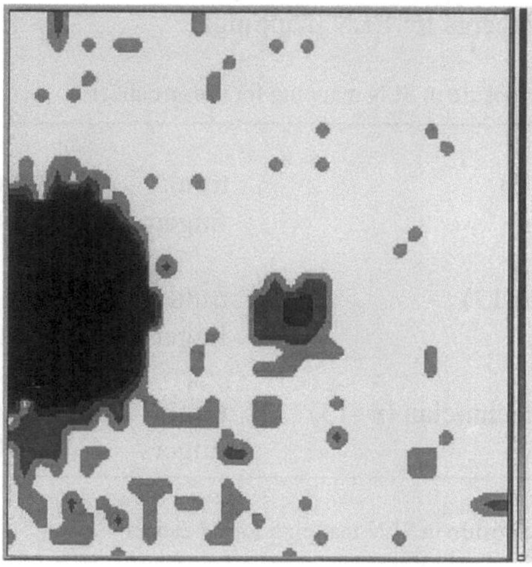

Ogawa and Motomura[16] recently proposed a new reconstruction method of sectional scintigraphic images without rotating gamma cameras. This method requires obtaining the data from various directions. Thus, a compact gamma camera with high flexibility is essential for practical application, and the semiconductor detector is thought to be suitable for this purpose.

These developments in detecting devices would be helpful in the survey of SLNs of various organs.

RADIATION SAFETY ISSUES FOR THE MULTIDISCIPLINARY TEAM

Although radio-guided SLN mapping using ^{99m}Tc-labeled tracers is basically safe and acceptable for international regulation, it is important to reduce the radiation exposure to the patients and medical staffs. Also an explanation of actual data and safety of this procedure for all personnel involved in this project is required.

In 1996, the International Atomic Energy Association (IAEA) recommended that the acceptable excempt dose of ^{99m}Tc is 0.3 mCi.[17] We have confirmed that 0.3 mCi at the time of survey is sufficient for SLN mapping using hand-held gamma probe.

Actual data of radiation exposure to medical staffs in SLN mapping for breast cancer and gastrointestinal cancer are summarized in Tables 1 and

2. From these data, we can perform a sufficient number of cases of SLN mapping in a year without any adverse effect of radiation exposure. An announcement of this fact is important in the cooperation of multidisciplinary teams for SLN mapping.

Table 1. Radiation exposure in SLN mapping for breast cancer

Surgeon (n=16)	trunk	0–2 (1.1±0.4) μSv
	fingers	8–69 (34±12)
Pathologist (n=13)	trunk	0
	fingers	0–41 (4±11)
Pathological technician (n=13)	trunk	0–1 (0.1±0.3)
	fingers	0–84 (8±22)

Table 2. Radiation exposure in SLN mapping for GI cancer

Endoscopist	trunk	0–1μSv
	fingers	96.5
Surgeon	trunk	1–5 (2.1±1.2)
	finger	3–125 (62±42)
Pathologist	trunk	0
	finger	0–21 (8±10)
Pathological technician	trunk	0
	finger	0–64 (25±28)

DEVELOPMENT OF NEW TYPES OF GAMMA PROBE FOR LAPAROSCOPIC/THORACOSCOPIC SLN BIOPSY

For the universal application of SLN technology to minimally invasive surgery for various solid tumors, a combination with endoscopic surgery is essential. There are several technical issues to be solved in this point of view. Laparoscopic SLN sampling is not always easy to perform because of the shine-through effect from the primary lesion as an injection site. Surgeons have to pay attention to avoid the shine-through effect from the primary lesion by handling of the gamma probe as indicated in Figure 9. In comparison with the sufficient collimation of a normal gamma probe

(Navigator, Tyco Healthcare Japan Inc., Tokyo, Japan) with a shielding device (Top Gun, Tyco Healthcare Japan Inc.), collimation of currently available laparoscopic and thoracoscopic probes is not satisfactory. There is a serious limitation of maneuverability of laparoscopic gamma probes because the axis of gamma probes is rigidly fixed on the abdominal wall by entry trocar. From these limitations, it is relatively difficult to get information on the depth of SLNs located in deep portions of the dense fat tissue as shown in Figure 10. To overcome these problems, development of a new type of gamma probe with a flexible shaft would be required.

Figure 9. Laparoscopic detection of SLNs in radio-guided method. In laparoscopic probing procedure, handling of gamma probe to avoid shine-through from primary lesion is crucial.

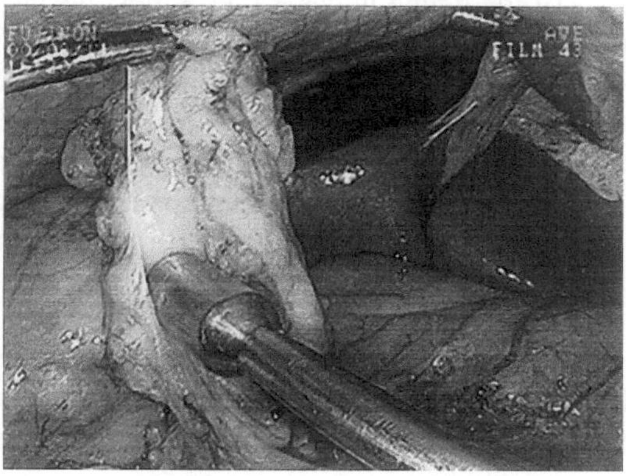

Figure 10. Limitations in laparoscopic gamma probing. There is a serious limitation of maneuverability of laparoscopic gamma probes because the axis of gamma probe is rigidly fixed on the abdominal wall by entry trocar.Thus, it is relatively difficult to get information on the depth of SLNs located in deep portions of the dense fat tissue.

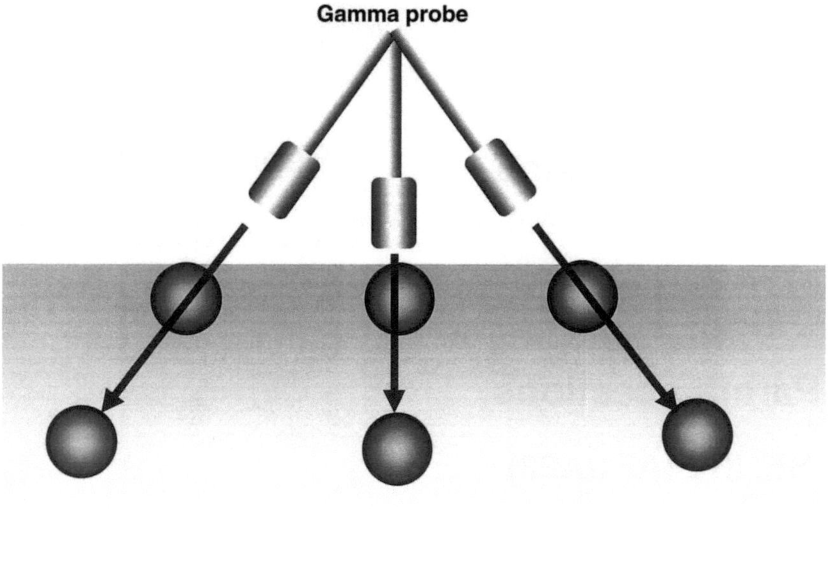

AN OPTIMAL PROCESSING PROCEDURE OF HARVESTED SLN FOR PATHOLOGICAL AND MOLECULAR BIOLOGICAL EXAMINATION

Although the focused pathological examination of SLNs contributed to the effective and accurate staging for various solid tumors, an optimal processing procedure of harvested SLNs is still controversial, particularly in an intraoperative setting. Current protocol used in our institute is indicated in Figure 11. The introduction of immunohistochemistry using anticytokeratin antibody (AE1/AE3) improved the sensitivity of intraoperative assessment of micrometastasis as shown in Figure 12. In a previous study,[18] latent micrometastases and isolated tumor cells were identified in 15% of the lymph nodes RT-PCR positive and histologically negative for routine examination. Recently, we introduced intraoperative real-time RT-PCR to detect CK19mRNA and CK20mRNA. Processing the sample, including extraction of RNA and real-time RT-PCR, still takes between 60 and 80 min. Also we have to pay attention for false-positive results in RT-PCR because of several factors. A more rapid and quantitative system of real-time RT-PCR would provide useful information for the evaluation of SLNs in addition to the routine examination of H&E and IHC. Although intensive support from pathologists is essential for successful SLN biopsy, complementary information from molecular biological analysis would be required for much safer clinical application.

Figure 11. Processing of SLNs at Keio University Hospital.

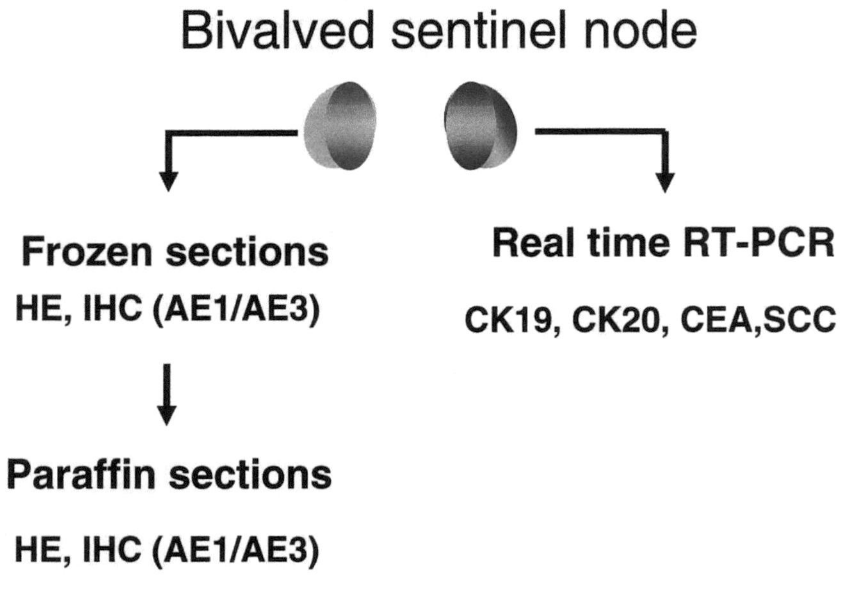

Figure 12. Intraoperative histological examination of SLNs. Immunohistochemistry using anti-cytokeratin antibody (B) is useful to identify metastasis in SLNs in comparison with routine H&E staining (A).

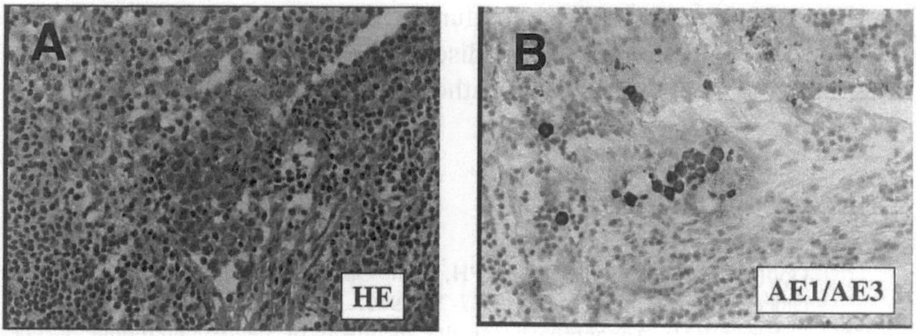

SLN AS A TARGET FOR INVESTIGATION OF BASIC ONCOLOGY

The SLN concept would contribute not only to clinical practice but also to the basic science for the molecular mechanism of lymphatic spread and local antitumor immunology. Recently, several reports have demonstrated the downmodulation of immune functions in SLNs. Cochran et al. reported that the frequency of paracortical interdigitating dendritic cells (IDCs) was dramatically reduced in SLNs from melanoma patients and most IDCs lacked the complex dendrites associated with active antigen presentation.[19] This immune suppressive reaction might be attributed to the release of factors from primary melanoma and a mechanism of formation of micrometastasis. SLNs are the second important battlefield for malignant cells against host immune systems next to the primary site. It is important to investigate the process of the formation of micrometastasis in SLNs to understand the mechanism of cancer metastasis. There may be some suggestions for novel biological approaches using cytokine modification or immunomodulation. The crosstalk between basic science and clinical approach would be provided by actual SLNs from various organs and may introduce a breakthrough for clinical oncology. Surgical oncologists could provide precious resources of oncological and immunological investigations for pathologists and basic scientists.

CONCLUSIONS

The SLN concept has a great potential to change the patient care in the field of clinical oncology. For further development of individualized treatment for solid tumors, multidisciplinary teamwork with surgeons, nuclear medicine physicians, and pathologists would be required.

REFERENCES

1. Gould EA, Winship T, Philbin PH, et al: Observation on a "sentinel node" in cancer of the parotid. Cancer 13:77-78, 1960.
2. Cabanas RM: An approach for the treatment of penile carcinoma. Cancer 39:456-466,1977.
3. Morton DL, Wen DR, Wong JH, et al: Technical details of intraoperative lymphatic mapping for early stage melanoma. Arch Surg 127:392-399, 1992.
4. Giuliano AE, Kirgan DM, Guenther JM, et al:Lymphatic mapping and sentinel lymphadenectomy for breast cancer. Ann Surg 220:391-401, 1994.
5. Saha S, Wiese D, Badin J, et al: Technical details of sentinel lymph node mapping in colorectal cancer and its impact on staging. Ann Surg Oncol 7:82-84, 2000.
6. Hiratsuka M, Miyashiro I, Ishikawa O, et al: Application of sentinel node biopsy to gastric cancer surgery. Surgery 129:335-340, 2001.
7. Kitagawa Y, Fujii H, Mukai M, et al: Intraoperative lymphatic mapping and sentinel lymph node sampling in esophageal and gastric cancer. Surg Oncol Clin North Am 11:293-304, 2002.
8. Fujii H, Kitagawa Y, Kitajima M, Kubo A: Sentinel nodes of malignancies originating in the alimentary tract. Ann Nucl Med 18:1-12, 2004.
9. Fujii H, Yamashita H, Nakahara T, Ikeda T, Kitagawa Y, Iwasaki R, et al: Outlining the body contours with scattered photons in lymphoscintigraphy for sentinel nodes. Ann Nucl Med 14: 401-404, 2000.
10. Yokoyama K: Imaging techniques for radio-guided sentinel node detection (abstract). In Proceedings of SN2002, p. 127.
11. Mori I, Takayama T, Motomura N: The CdTe detector module and its imaging performance. Ann Nucl Med 15: 487-494, 2001.
12. Yokoyama K, Tonami N, Tsugawa K, Kinami S, Miwa K: Sentinel node detection with radiocolloids (in Japanese with English abstract). Jpn J Clin Radiol 46: 1373-1381, 2001.
13. Fujii H, Kitagawa Y, Ikeda T, Ogawa K, Kunieda E, Nakamura K, et al: Sentinel node imaging using an imaging probe with semiconductor detector (Japanese with English abstract). Jpn J Clin Radiol 47: 1725-1733, 2002.
14. Anzai I, Inoue T, Ito T, Shimizu M, Ryuo H, Takeuchi Y: Analysis of tomographical information of tracer distribution by using a CdZnTe semiconductor-based gamma counter equipped with using coded aperture (in Japanese). Radioisotopes 51: 505-508, 2002.
15. Tsuchimochi M, Sakahara H, Hayama K, Funaki M, Ohno R, Shirahata T, et al: A prototype small CdTe gamma camera for radioguided surgery and other imaging applications. Eur J Nucl Med Mol Imaging (Epub ahead of print), 2003.

16. Ogawa K, Motomura N: Proposing a new myocardial SPECT system. Conference Record of IEEE Nuclear Science and Medical Imaging Conference. (CD-ROM), 2002.
17. IAEA: International Basic Safety Standards for Protection against Ionizing Radiation and for the Safety of Radiation Sources (IAEA Safety Series No. 115). IAEA, Vienna, 1996.
18. Matsuda J, Kitagawa Y, Fujii H, et al: Significance of metastasis detected by molecular techniques in sentinel nodes of patients with gastrointestinal cancer. Ann Surg Oncol 11:250S-254S, 2004.
19. Lana AM, Wen DR, Cochran AJ. The morphology, immunophenotype and distribution of paracortical dendritic leukocytes in lymph nodes regional to cutaneous melanoma. Melanoma Res 11: 401-410, 2001.

Chapter 14

SELECTIVE SENTINEL LYMPHADENECTOMY: PROGRESS TO DATE AND PROSPECTS FOR THE FUTURE

John F. Thompson[1,3], Roger F. Uren[1,4], Richard A. Scolyer[1,2], Jonathan R. Stretch[1,3]

[1]Sydney Melanoma Unit and the [2]Department of Anatomical Pathology, Royal Prince Alfred Hospital, Camperdown, NSW, 2050, Australia. Disciplines of [3]Surgery and [4]Medicine, The University of Sydney, Sydney, NSW, 2006

Abstract: The sentinel node (SN) concept was clearly outlined by Virchow in the mid-nineteenth century, and Braithwaite used the term "glands sentinel" in 1923. However, it was not until Morton, Cochran et al. published their landmark report in 1992 that the clinical relevance of the SN was fully appreciated. Since then, the validity of the concept has been confirmed in studies undertaken at a number of centers worldwide. It has become clear that SN status accurately reflects the status of the entire regional node field, not only in patients with melanoma but also in those with breast cancer and a wide range of other primary malignancies. New insights into lymphatic anatomy have been gained by preoperative lymphoscintigraphy, and the original blue dye mapping technique for SN identification has been supplemented by intraoperative use of a hand-held gamma probe to identify radioactivity in colloid particles injected at the primary tumor site. It has become clear that all three methods are required to achieve optimal accuracy of SN identification.

Although SN assessment provides very important prognostic information, the results of randomized trials must be awaited to determine whether selective sentinel lymphadenectomy, with full regional node dissection if a positive SN is found, is of any therapeutic value. It is possible that SN positivity is merely a marker of disease that has the potential for hematogenous dissemination and systemic metastasis. As follow-up times extend, reported false-negative SN rates are increasing, and ways to reduce these false-negative rates are therefore being actively sought. Attempts are being made to increase the accuracy of SN identification, and to confirm true SN identity both at the time of surgery and retrospectively. The ultimate objective is to develop minimally invasive and even non-invasive methods of SN assessment. Proton magnetic resonance spectroscopy is one technique that might make it possible to achieve this goal, and avoid the present morbidity and cost of operative SN removal.

Key words: sentinel node, history, lymphoscintigraphy, pathology, surgery

THE PAST

History of the sentinel node concept

Among his many important contributions to present-day understanding of the pathophysiology of a wide range of human diseases, the celebrated German pathologist and statesman Rudolf Virchow (1821–1902) very clearly described the sentinel node (SN) concept in his lectures. Undoubtedly one of the greatest minds in medicine of the 19th century, he pointed out that tissue fluid (lymph), which in disease states may contain bacteria or tumor cells, drains from a particular body location to a specific lymph node, before onward passage to other lymph nodes and eventually to systemic sites.[1]

Fifty years later, in the early 20th century, the process by which lymphatic drainage to specific nodes occurred was examined in great detail by Braithwaite,[2] whose studies involved tracing the passage of vital dye injected at various body sites to draining lymph node fields. These investigations were performed first in the cat, then in man. Braithwaite appears to have been the first to use the word "sentinel" in reference to a node receiving direct lymphatic drainage from a particular site. This work by Braithwaite, describing "glands sentinel", was reported in 1923, but attracted little attention at the time. The concept was revisited by Gould et al., who in 1960 described direct lymphatic drainage in patients with parotid malignancy to a "sentinel node" at the confluence of the anterior and posterior facial veins.[3] They undertook frozen section examination of the SN at the time of parotidectomy. If micrometastatic disease was found, a radical neck dissection was performed, but if the SN was negative only the parotidectomy was undertaken. A few years later, in 1966, Sayegh et al.[4] reported the results of their studies of lymphatic drainage using lymphangiography to elucidate lymphatic drainage pathways from the testis. They used the term "sentinel node" to describe the "primary" node to which direct lymphatic drainage occurred. In 1977, Cabanas reported clinical studies in patients with primary tumors not only of the testis, but also of the penis, anus, rectum, breast, and skin.[5] He indicated that there was a "sentinel node" in a relatively constant position draining the penis, although he did not perform lymphatic mapping to specifically identify that SN in each patient. He demonstrated in his series of 250 patients that the SN concept held true for a range of quite different tumor types.

Although a number of individuals had thus recognized the pathophysiological processes that made disease in an SN a marker of tumor spread to a regional node field, the potential clinical application of lymphatic mapping and selective sentinel lymphadenectomy was not fully appreciated until Morton, Cochran, and colleagues from the John Wayne Cancer Institute in Santa Monica began undertaking studies in the early 1980s. Like Braithwaite some 60 years earlier, they used a feline model initially,[6] and then went on to demonstrate that the situation in man was similar. It is interesting to note that their landmark report published in 1992,[7] destined to become one of the most often quoted papers in the surgical literature over the subsequent decade, was initially rejected for publication by several prominent journals. However, the elegant simplicity and logic of the SN concept was quickly appreciated by others, and a number of validation studies were commenced.

Validation studies

Within three years of the 1992 publication by Morton et al., two major validation studies had been completed and reported confirming the SN hypothesis that had been proposed, namely, that SN status in melanoma patients accurately reflected the status of the entire regional node field. One was a study performed by Reintgen et al. in the United States,[8] involving 42 patients, and the other was undertaken by Thompson et al.[9] in Australia, involving 118 patients. Both studies produced results that were remarkably similar to those originally reported by Morton et al., indicating very clearly that sentinel lymph node status was an accurate indicator of the presence of metastatic melanoma in a regional lymph node field.

In each of these confirmatory studies, as in the original study at the John Wayne Cancer Institute, SNs were identified by injecting blue dye intradermally at the primary melanoma site, then tracing blue-stained afferent lymphatics to blue-stained SNs in regional node fields. After the SN or SNs had been removed from each patient, a full completion regional lymph node dissection was performed, allowing all the other nodes in the node field to be examined carefully for micrometastatic disease. This process enabled the accuracy of SN examination as an indicator of the status of the entire node field to be assessed. In the study by Reintgen et al., 8 of the 42 patients were found to have micrometastatic melanoma in an SN, and in 7 of them the SN was the exclusive site of disease. None of the other patients in the series was found to have metastatic disease in either SNs or non-SNs. In the study by Thompson et al., micrometastatic melanoma was found in 22 of 118 patients. In 18 of these patients, the SN was the only site of disease. In 2 of the 118 patients a positive node was found in the completion lymph node dissection specimen, after an SN removed from that patient had been reported as negative. In each case, however, the positive node that was found in the completion node dissection specimen appeared to have been an additional SN that had been overlooked because of deficiencies in technique, and not because the concept that metastatic melanoma cells spread first to SNs was flawed. With the benefit of hindsight, it is remarkable that such good results were obtained in the three studies, because preoperative lymphoscintigraphy was not undertaken in every patient, nor was a hand held-gamma probe routinely employed to assist in SN identification. Nevertheless, the results of the confirmatory studies were as impressive and convincing as those originally reported from the John Wayne Cancer Institute. Similar validation studies from other centers were subsequently reported, all with very similar results, and all strongly supporting the original hypothesis that SN status accurately reflects the status of the entire node field in patients with melanoma.[10]

At the time that the SN biopsy procedure was first introduced in the early 1990s, the routine treatment recommendation in many major melanoma treatment centers around the world was for an elective lymph node dissection (ELND) for patients with primary tumors exceeding 1.5 mm in Breslow thickness. However, clinical trials failed to demonstrate any convincing improvement in overall survival,[11-14] and there was concern about the troublesome long-term morbidity in the form of lymphedema that regularly resulted from ELND. Routine ELND was therefore abandoned as a treatment option in most centers. It is thus unlikely that further SN validation studies of the type described above will ever be undertaken, but at least as far as melanoma is concerned, there is consensus that the SN hypothesis as proposed by Morton, Cochran, and colleagues has been very adequately demonstrated to be correct. There is also an accumulating body of evidence, presented elsewhere in this book, that the concept is valid for a wide range of other tumors that can metastasize via lymphatics to regional lymph nodes.

THE PRESENT

New insights into lymphatic anatomy and nodal metastasis

Although it is only a little over a decade since the enormous clinical relevance of the SN concept was first appreciated, major advances in our understanding of the process of metastasis via lymphatics have been made during that period, and a number of important refinements of the technique for selective sentinel lymphadenectomy have been introduced. Probably the most important of these advances has been the recognition that lymphatic drainage patterns are much more variable than had previously been appreciated, making high-quality preoperative lymphoscintigraphy an important component of the SN biopsy procedure. At the Sydney Melanoma Unit (SMU), over 3300 preoperative lymphoscintigrams have now been performed in melanoma patients, and a number of previously unsuspected lymphatic drainage pathways have been discovered.[15-17] For example, it has been found that in 26% of patients with melanomas on the back, there is an SN in the triangular intermuscular space, lateral to the scapula.[18] If high-quality preoperative lymphoscintigraphy is not performed, SNs in this location will be mistaken for axillary SNs, or missed completely, greatly increasing the possibility that a positive SN will not be found, if lymph node metastasis has in fact occurred. Another situation in which preoperative lymphoscintigraphy is of critical importance is when an interval node, which is an SN and therefore could contain micrometastatic disease, is present.[19] Such nodes are unlikely to be detected if only blue dye mapping is used.

In many patients, lymphatic drainage is to a site or node field that would not have been predicted clinically. Drainage to node fields on the opposite side of the body is regularly observed, shattering long-held beliefs about lymphatic drainage pathways originally proposed by Sappey and his associates in the mid-nineteenth century.[17,20] Primary melanomas of the head and neck demonstrate particularly unpredictable lymphatic drainage, with up to one third of them having SNs in sites that would not have been predicted clinically.[21] These findings are of considerable importance, since it is clear that an SN in an aberrant location is just as likely to contain micrometastatic disease as a SN in an predicted site.[18,19] Lymphatic drainage patterns, both normal and abnormal, are discussed in greater detail in Chapter X of this book and elsewhere.[16, 17, 22]

Value of a gamma probe intraoperatively

Another important advance in the past 10 years has been the development of hand-held gamma probes for use intraoperatively. These devices have allowed SNs to be found more quickly and with less dissection, as well as increasing reliability by permitting the entire node field to be checked for retained foci of isotope, once all SNs are thought to have been removed. A number of studies have now demonstrated that accuracy rates for SN identification are greater if a triple modality technique is used, i.e., preoperative lymphoscintigraphy, injection of blue dye immediately preoperatively, and use of a hand-held gamma probe intraoperatively.[10, 17, 23]

Prognostic importance of sentinel node status

A great frustration at the present time is that results are not yet available from large-scale clinical trials that were designed to demonstrate whether or not selective sentinel lymphadenectomy, with complete regional lymph node dissection if a positive SN is found, improves survival outcome. Although nearly a decade has passed since major trials such as the Multicenter Selective Lymphadenectomy Trial[24] and the Sunbelt Melanoma Trial[25] were initiated, it is likely to be several more years before definitive results are available. It is already very clear, however, that SN status is an extremely important prognostic indicator. Even with relatively short follow-up periods, the difference in outcome for patients who are SN positive compared with those who are SN negative is large. A recent analysis of our own results from the SMU, for example, has shown that with a median follow-up period of 5 years, 85.5% of patients with negative SNs are alive and disease free, compared to 43.5% of those with positive SNs (unpublished data). Results reported from numerous other centers have been remarkably similar.[10, 26-29]

The prognostic importance of microscopic deposits of metastatic tumor in macroscopically normal SNs was recognized by the Melanoma Staging Committee of the American Joint Committee on Cancer (AJCC) when, in 2000, it recommended a revision of the AJCC staging system.[30] The Committee proposed that, for the first time, melanoma patients with disease in regional lymph nodes (i.e., with Stage III disease) should be separated into two substages (a and b), depending on whether the nodal disease was microscopic (IIIa) or macroscopic (IIIb). Substantial differences in prognosis were demonstrated for patients with Stage IIIa and Stage IIIb disease according to this system. A new AJCC staging system incorporating these changes has now been introduced[31] and, having been adopted by the International Union Against Cancer (UICC), is now the accepted melanoma staging system worldwide.

Pathologic assessment of sentinel nodes

A present difficulty is that there is no standardized procedure for the pathologic assessment of SNs. Cochran et al. have stated that, because most melanoma micrometastases occur in the central plane of the lymph node, bivalving the SN through the hilum and its longest dimension, then examining up to 10 tissue sections from this central plane (stained both with hematoxylin and eosin (H&E) and immunohistochemically for S100 and HMB45) is sufficient.[32] Alternative procedures have involved parallel slicing of the SN, not necessarily through the hilum, and examining a section from each slice.[33] Using either of these procedures, the detection rate of melanoma micrometastasis in SNs varies from 15 to 25%, with an average of about 17%.[33-35] Others have suggested that the use of a more comprehensive protocol involving the microscopic examination of up to 20 sections, taken at different levels through the node and stained with H&E and with various immunohistochemical markers, increases the detection rate of melanoma micrometastasis in SNs (to 34% in one study).[36] At the SMU we use a modification of the Cochran method for pathologic examination of SNs, staining 2 sections with H&E and 2 sections immunohistochemically for S100 and HMB45, respectively. On the basis of our results, we believe that routinely performing more intensive histopathologic examination of SNs is difficult to justify from a cost-benefit perspective.[35] Between March 1992 and June 2001, of 1152 patients who had undergone SN biopsy for primary melanomas at the SMU, 976 were diagnosed with negative SNs by initial pathologic examination, and follow-up was available in 957. Of these, 26 (2.7%) developed regional lymph node recurrence during a median follow-up period of 35.7 months. More detailed pathologic examination of the SNs of 22 of the patients with a false-negative SNB revealed melanoma micrometastasis in only 7 of them. As discussed in more detail below, there are probably other reasons for failure of the selective sentinel lymphadenectomy procedure apart from failure to detect micrometastatic disease pathologically.

Role of RT-PCR

SNs have also been assessed for the presence of melanoma micrometastases using the reverse transcriptase polymerase chain reaction (RT-PCR). This has been performed using a variety of probes, most commonly tyrosinase and melan-A (MART-1) and occasionally gp100 (HMB45). Use of this highly sensitive technique has resulted in the detection of much higher rates of metastatic disease (up to 70%) than those detected by histopathologic evaluation. However, it is suspected that this technique is too sensitive, leading to a significant false-positive rate. It has been speculated that the cause of these false-positive cases might be intranodal melanophages, nerves, or benign nevus cells.[32] The use of multimarker quantitative RT-PCR appears to significantly reduce the false-positive rate of this technique and its use in combination with histopathologic evaluation of SNs (including immunohistochemistry) may improve the accuracy of SN evaluation.[29]

Reliability of sentinel node identification, removal, and assessment

An emerging concern in relation to the selective sentinel lymphadenectomy procedure is the disturbingly high rate of false-negative results that have been reported from a number of centers around the world. Despite claimed rates for SN identification approaching 100%, false-negative rates exceeding 10% are now being reported,[21,37], representing the late appearance of metastatic disease in a node field from which an SN reported to be negative has previously been removed. In some cases, these regional node field recurrences occur at the same time as widespread systemic disease becomes apparent. However, detailed analysis of available data suggests that other late failures occur for a variety of reasons related to incorrect or incomplete SN identification—because the preoperative lymphoscintigram had not been performed or interpreted correctly, because the surgeon failed to identify and remove all SNs, or because the pathologist failed to locate or identify micrometastatic deposits that were present in the SNs.[38] An examination of possible reasons for a false-negative SN biopsy result in patients of the SMU suggests that approximately one third were attributable to a failure of nuclear medicine, approximately one third to a surgical failure, and the remaining third to a failure of the histopathologic process.[39] In other institutions the reasons for failure may be distributed differently, depending on the skill, experience, and commitment of the nuclear medicine physicians, surgeons, and pathologists, respectively, at that institution.

When centers report "success rates" for SN identification approaching 100%, caution must be exercised in the interpretation of this information. In most cases it simply represents the proportion of patients in whom *at least one* blue and/or hot node was found and removed. Indeed, in some series no attempt has been made to find more than one SN in any lymph node field, because of an erroneous interpretation of the definition of an SN originally proposed by Morton, Cochran et al., i.e., that it is the "first" node on a lymphatic drainage pathway from a given primary tumor site.[7] Because of the confusion this definition has caused, we believe that it is better to define an SN as "any lymph node receiving direct lymphatic drainage from a primary tumor site."[40] This clearly allows for the possibility of there being more than one SN in a node field. The situation is well illustrated by the results of a recent study at the SMU, in which a critical analysis was undertaken of 362 patients with head and neck melanomas who underwent lymphatic mapping and a selective sentinel lymphadenectomy procedure.[21] In 99.3% of these patients, at least one node considered to be an SN was identified, but in only 70% of the patients was every node reported as a probable SN by the nuclear medicine physician at the time of preoperative lymphoscintigraphy found and removed. In our study, all but one of the patients had at least one node identified and removed during surgery, which could therefore be reported as a 99.3% success rate (i.e., 135/136). Although the head and neck is undoubtedly the most difficult area of the body in which to identify and remove SNs, similar problems undoubtedly occur for melanomas that drain to the axilla or the groin, as well as for melanomas that drain to SNs in sites outside recognized node fields. Melanomas located on the lower back, the lower abdomen, or a lower limb, for example, may drain directly to SNs in the external iliac and obturator regions. These nodes can easily be misinterpreted as second tier nodes on preoperative lymphoscintigraphy and may be difficult to locate at the time of sentinel node surgery.

When considering the question of false-negative rates, it is important that the correct method of calculating these rates is used. The number of patients who recur in a node field must be related to the total number of SN-positive patients, rather than to the total number of patients undergoing selective sentinel lymphadenectomy (the majority of whom will be SN negative). In the original SMU validation study mentioned previously,[9] for example, only 2 of 118 patients had an additional positive lymph node found when completion lymph node dissection was performed (2/118 = 1.9%). However, when this number of patients is related to the total number of patients ultimately shown to have micrometastatic melanoma in a regional node (22 patients), the actual false-negative rate for the procedure becomes 9% (2/22). In the SMU review of 136 head and neck patients having a selective sentinel lymphadenectomy, mentioned above, 14 patients were initially reported to be SN positive. However, recurrence in a node field from which an SN reported to be negative had been removed occurred in 11 patients. Thus, 25 patients were ultimately found to have metastatic disease in the node field. This represents a false-negative rate of 44% (11 of 25), using the method of calculation described above.[21] There are good reasons to believe that several of these node field recurrences did not occur because of a failure to identify the correct nodes as SNs and remove them, or because of a deficiency of the SN concept. The most compelling explanation is generalized hematogenous spread, as evidenced by the simultaneous appearance of widespread systemic metastases. Nevertheless, false-negative rates of this order of magnitude are clearly of concern, and strenuous efforts must therefore be made to reduce them.

General applicability of sentinel node technology

While much of the early work on lymphatic mapping and selective sentinel lymphadenectomy was undertaken in patients with melanoma, there are now many reports in the literature describing lymphatic mapping and SN assessment for breast cancer, and smaller numbers of publications reporting use of the technique for other tumors, including squamous cell and Merkel cell carcinomas of the skin, upper gastrointestinal and colorectal cancers, genitourinary cancers, lung cancer, and thyroid cancer. The role of SN assessment in the management of patients with these various tumor types is discussed in other chapters of this book. The present position appears to be that staging by SN identification, removal, and examination may be useful for any malignant tumor that has the potential to spread to regional lymph nodes via lymphatics. It must be borne in mind, however, that some of these other tumors, like thick melanomas, may spread preferentially via the bloodstream, in which case the value of regional lymph node staging will be reduced, and may even be negligible.

THE FUTURE

Pathologic assessment of sentinel nodes

It is the current policy of most large melanoma treatment centers worldwide to perform a completion lymph node dissection (CLND) if metastatic cells are found in an SN. However, among patients with positive SNs, further nodal involvement in CLND specimens is identified in only 8–30% of cases.[33,41] It is logical to assume that patients with metastatic melanoma confined to their SN do not benefit from this further surgery. The ability to predict who is *not* likely to have further nodal involvement in a CLND would therefore allow such major surgery and its inherent short-term and long-term morbidity to be avoided in these patients.

Characteristics of both the primary tumor and the tumor deposits in SNs have been assessed in a number of studies that have sought to identify patients with a low probability of having disease in non-SNs. These studies have yielded conflicting results.[42-44] The various factors assessed have included features of the primary tumor (such as its thickness, ulcerative state, mitotic rate, Clark level of invasion, and histologic subtype), patient characteristics (such as age and gender), and features of the positive SNs (such as their number and the distribution and volume of tumor deposits within them).

Consistent with the concept of an orderly progression of lymph node metastases, it appears that the risk of spread of tumor from SNs to non-SNs depends mostly on the extent of SN involvement. That is, the risk of spread to non-SNs is likely to be greater when there are macrometastases containing tens of thousands of tumor cells within the SN compared with the risk when only a few tumor cells are present. However, the challenge lies in identifying with a high degree of accuracy which measurement of tumor burden or combination of other factors best predicts an acceptably low probability of metastatic tumor being present in non-SNs.

Starz et al. recently suggested that micromorphometric features of SNs, in particular centripetal thickness (defined as the maximum distance of melanoma cells from the inner margin of the SN capsule as measured using an ocular micrometer) may be useful in predicting further nodal involvement in CLND specimens.[33] They found non-SN involvement in CLND specimens in 9 of 15 patients (60%) with an SN centripetal thickness of > 1 mm but in only 2 of 25 patients (8%) with a centripetal thickness of ≤ 1 mm. They suggested that the centripetal thickness of melanoma deposits in SNs may also provide additional prognostic information, complementing the TNM staging system for primary cutaneous melanoma. In a subsequent, larger study from the SMU, various pathological features of positive SNs were assessed (unpublished data). It was found that the presence of non-SN metastases was significantly correlated with centripetal thickness > 2 mm, deposit size > 10 mm^2 as measured microscopically in histologic tissue sections, effacement of nodal architecture, and the presence of melanoma cells in perinodal lymphatic vessels. Cochran and colleagues have found that relative tumor area in the SN (as determined by computer-assisted image analysis), Breslow thickness of the primary tumor, and density of dendritic leukocytes in the nodal paracortex were each highly significant predictors of non-SN positivity.[45] Furthermore, they used these features to develop an algorithm that may be applied to assess the risk of non-SN positivity for individual patients and to guide their management.

More work is clearly necessary to optimally define the most accurate and practical method of predicting which patients have a low probability of metastatic tumor in non-SNs, and using this information to select patients who can be spared a CLND. It is hoped that this matter will be clarified in future trials of selective sentinel lymphadenectomy. Until this further information is available, however, there is general consensus that the most appropriate course of action is to recommend a CLND for every patient found to have a positive SN. Although it remains possible that even removal of all metastatic disease in regional lymph nodes will have no effect on survival, if SN positivity merely indicates the potential for hematogenous dissemination and systemic metastasis, the process should at least minimize the risk of severely troublesome node field recurrence.

Improving and validating the accuracy of SN identification

It is clear that the accuracy of detection of nodal micrometastases still needs to be improved, and studies seeking to improve accuracy rates are proceeding on a number of fronts.[29] Retrospective attempts to determine why false-negative SN results occurred have been thwarted by the lack of an objective method of confirming the identity of an SN after it has been removed. To overcome this problem and confirm SN identity, Haigh et al. undertook a study in melanoma patients in which carbon particles were injected intradermally at the primary tumor site, allowing the presumptive SN to be examined for the presence of carbon particles in it.[46] The presence of carbon particles was taken to indicate direct lymphatic drainage from the primary melanoma site, confirming the node's identity as an SN. At the SMU we have employed a technique that is similar in principle, but has the great advantage that it can be used on existing archival tissue. It involves using inductively coupled plasma mass spectrometry (ICP-MS) to identify antimony particles in nodes.[47] The antimony is derived from the antimony sulfide colloid particles used for preoperative lymphoscintigraphy at our institution, and it should therefore be found in high concentrations in SNs but not in non-SNs, like the carbon particles used by Haigh et al. The highly sensitive and accurate ICP-MS technique has revealed high antimony levels in definite SNs (containing micrometastatic disease) and low antimony levels in non-SNs (see Figure 1). When 20 patients classified as having false- negative SNs were assessed, 5 were found to have very low levels of antimony, indicating that the nodes removed from these patients had probably not been true SNs, and providing a likely explanation for the regional node field recurrences.[38] It is probably relevant that 4 of the 5 patients were treated early in the SMU experience of SN biopsy, when only blue dye identification was being used, and before routine use of an intraoperative gamma probe had been introduced. In more recent studies at the SMU we have been attempting to analyze antimony concentrations in fine needle aspiration biopsy specimens obtained from lymph nodes, and have found that the technique is sufficiently sensitive to permit differentiation between SNs and non-SNs on the basis of a fine needle aspirate.

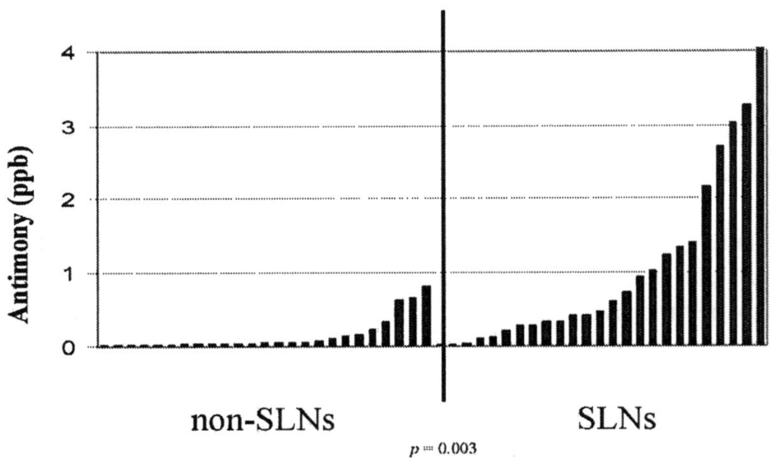

Figure 1. Antimony concentrations (ppb) in 50 um-thick tissue sections of 24 pairs of sentinel nodes (SLNs) and nonsentinel nodes (non-SLNs) removed from one regional node field during the same operation from individual patients.

Assessment of sentinel nodes using proton magnetic resonance spectroscopy

In parallel with the studies outlined above, we have been assessing the value of proton magnetic resonance spectroscopy (MRS) to examine fine needle aspirates of SNs and non-SNs. We have already demonstrated that, as with other types of tumor including breast, prostate, and colon cancer,[48, 49]

MRS can identify the presence of tumor by spectrographic analysis of tissue samples.[50] We have found that it is possible to examine fine needle aspiration biopsy specimens from SNs and non-SNs using MRS, and to use the results to predict the presence of micrometastatic disease with a sensitivity of 97.3%, a specificity of 90.2%, and an overall accuracy of 94.7%. Key features of the spectrum when melanoma cells are present are peaks for metabolites such as choline and taurine (see Figure 2). If validation studies confirm these initial findings, the possibility of using this technique in clinical practice will be assessed. There are several ways in which it could prove useful. It may, for example, provide a less expensive and possibly more accurate alternative to RT-PCR for the examination of SNs to determine whether or not they contain micrometastatic disease.

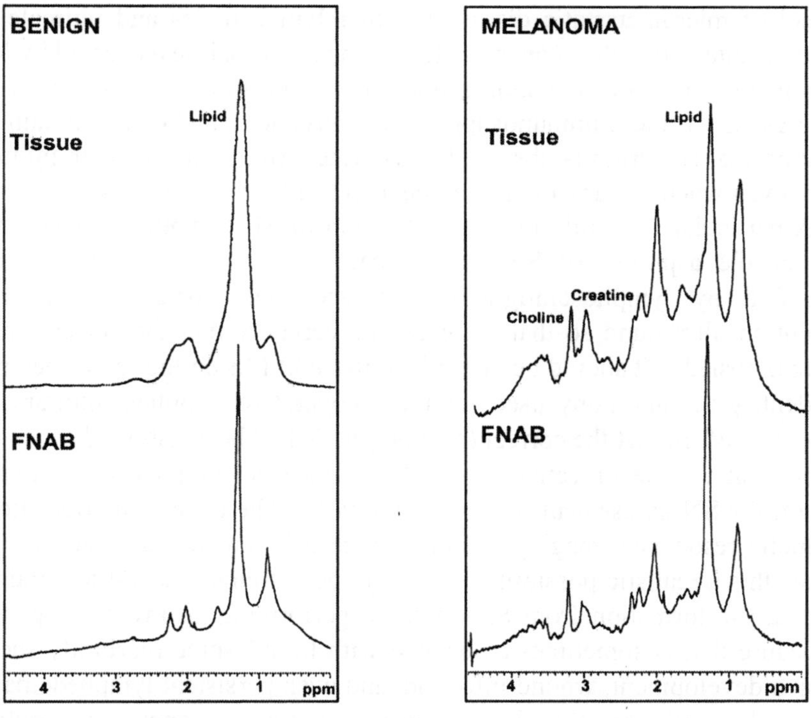

Figure 2. Proton MR spectra of tissue and FNA biopsies of lymph nodes containing metastatic melanoma and control benign lymph nodes from melanoma patients. Note the choline peaks in both tissue and FNAB specimens from nodes containing melanoma. (Reproduced with permission from *Melanoma Research.*)

An important observation has been that when using MRS to examine node aspirates, it does not appear to be necessary for the aspirated material to contain tumor cells for an abnormal spectrum to be produced.[50] In other words, it appears that the biochemical abnormalities associated with metastatic tumor are widely dispersed throughout nodes containing even very small micrometastatic foci. This is consistent with the concept that the microenvironment in an SN, which leads to and is associated with micrometastasis, is different from that in a non-SN. The process is probably immunologically mediated, since dramatic and profound immunosuppression of the SN as a result of its direct exposure to immunosuppressive factors from the primary tumor has been demonstrated.[29] It is postulated that once metastases have successfully implanted in the SN and begun to grow, they in turn produce more (and possibly different) immunosuppressive factors that eventually lead to the spread of micrometastatic disease to other lymph nodes and ultimately to systemic sites. It is thus conceivable that the abnormalities detected by MRS examination of nodes containing micrometastatic tumor foci are related to the presence of these immunosuppressive substances, and could explain why an abnormal spectrum is observed in aspirates from nodes containing tumor cells, even when no tumor cells can be identified in the aspirates.

A particularly useful clinical application of MRS would be to examine fine needle aspirates of SNs that remain in situ (after they have been identified by lymphoscintigraphy and accurately localized with high-resolution ultrasound so that there can be certainty that the correct area is being biopsied). It should be possible to use ICP-MS on the same specimens to identify the antimony used for the preoperative lymphoscintigram, and thereby confirm that the correct (sentinel) node had been assessed.

Ultimately, the objective would be to have a completely noninvasive system for SN assessment in vivo using MRS. The advent of sophisticated magnetic resonance imaging machines with 3 T magnets and surface coils makes this a realistic possibility. It would be extremely useful to obtain the necessary information from SNs without performing an invasive operative procedure that is sometimes associated with troublesome morbidity such as seroma development, wound infection, and even persistent lymphedema of a limb. As well, the considerable cost of a surgical operation would be avoided and operating room utilization reduced, with further economic benefits. In Sydney, assessment of the validity of MRS for assessing SNs is proceeding in patients with melanoma and breast cancer, but it is likely to be equally useful in patients with other forms of malignancy.

What Lies Ahead?

As previously indicated, results are still awaited from large, well-designed trials that were designed to ascertain whether SN examination, with complete regional node clearance if a positive SN is found, improves ultimate survival outcome in patients with melanoma and breast cancer. As we and others (including Morton) have suggested, it seems scientifically inappropriate to insist that SN removal and examination should be regarded as the "standard of care" until the results of these trials are available.[51-55] This is because no effect on ultimate outcome has yet been demonstrated, nor has the morbidity of the SN procedure been well documented in large randomized studies.

On the other hand, it seems equally inappropriate, on scientific grounds, to abandon selective sentinel lymphadenectomy at this stage (as some have insisted should be done[51-53]). This is because there are a number of definite benefits that accrue for patients if SN assessment is performed. First, much more accurate staging is achieved, allowing a more reliable prognostic estimate than would otherwise be possible. This knowledge is of great importance to most patients. Second, SN positive patients (who are thus identified as being at higher risk) can be offered any adjuvant therapy considered likely to be effective, or participation in adjuvant therapy trials (with more confident assignment to appropriate stratification categories). And third, complete regional node clearance in SN-positive patients should minimize the risk of troublesome node field recurrence, even if systemic metastasis occurs.

Further trials are required, and some are currently in advanced stages of planning, to determine whether every melanoma patient found to be SN positive requires a complete regional node field clearance. Meanwhile, methods of achieving more accurate SN identification and thereby reducing false-negative rates are being assessed, and techniques for minimally invasive and, ultimately, noninvasive in vivo SN evaluation, such as proton MRS, are being investigated.

Finally, it should be noted that the SN concept is now finding widespread application in patients with tumors other than melanoma and breast cancer. SN assessment appears to provide similarly accurate staging in gastrointestinal cancers, for example.[56, 57] For this disease, as for melanoma and breast cancer, knowledge of SN status has the potential to spare patients unnecessary nodal surgery, while identifying those in whom radical surgical clearance of lymph nodes and adjuvant postoperative therapy are most likely to be beneficial. It is probable that similar benefits will accrue with most tumors that spread primarily via lymphatics. Several of these are discussed in other chapters of this book. The practical value of SN assessment for all these tumor types will doubtless become clear over the next few years, as the results of appropriately designed studies become available.

REFERENCES

1. Virchow R. Lecture IX: Pyaemia and leucocytosis. Cellular pathology as based upon physiology and pathological history. New York: Dover Publications, Inc., 1971. pp. 211-29.
2. Braithwaite LR. The flow of lymph from the ileocaecal angle, and its possible bearing on the cause of duodenal and gastric ulcer. Br J Surg 1923; 11:7-26.
3. Gould EA, Winship T, Philbin PH, Kerr HH. Observations on a "sentinel node" in cancer of the parotid. Cancer 1960; 13:77-8.
4. Sayegh E, Brooks T, Sacher E, Busch F. Lymphangiography of the retroperitoneal lymph nodes through the inguinal route. J Urol 1966; 95:102-7.
5. Cabanas RM. An approach for the treatment of penile carcinoma. Cancer 1977; 39:456-66.
6. Wong JH, Cagle LA, Morton DL. Lymphatic drainage of skin to a sentinel lymph node in a feline model. Ann Surg 1991; 214:637-41.
7. Morton DL, Wen DR, Wong JH, Economou JS, Cagle LA, Storm FK, Foshag LJ, Cochran AJ. Technical details of intraoperative lymphatic mapping for early stage melanoma. Arch Surg 1992; 127:392-9.
8. Reintgen D, Cruse CW, Wells K, Berman C, Fenske N, Glass F, Schroer K, Heller R, Ross M, Lyman G, et al. The orderly progression of melanoma nodal metastases. Ann Surg 1994; 220:759-67.
9. Thompson JF, McCarthy WH, Bosch CM, O'Brien CJ, Quinn MJ, Paramaesvaran S, Crotty K, McCarthy SW, Uren RF, Howman-Giles R. Sentinel lymph node status as an indicator of the presence of metastatic melanoma in regional lymph nodes. Melanoma Res 1995; 5:255-60.
10. Reintgen D, Ross MI, Essner R. Sentinel lymph node biopsy: results to date. *In* Thompson JF, Morton DL, Kroon BB, eds. Textbook of Melanoma. London: Martin Dunitz, 2004. pp. 365-72.
11. Sim FH, Taylor WF, Ivins JC, Pritchard DJ, Soule EH. A prospective randomized study of the efficacy of routine elective lymphadenectomy in management of malignant melanoma. Preliminary results. Cancer 1978; 41:948-56.
12. Veronesi U, Adamus J, Bandiera DC, Brennhovd O, Caceres E, Cascinelli N, Claudio F, Ikonopisov RL, Javorski VV, Kirov S, Kulakowski A, Lacour J, Lejeune F, Mechl Z, Morabito A, Rode I, Sergeev S, van Slooten E, Szczygiel K, Trapeznikov NN, Wagner RI. Delayed regional lymph node dissection in stage I melanoma of the skin of the lower extremities. Cancer 1982; 49:2420-30.
13. Balch CM, Soong SJ, Bartolucci AA, Urist MM, Karakousis CP, Smith TJ, Temple WJ, Ross MI, Jewell WR, Mihm MC, Barnhill RL, Wanebo HJ. Efficacy of an elective regional lymph node dissection of 1 to 4 mm thick melanomas for patients 60 years of age and younger. Ann Surg 1996; 224:255-63.
14. Cascinelli N, Morabito A, Santinami M, MacKie RM, Belli F. Immediate or delayed dissection of regional nodes in patients with melanoma of the trunk: a randomised trial. WHO Melanoma Programme. Lancet 1998; 351:793-6.
15. Thompson JF, Uren RF, Shaw HM, McCarthy WH, Quinn MJ, O'Brien CJ, Howman-Giles RB. Location of sentinel lymph nodes in patients with cutaneous melanoma: new insights into lymphatic anatomy. J Am Coll Surg 1999; 189:195-204.

16. Uren RF, Thompson JF, Howman-Giles R. Lymphatic drainage of the skin and breast: locating the sentinel lymph nodes. Amsterdam: Harwood Academic Publishers, 1999.
17. Uren RF, Hoefnagel CA. Lymphoscintigraphy. *In* Thompson JF, Morton DL, Kroon BB, eds. Textbook of Melanoma. London: Martin Dunitz, 2004. pp. 339-64.
18. Uren RF, Howman-Giles R, Thompson JF, Quinn MJ, O'Brien C, Shaw HM, Bosch CM, McCarthy WH. Lymphatic drainage to triangular intermuscular space lymph nodes in melanoma on the back. J Nucl Med 1996; 37:964-6.
19. Uren RF, Howman-Giles R, Thompson JF, McCarthy WH, Quinn MJ, Roberts JM, Shaw HM. Interval nodes: the forgotten sentinel nodes in patients with melanoma. Arch Surg 2000; 135:1168-72.
20. Sappey M. Injection, preparation et conservation des vaisseaux lymphatiques: These pour le doctorate en medecine, No.241. Paris: Rignoux Imprimeur de la Faculte de Medecine, 1843.
21. de Wilt JHW, Thompson JF, Uren RF, McCarthy WH, O'Brien CJ, Quinn MJ, Shannon KF, Ka VSK, Scolyer RA. Correlation between preoperative lymphoscintigraphy and metastatic nodal disease sites in 362 patients with cutaneous melanomas of the head and neck. Ann Surg 2004; 239:544-52.
22. Thompson JF, Uren RF, Coventry BJ, Chatterton BE. Lymphoscintigraphy. *In* Balch CM, Houghton AN, Sober A, Soong S-J, eds. Cutaneous Melanoma. St Louis: Quality Medical Publishing, Inc., 2003. pp. 329-52.
23. Essner R, Thompson JF, Nieweg OE. The sentinel lymph node biopsy procedure: identification with blue dye and a gamma probe. *In* Thompson JF, Morton DL, Kroon BB, eds. Textbook of Melanoma. London: Martin Dunitz, 2004. pp. 328-38.
24. Morton DL, Thompson JF, Essner R, Elashoff R, Stern SL, Nieweg OE, Roses DF, Karakousis CP, Mozzillo N, Reintgen D, Wang HJ, Glass EC, Cochran AJ. Validation of the accuracy of intraoperative lymphatic mapping and sentinel lymphadenectomy for early-stage melanoma: a multicenter trial. Ann Surg 1999; 230:453-63; discussion 463-5.
25. McMasters KM. The Sunbelt Melanoma Trial. Ann Surg Oncol 2001; 8:41S-3S.
26. Cascinelli N, Belli F, Santinami M, Fait V, Testori A, Ruka W, Cavaliere R, Mozzillo N, Rossi CR, MacKie RM, Nieweg O, Pace M, Kirov K. Sentinel lymph node biopsy in cutaneous melanoma: the WHO Melanoma Program experience. Ann Surg Oncol 2000; 7:469-74.
27. Gershenwald JE, Colome MI, Lee JE, Mansfield PF, Tseng C, Lee JJ, Balch CM, Ross MI. Patterns of recurrence following a negative sentinel lymph node biopsy in 243 patients with stage I or II melanoma. J Clin Oncol 1998; 16:2253-60.
28. Harlow SP, Krag DN. Sentinel lymph node—why study it: implications of the B-32 study. Semin Surg Oncol 2001; 20:224-9.
29. Morton DL, Hoon DS, Cochran AJ, Turner RR, Essner R, Takeuchi H, Wanek LA, Glass E, Foshag LJ, Hsueh EC, Bilchik AJ, Elashoff D, Elashoff R. Lymphatic mapping and sentinel lymphadenectomy for early-stage melanoma: therapeutic utility and implications of nodal microanatomy and molecular staging for improving the accuracy of detection of nodal micrometastases. Ann Surg 2003; 238:538-49; discussion 549-50.
30. Balch CM, Buzaid AC, Atkins MB, Cascinelli N, Coit DG, Fleming ID, Houghton A Jr, Kirkwood JM, Mihm MF, Morton DL, Reintgen D, Ross MI, Sober A, Soong SJ, Thompson JA, Thompson JF, Gershenwald JE, McMasters KM. A new American Joint Committee on Cancer staging system for cutaneous melanoma. Cancer 2000; 88:1484-91.
31. Balch CM, Buzaid AC, Soong SJ, Atkins MB, Cascinelli N, Coit DG, Fleming ID, Gershenwald JE, Houghton A Jr, Kirkwood JM, McMasters KM, Mihm MF, Morton DL, Reintgen DS, Ross MI, Sober A, Thompson JA, Thompson JF. Final version of the

American Joint Committee on Cancer staging system for cutaneous melanoma. J Clin Oncol 2001; 19:3635-48.

32. Cochran AJ. Surgical pathology remains pivotal in the evaluation of 'sentinel' lymph nodes. Am J Surg Pathol 1999; 23:1169-72.
33. Starz H, Balda BR, Kramer KU, Buchels H, Wang H. A micromorphometry-based concept for routine classification of sentinel lymph node metastases and its clinical relevance for patients with melanoma. Cancer 2001; 91:2110-21.
34. Messina JL, Glass LF, Cruse CW, Berman C, Ku NK, Reintgen DS. Pathologic examination of the sentinel lymph node in malignant melanoma. Am J Surg Pathol 1999; 23:686-90.
35. Li LX, Scolyer RA, Ka VS, McKinnon JG, Shaw HM, McCarthy SW, Thompson JF. Pathologic review of negative sentinel lymph nodes in melanoma patients with regional recurrence: a clinicopathologic study of 1152 patients undergoing sentinel lymph node biopsy. Am J Surg Pathol 2003; 27:1197-202.
36. Cook MG, Green MA, Anderson B, Eggermont AM, Ruiter DJ, Spatz A, Kissin MW, Powell BW. The development of optimal pathological assessment of sentinel lymph nodes for melanoma. J Pathol 2003; 200:314-9.
37. Nieweg OE, Estourgie SH. Summary of the Third International Sentinel Node Conference 16-18 November 2002, Yokohama. Eur J Nucl Med Mol Imaging 2003; 30:483-7.
38. Scolyer RA, Thompson JF, Li LX, Beavis A, Dawson M, Doble P, Ka VSK, McKinnon JG, Soper R, Uren RF, Shaw HM, Stretch J, McCarthy SW. Failure to remove "true" sentinel nodes can cause failure of the sentinel node biopsy technique. Evidence from antimony quantification of false negative sentinel nodes from melanoma patients. Ann Surg Oncol *In Press*.
39. Ka VSK, McKinnon JG, Scolyer RA, Li LX, Uren RF, Thompson JF. Analysis of reasons for false negative sentinel node biopsies in patients with melanoma. Ann Surg Oncol *In Press*.
40. Uren RF, Howman-Giles RB, Shaw HM, Thompson JF, McCarthy WH. Lymphoscintigraphy in high-risk melanoma of the trunk: predicting draining node groups, defining lymphatic channels and locating the sentinel node. J Nucl Med 1993; 34:1435-40.
41. Joseph E, Brobeil A, Glass F, Glass J, Messina J, DeConti R, Cruse CW, Rapaport DP, Berman C, Fenske N, Reintgen DS. Results of complete lymph node dissection in 83 melanoma patients with positive sentinel nodes. Ann Surg Oncol 1998; 5:119-25.
42. Salti GI, Das Gupta TK. Predicting residual lymph node basin disease in melanoma patients with sentinel lymph node metastases. Am J Surg 2003; 186:98-101.
43. Reeves ME, Delgado R, Busam KJ, Brady MS, Coit DG. Prediction of nonsentinel lymph node status in melanoma. Ann Surg Oncol 2003; 10:27-31.
44. Wagner JD, Davidson D, Coleman JJ 3rd, Hutchins G, Schauwecker D, Park HM, Havlik RJ. Lymph node tumor volumes in patients undergoing sentinel lymph node biopsy for cutaneous melanoma. Ann Surg Oncol 1999; 6:398-404.
45. Cochran AJ, Wen DR, Huang R-R, Wang H-J, Elashoff R, Morton DL. Prediction of metastatic melanoma in non-sentinel nodes and clinical outcome based on the primary melanoma and the sentinel node. Mod Pathol *In press*.
46. Haigh PI, Lucci A, Turner RR, Bostick PJ, Krasne DL, Stern SL, Morton DL. Carbon dye histologically confirms the identity of sentinel lymph nodes in cutaneous melanoma. Cancer 2001; 92:535-41.
47. Dawson M, Doble P, Beavis A, Li LX, Soper R, Scolyer RA, Uren RF, Thompson JF. Antimony by ICP-MS as a marker for sentinel lymph nodes in melanoma patients. Analyst 2003; 128:217-9.

48. Mountford CE, Lean CL, Hancock R, Dowd S, Mackinnon WB, Tattersall MH, Russell P. Magnetic resonance spectroscopy detects cancer in draining lymph nodes. Invasion Metastasis 1993; 13:57-71.
49. Mackinnon WB, Barry PA, Malycha PL, Gillett DJ, Russell P, Lean CL, Doran ST, Barraclough BH, Bilous M, Mountford CE. Fine-needle biopsy specimens of benign breast lesions distinguished from invasive cancer ex vivo with proton MR spectroscopy. Radiology 1997; 204:661-6.
50. Lean CL, Bourne R, Thompson JF, Scolyer RA, Stretch J, Li LX, Russell P, Mountford C. Rapid detection of metastatic melanoma in lymph nodes using proton magnetic resonance spectroscopy of fine needle aspiration biopsy specimens. Melanoma Res 2003; 13:259-61.
51. Medalie NS, Ackerman AB. Sentinel lymph node biopsy has no benefit for patients with primary cutaneous melanoma metastatic to a lymph node: an assertion based on comprehensive, critical analysis: part I. Am J Dermatopathol 2003; 25:399-417.
52. Medalie NS, Ackerman AB. Sentinel lymph node biopsy has no benefit for patients with primary cutaneous melanoma metastatic to a lymph node: an assertion based on comprehensive, critical analysis: part II. Am J Dermatopathol 2003; 25:473-84.
53. Thomas JM, Patocskai EJ. The argument against sentinel node biopsy for malignant melanoma. BMJ 2000; 321:3-4.
54. Thompson JF, Uren RF. What is a 'sentinel' lymph node? Eur J Surg Oncol 2000; 26:103-4.
55. Pharis DB, Zitelli JA. The management of regional lymph nodes in cancer. Br J Dermatol 2003; 149:919-25.
56. Kitagawa Y, Fujii H, Mukai M, Kubo A, Kitajima M. Current status and future prospects of sentinel node navigational surgery for gastrointestinal cancers. Ann Surg Oncol 2004; 11:242S-4S.
57. Song X, Wang L, Chen W, Pan T, Zhu H, Xu J, Jin M, Finley RK 3rd, Wu J. Lymphatic mapping and sentinel node biopsy in gastric cancer. Am J Surg 2004; 187:270-3.

Index

D

E

N

O

P

Q

R

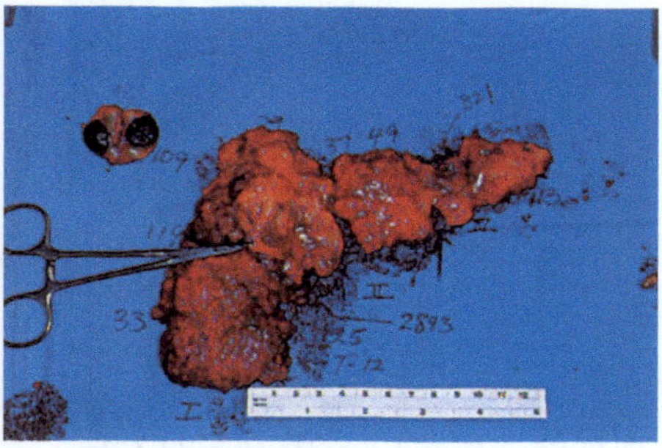

1) *Chapter 3, Figure 3, Page 65, Stanley P. L. Leong*

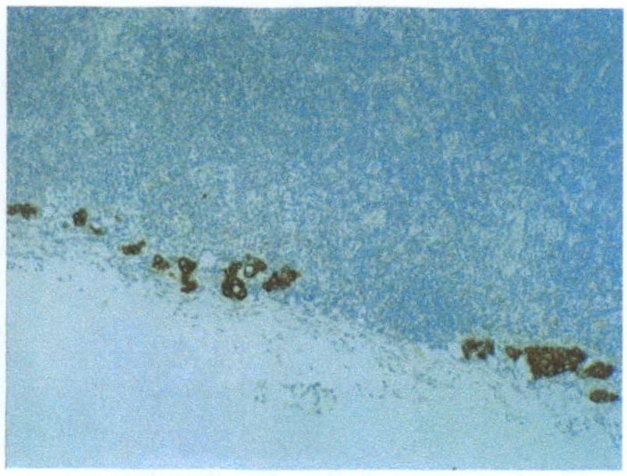

2) *Chapter 4, Figure 4, Page 83, Charles E. Cox et al*

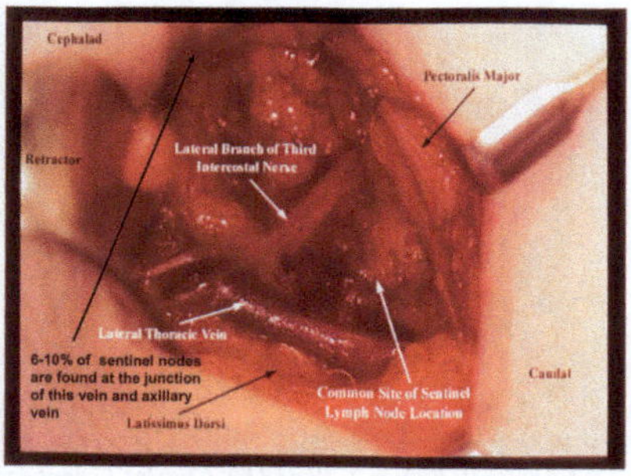

3) *Chapter 4, Figure 6, Page 87, Charles E. Cox et al*

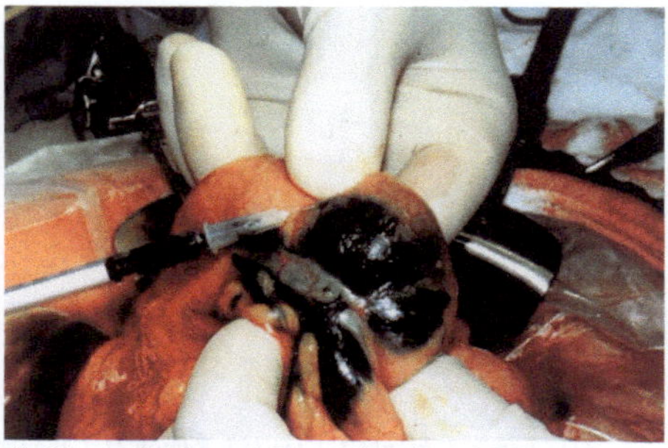

4) *Chapter 5, Figure 1, Page 117, Sukamal Saha et al*

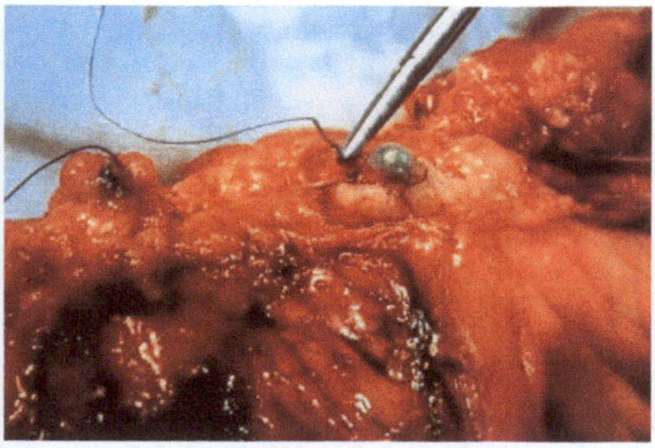

5) *Chapter 5, Figure 2, Page 117, Sukamal Saha et al*

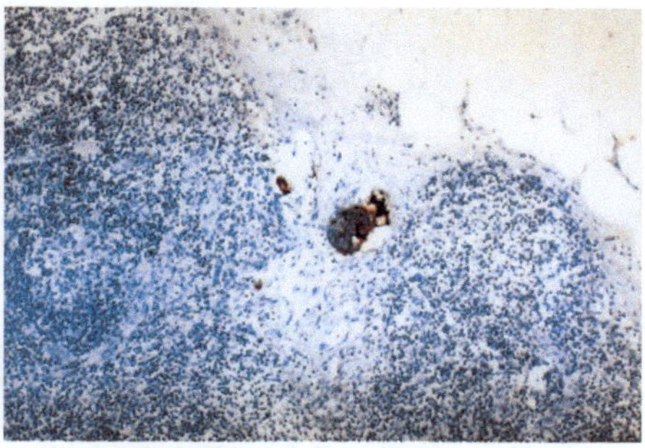

6) *Chapter 5, Figure 4, Page 118, Sukamal Saha et al*

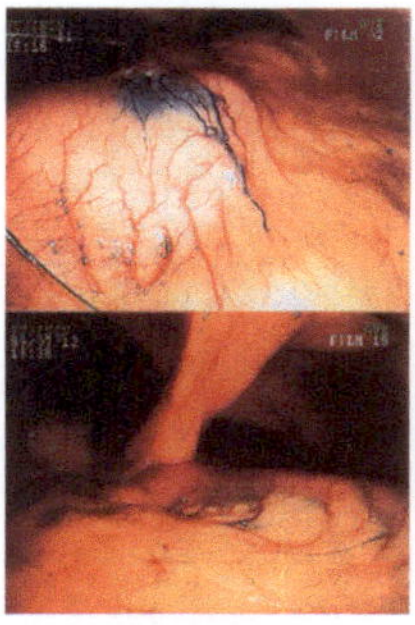

7) *Chapter 6, Figure 2, Page 128, Yuko Kitagawa et al*

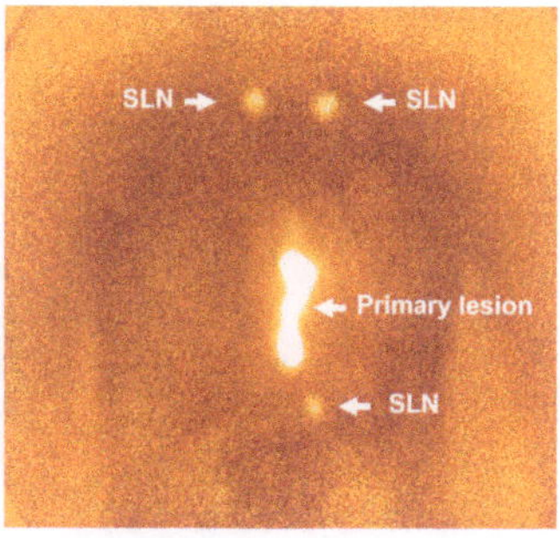

8) *Chapter 6, Figure 7, Page 134, Yuko Kitagawa et al*

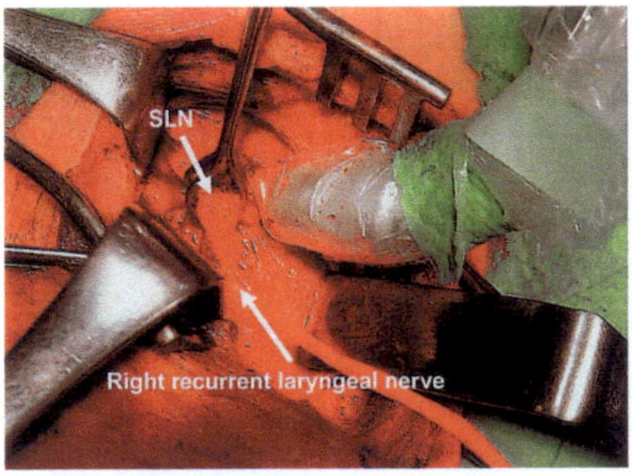

9) Chapter 6, Figure 8, Page 134, Yuko Kitagawa et al

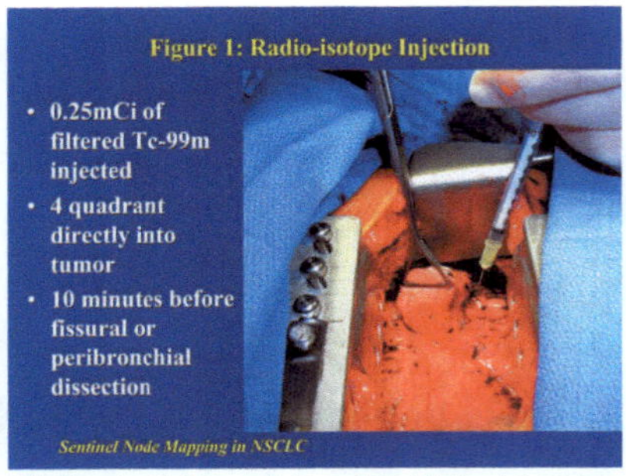

10) Chapter 7, Figure 1, Page 144, Michael J. Liptay

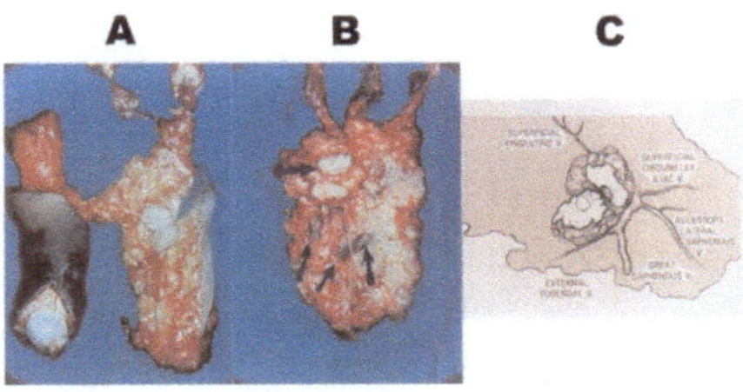

11) Chapter 8, Figure 3, Page 155, Ramon M. Cabanas

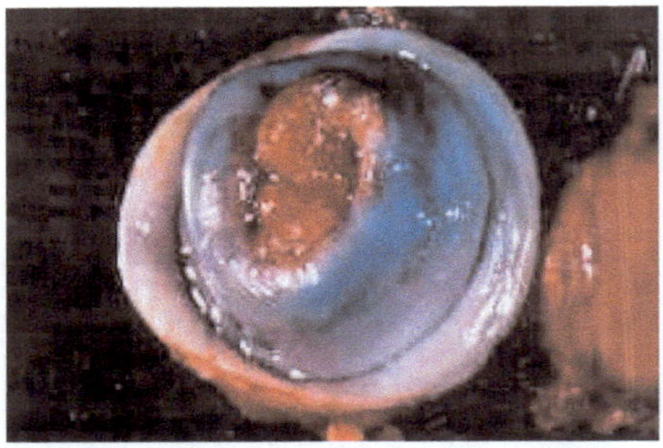

12) Chapter 9, Figure 2, Page 180, Charles Levenback

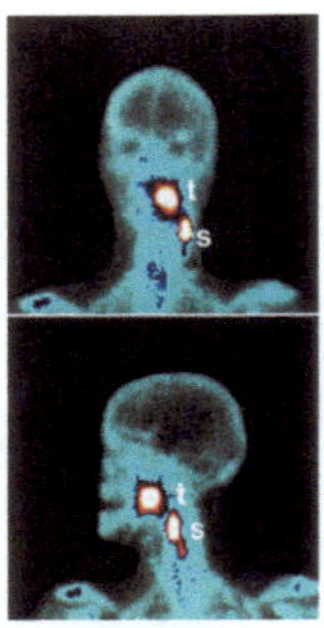

13) Chapter 10, Figure 2, Page 191, Jochen A. Werner

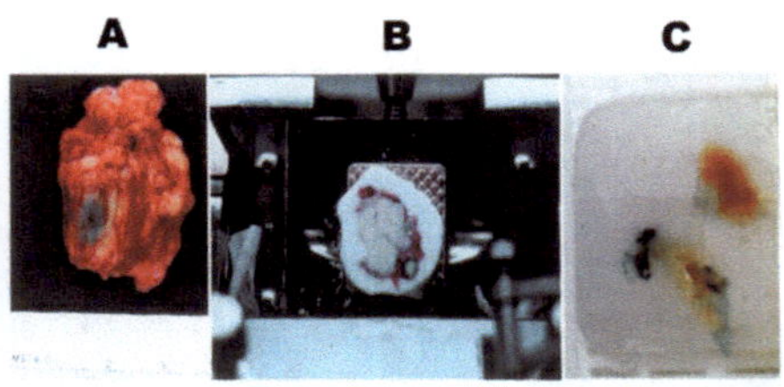

14) Chapter 11, Figure 1, Page 209, Alistair J. Cochran et al

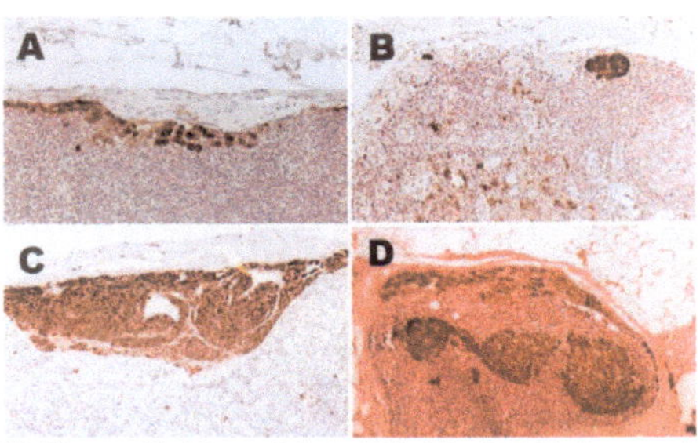

15) Chapter 11, Figure 5, Page 214, Alistair J. Cochran et al

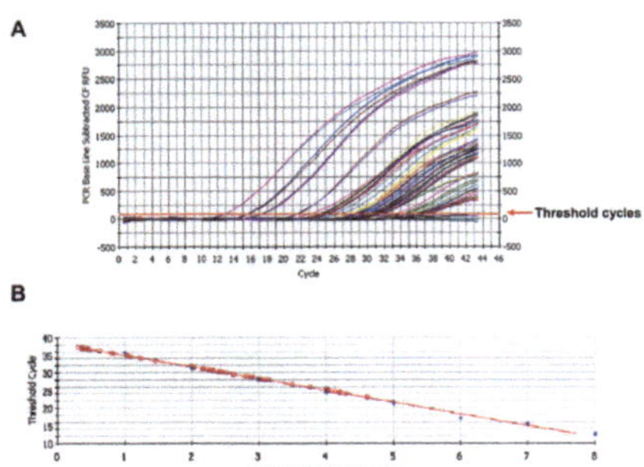

16) Chapter 12, Figure 3, Page 227, Dave S.B. Hoon et al

MIX
Papier aus verantwortungsvollen Quellen
Paper from responsible sources
FSC® C105338

If you have any concerns about our products,
you can contact us on
ProductSafety@springernature.com

In case Publisher is established outside the EU,
the EU authorized representative is:
Springer Nature Customer Service Center GmbH
Europaplatz 3, 69115 Heidelberg, Germany

Printed by Libri Plureos GmbH
in Hamburg, Germany